Outsmart
your
Cancer

Outsmart *your* Cancer

Alternative Non-Toxic Treatments *That Work*

TANYA HARTER PIERCE

THOUGHTWORKS PUBLISHING

Stateline, Nevada
2004

First printing 2004
2nd printing 2005
3rd printing 2006

ISBN 0-9728867-3-7
LCCN 2003104206

ATTENTION CORPORATIONS, UNIVERSITIES, COLLEGES, AND PROFESSIONAL ORGANIZATIONS: Quantity discounts are available on bulk purchases of this book for educational, gift purposes, or as premiums for increasing magazine subscriptions or renewals. Special books or book excerpts can also be created to fit specific needs. For information, please contact Thoughtworks Publishing, P.O. Box 4949, Stateline, NV 89449; (888) 679-2669.

Disclaimer

The author, Tanya Harter Pierce, is *not* a physician and *none* of the information in this book should be construed as "medical advice." In this book, the author is merely presenting her findings, as would an investigative journalist. Thus, the material in this book should be used for educational and informational purposes only. Each person must make his or her own decisions about treatment. Prior to making those decisions, it is recommended that anyone who has cancer, or suspects he or she may have cancer, should consult with a qualified physician.

A conscientious effort has been made to only present information that is accurate and truthful. However, the author cannot be held responsible for inaccuracies that may be found in her source material. Moreover, it is not a comprehensive survey of *all* non-toxic cancer treatments available, but rather those treatment approaches and issues the author has deemed most important for readers to know about in their search for ways to regain their health.

Note: The alternative non-toxic approaches presented in this book are not approved by the FDA as treatments for cancer.

Acknowledgments

My abundant and never-ending gratitude goes to my husband, David Pierce. Without his total support and belief in me, I would not have been able to write this book. He not only supported me in a myriad of personal ways, but also gave me excellent editorial input on every chapter.

I also want to thank my brother, Craig, who introduced me to many important sources of alternative cancer treatment information, and to express warm gratitude to my sisters, Margo and Kathy, and my mother, Bonnie, for their enthusiasm and encouragement about my project. And I sincerely thank the many medical professionals and other experts who graciously reviewed or provided important input to specific sections of this book.

Finally, I deeply appreciate and applaud the efforts of *all* the pioneering physicians, dentists, patients, researchers, and authors who went before me and wrote books, articles, and Internet postings to share their experiences and knowledge of alternative cancer therapies. To *all* of them I say, "Your commitment and courage will never be forgotten!"

Table of Contents

For additional information and new
cancer recovery testimonials please visit:

www.OutsmartYourCancer.com

Introduction

The writing of this book came about quickly and unexpectedly. I was suddenly jolted into cancer treatment research when one of my own family members was diagnosed with cancer and conventional medicine could not offer the likelihood of a long-term cure. What I discovered in my search for information *amazed me*. The alternative treatments were fascinating to read about, and I was quite startled that I had not heard much, or even *anything*, about these non-toxic approaches. This was particularly surprising to me since I was one of those people who had spent many years researching various alternative treatments for my own chronic health challenges. When I found out about the effectiveness and frequently *incredible* recoveries that alternative, non-toxic cancer treatments are often able to achieve, I was stunned!

Why hadn't I heard of these treatment approaches? Why hadn't I read about them? Why was it so hard to find this information? At first, I did not have answers to these questions, but the one thing I knew was that people with cancer should *not* have to spend the amount of time I did to find this information for themselves!

Initially, I was not going to write a book at all. I was just going to do my research like an investigative journalist, then put a small pamphlet together that I could give out to friends and family. But the stacks of information on my desk kept getting bigger and bigger, so I finally decided to turn what I had learned into a full-length book. My goal was to present the material in ways that readers could easily understand, and to answer such questions as, "What are the most common alternative cancer treatments?" . . . "How effective are they?" . . . "How do they work?" . . . "Where can I obtain these treatments?" . . . and . . . "Why doesn't my doctor tell me about these options?" These questions, and more, are answered in the following pages.

One thing that surprised me, and I think may surprise many people, is the reality that alternative approaches to cancer do *not* just involve taking supplements from the local health food store to strengthen one's immune system. The successful alternative approaches I found out about do much more than that! In fact, they tend to involve such specific actions on cancer cells that some of the alternative approaches cannot be done along with other approaches because they would counteract each other.

I also wanted to share with readers that the way these approaches work has already been backed up by rigorous scientific research performed by highly respected physicians, brilliant biochemists, and Nobel prize-winning scientists! I chose to present the approaches in a somewhat chronological order, starting with the alternative treatments that were developed first, and to include some of the history of each one. I learned that a historical overview is important to understanding and accepting the validity of these methods.

Effective alternative, non-toxic approaches to cancer *are* obtainable today. This is clearly evident from a multitude of documented real-life recoveries. During my own search, I spoke to over a hundred people who had recovered from their cancer using the alternative treatments presented in this book. In many of the treatment chapters, you will read multiple recovery stories for yourself. Some of these stories were borrowed from other publications with permission. Most, however, are case histories resulting from interviews I conducted personally with cancer survivors.

All of the alternative approaches to cancer discussed in this book are methods that could have been accepted into mainstream medicine and practiced by oncologists and cancer clinics around the world. Unfortunately, that has not happened. In the following chapters, you will learn many of the reasons why.

Though I cannot counsel you as to which decision you should make for your own particular medical situation, my hope is that this book will save you valuable time in your own search for answers. And, if you have been told that conventional medicine has no treatment that can offer you a long-term cure, then it will provide you with much-needed hope.

I sincerely wish you the very best on your path to recovery!

Tanya Harter Pierce

Section I

Understanding Cancer

CHAPTER 1

The Cancer Reality Today

I f you are facing a cancer diagnosis, the first thing you should know is that there *is* hope in the world of alternative, non-toxic treatments. And I am referring to very *real* hope—not the "false hope" that is so often offered in the guise of chemotherapy and radiation. Tens of thousands of people have used alternative, non-toxic treatments to overcome their cancer and then gone on to live normal, healthy lives!

The second thing you should know is that you are *far* from alone. Right now, one in every two to three Americans will develop life-threatening cancer at some point in their lives! This estimate comes primarily from the official American Cancer Society figures of 1996, which predicted that 40 percent of all Americans will develop life-threatening cancer. This statistical estimate has been confirmed by other researchers as well, many of whom believe the 40 percent figure to be *conservative*. Overall, cancer rates have been rising at an alarming rate for the past 100 years. In recent years, the rate of lung cancer incidence has been going down due to fewer people smoking, but the rates of virtually all other types of cancer are still increasing!

I understand that whenever a person finds themselves facing a cancer diagnosis, time is of the essence. There are urgent decisions to make, and you need treatment information fast. You may have various doctors, relatives, or friends pushing you to quickly get your surgery, chemotherapy, and/or radiation. They may even say things like, "If you don't do this now, you will die!" If this is happening to you, try to remember that these people are pushing you because they care about you and are, themselves, scared. And they are right when they say that you need to take action *very soon*.

But you deserve to know that everyone in America is strongly influenced—even brought up all their lives—to think that the conventional treatments are the only answers to cancer. Surgery, chemotherapy, and radiation are commonly called "the Big Three" of mainstream cancer medicine, and even most doctors think these are the only answers.

Unfortunately, there are serious problems with these conventional treatment approaches. Of the three, surgery is definitely the most effective. Surgery can sometimes bring about long-term recovery when cancer is caught early and is in an area where the *entire* cancerous area can be cut out. This is particularly true for early cancers where an entire organ or body part can be removed, such as a kidney, thyroid gland, testicle, or uterus. But for the majority of cases, the cancer has *already metastasized* (or spread to other areas of the body) by the time a person is diagnosed. And, for those cases, surgery cannot get all of the cancer cells. Many researchers believe that surgery can even *promote* metastasis in some cases.

Chemotherapy and radiation have even *worse* long-term recovery rates than surgery. This is largely because they resort to toxic methods of "bludgeoning" a person's cancer to death. These toxic treatments harm healthy parts of a person's body along with the cancer, thereby making long-term recovery difficult.

The good news is that, even if you have been diagnosed with cancer that has metastasized, there *are* alternatives to conventional treatments. And they often have better track records, in general, than what mainstream medicine is offering. I know many people who were told by their conventional doctors that their late-stage or metastasized cancer was incurable, only to *completely* recover later by using a non-toxic, alternative approach! In fact, you may find after reading this book that your biggest difficulty is not in finding a good alternative treatment approach to cancer, but in deciding which one to use.

There are very important reasons why alternative treatments for cancer often have better track records than conventional ones. Most importantly, alternative, non-toxic approaches work in ways that do *not* harm normal, healthy cells of the body. They do this by focusing on those aspects of cancer cells that are *significantly different* from healthy cells. These approaches also treat cancer as a "whole-body" disease, which means they work *with* a person's immune system to attack the cancer cells everywhere, even the "free-floating" individual cells. This is different from mainstream practices, which focus primarily on just treating tumors (which represent most of the cancer cells in a person's body, but not all). In the world of alternative treatments for cancer, tumors are generally considered "symptoms" of the cancer, and treatment is focused on both the "cause" as well as the "symptoms."

In other words, conventional medicine tries to *bludgeon* your cancer to death with treatments that can be extremely harmful to your body, while alternative methods use non-toxic approaches to *Outsmart Your Cancer!*

Benefits of Non-Toxic Approaches

The most obvious benefit of using a non-toxic approach to cancer is that, by doing so, a person does not damage healthy parts of his or her body while trying to recover from illness. Surgery, chemotherapy, and radiation can damage virtually any cells they come in contact with and may have extremely serious long-term side effects on the body such as liver, kidney, nerve, and heart damage. These side effects can often be life-threatening in and of themselves.

Besides general bodily damage that can be caused, many cancer patients are not even told by their doctors that some common conventional treatments for cancer are themselves *carcinogenic*. The fact is that some chemotherapy agents are known carcinogens, and the chemotherapy treatment given to many patients to put their cancer into remission may directly cause a *secondary* cancer in that person a few years later. Radiation can also cause cancer, which has been well-known since radiation techniques were first developed. Though surgery is not considered carcinogenic, it may cause the spread of cancer to other parts of the body.

Moreover, at some point, the use of a toxic treatment for cancer may enable the cancer to spread *even faster* in a person's body. This is because that person's immune system and other natural defense mechanisms have been so weakened by the treatment itself, the body can no longer fight off the cancer. So it only makes sense that using a toxic treatment for cancer can work *against* long-term recovery by giving the body more damage to recover from.

But there is another benefit of non-toxic approaches that is critical to long-term recovery from cancer, yet is not usually talked about. This is the benefit that comes from *continual use* of a treatment. The importance of this particular benefit cannot be overstated. Conventional toxic approaches, such as chemotherapy and radiation, do not allow for continual use because they are so toxic, continual use would kill the patient before the cancer could! For this reason, toxic treatments are always administered with doses spaced out. This necessity to space out the administration of a toxic treatment is not optimally effective since one of cancer's best abilities is to grow new cells *fast*. Thus, in-between toxic treatment administrations, while the patient's body is recovering from the treatment, the cancer cells are recovering too. And those cancer cells that grow back the fastest are those cells that have some amount of "resistance" to the treatment. In other words, the treatment itself selects for the proliferation of resistant cancer cells in a person's body. This type of resistance has become more and more evident with the use of antibiotics causing antibiotic-resistant bacteria. In the case of chemotherapy use, this type of dynamic may result in what are called "multi-drug-resistant" cancer cells, or MDR cells.

With non-toxic treatments, however, these vicious dynamics are avoided. Non-toxic approaches do not harm the body and therefore do allow for continual use. When a cancer treatment is non-toxic and can be administered continually every day, resistant cells are not selected and allowed to proliferate. In fact, a non-toxic approach can be done every single day for months or years. This allows the treatment approach to work in the body "24/7" and *never* gives the cancer cells a chance to grow back in ever more virulent forms.

Also, non-toxic approaches can often be continued for years *after* one has achieved remission, if a person chooses to. This gives people a way to help ensure their cancer does not come back!

The Bigger Picture

To sum up the bigger picture of conventional versus alternative cancer treatments today, I have come up with what I call the "three basic truths." They are:

1. Conventional treatments have failed

2. Successful alternative treatments abound

3. The "disbelief factor" is alive and well

First Basic Truth — Conventional Treatments Have Failed

It is commonly accepted by many reputable cancer researchers that the conventional "war on cancer" has failed. In fact, it has failed *so* miserably that the conventional cancer industry has had to resort to "fudging" their cure-rate statistics so the public will continue to think they are doing a good job! (By "cancer industry," I mean the part of organized medicine devoted to cancer research, treatment, and education, which is led primarily by the National Cancer Institute [NCI], the American

Cancer Society [ACS], the Food and Drug Administration [FDA], the American Medical Association [AMA], a few large centers throughout the country such as Memorial Sloan-Kettering Cancer Center in New York, and various pharmaceutical companies that produce cancer drugs.)

Once we clear away the fudged statistics and get down to the true reality, however, we find that current conventional medical treatments for cancer can only bring about *real* cures (long-term survival) for a very small percentage of cancer patients. People with primary cancer (cancer that has not yet metastasized) have the best chance of survival with conventional treatments, which may be able to achieve about a 10 to 15 percent long-term recovery rate if the cancer is caught early and is in an area of the body that is amenable to total surgical removal. But most cancer patients are not lucky enough to be diagnosed with primary cancer. In the United States, between two-thirds and three-fourths of *all* cancer patients have cancer that had *already metastasized* by the time they were first diagnosed. And when it comes to conventional medical treatments for metastasized cancer, many researchers agree that the long-term survival rate for these patients is less than 1 percent. (Some researchers claim that it is as low as one-tenth of a percent.) When it comes to the long-term effectiveness of chemotherapy, in general, some highly respected cancer researchers believe it is effective in only 2 to 3 percent of all cancers.

You might say, "Wait a minute; I heard that 40 to 50 percent of all cancer cases today are being cured by mainstream medicine. I also heard that *most* cancers, when caught early enough, are curable." Well, I believe that you heard that because these are the typical types of figures the cancer industry likes to advertise. But the truth is that when you hear a statistic like "40 to 50 percent cure rate" or "most cancers are curable if caught early," you are being presented statistics that have been incredibly *fudged and manipulated*. I learned about the official fudging tactics from a variety of sources, but primarily from the in-depth work done by two prominent cancer researchers: Ralph W. Moss, Ph.D., and Lorraine Day, M.D.

Ralph Moss is a highly renowned cancer researcher who has written numerous in-depth books including: *The Cancer Industry, Questioning Chemotherapy,* and *Cancer Therapy: The Independent Consumer's Guide to Non-Toxic Treatment and Prevention.* Moss began his cancer research when he was hired as a science writer at New York's Memorial Sloan-Kettering Cancer Center in 1974. There, he was able to observe the workings of the cancer industry from the inside. But according to Moss, his employment at Memorial Sloan-Kettering ended when he would not go along with the advertising of misleading information to the public. Over the years since then, he has diligently researched the *real* truth for the public, which he has carefully quoted and documented in his books. In an ever-growing circle of people researching the truth about cancer treatments, Ralph Moss is considered to be a leading authority.

Dr. Lorraine Day is an orthopedic trauma surgeon who rose to the position of chief of orthopedic surgery at San Francisco General Hospital. In 1992, Dr. Day's life changed dramatically when she was diagnosed with breast cancer that had already metastasized. Though she was pressured by specialists to undergo a mastectomy followed by chemotherapy and radiation, she chose *not* to receive these treatments because she knew so much about the severe damage to her body they could cause. Instead, she immediately started looking into other ways to treat herself, and eventually was able to completely heal and overcome her advanced cancer by drastically changing her diet and through other natural steps.

Dr. Day details her amazing story and reveals the results of her own in-depth research into cancer treatments in her numerous videos which can all be purchased from her website (www.DrDay.com). One of Dr. Day's videos reveals the stark truth about conventional cancer treatments and their side effects and real cure rates. It is called *Cancer Doesn't Scare Me Anymore*, and I highly recommend it. (See ordering instructions at the end of this chapter.)

Taken primarily from research done by both Dr. Moss and Dr. Day, the six *big ways* official cancer cure rates and statistics have been "fudged" are the following:

1. **By the way "cure" is defined.** The current cancer authorities, such as the ACS, NCI, and FDA, have all chosen to define "cure" as *alive five years after diagnosis*.[1] This official definition does *not* mean "cancer free," nor does it mean "healed of your disease," which is what most people think the word "cure" means.

   To give you a better idea of what I am talking about, we can look at the true story of one female cancer patient. In this woman's battle against breast cancer, she did all the conventional approaches — surgery, radiation, and chemotherapy. Unfortunately, the woman did *not* survive, and died five years and two weeks after her diagnosis. To add insult to injury, her husband found out later that his beloved wife was listed as a "cure" on the official ledgers, because she had died two weeks *after* the five-year mark. Thus, because of the American Cancer Society's definition of "cure," many patients who live five years after their cancer diagnoses are listed as "cured"—*even though they still show evidence of having cancer, or even though they die from their cancer.*[2] Thus, the definition of "cure" is the first big fallacy of official cancer cure-rate statistics, and may be the biggest official fudging tactic used.

2. **By simply *not including* certain groups of people, or certain types of cancer.** This is one of the hardest fudging tactics to believe. It means that, at times, the official cancer authorities have been able to make their statistics look better than they really are by simply *not including* certain groups of people in their statistics who tend to show lower recovery rates than other groups. These groups might be less likely to recover for socio-economic or other reasons.

   I was shocked when I discovered this could include *all non-white Americans*. According to Ralph Moss, two prominent medical researchers who published their findings in the *New England Journal of Medicine* stated that the NCI "generally reports whites-only figures. Nonwhites . . . are kept in a separate category, untallied with the main group."[3] Moss states that "NCI's solution is to list them in separate (but equal) charts, and then to present the white charts as the norm."[4] Moreover, the NCI has also been known to greatly improve its advertised cancer cure rates by simply omitting *all lung cancer patients* from their statistics![5] (It seems that the NCI sees lung cancer as different from other cancers because of its connection to cigarette smoking.) Yet, according to the American Cancer Society, lung cancer is the *leading cause* of cancer death for both men and women. Thus, in some statistics, the National Cancer Institute simply does not include the type of cancer that causes more deaths than any other type. Both of the above tactics of omission can only be called "biased selection," and yet these statistics are presented as representative of all patients and *all* life-threatening cancers.

3. **By including types of cancer that are *not* life-threatening.** The cancer authorities were able to improve their publicized cure rates even more when they took this brilliant step years ago. This tactic involves *including* cancers in their statistics that are easily treatable and not life-threatening, such as simple skin cancers. According to Dr. Douglas Brodie, "Five-year survivals of non-melanoma skin cancers, local-

ized cancers of the cervix, and some other non-spreading (metastasiz-ing) cancers detected early in specific sites, have been 'curable' (that is, amenable to five-year absences of symptoms) since the days of Ptolemy."[6]

As will be covered in Chapter 19, ductal carcinoma in situ (DCIS) is now included in breast cancer statistics. DCIS is really more of a "pre-cancerous" state that many experts believe should not even be classified as cancer, and is 99 percent curable. Yet, DCIS now com-prises about 30 percent of all breast cancer diagnoses in the United States and is included in the cure-rate statistics for life-threatening breast cancer as well. Thus, easily treatable skin cancers and DCIS are types of *non*-life-threatening cancers that are included in statistics used to imply what a patient's chances of recovering from *life-threat-ening* cancers are. This tactic is like adding the risk of being killed by a bicycle or by someone on a skateboard when compiling the statisti-cal likelihood of being killed in a car crash!

4. **By allowing earlier detection to imply longer survival.** This tactic is subtle but important. Over the decades, one of the aspects of cancer medicine that *has* improved because of improved technology is that of earlier detection. Advances in technology have allowed doctors and researchers to detect cancer on average about six months earlier than they used to be able to detect it. With the definition of cure be-ing "alive five years after diagnosis," earlier detection has, by itself, added many new patients to the conventional "cure" list.

    What is *not* accurate, however, is to claim that these improved statis-tics reflect *improved life expectancy* because of better treatment meth-ods. In other words, because tumors are getting diagnosed at earlier stages than before, and because of the way that "cure" is officially de-fined as a time deadline following diagnosis, long-term survival rates may *look* better now than they did years ago, but the reality is that no improvement in long-term survival has occurred at all.

5. **By deleting patients from studies who die too soon.** This is a partic-ularly treacherous way the cancer industry manipulates statistics. What this means is that it has become an acceptable practice in offi-cial cancer studies with human patients to simply "drop" a patient from the records if he or she dies from cancer before the treatment protocol is considered to have been completed. According to Dr. Lor-

raine Day, this means that "if a cancer patient dies on day 89 of a prescribed 90-day course of chemotherapy, he or she would just disappear from the list of treated patients and would not be listed as a failure."[7] Yet, if a patient in the control group (those *not* getting the specified treatment) dies at *any* time, that patient is listed in the study as a death from cancer. This is a double standard that shows an institutional lack of integrity and is definitely *not* consistent with true scientific method.

6. **By using an adjustment called "relative survival rate."** This was a variant on the five-year survival statistic that the official cancer industry created and adopted in the 1980s to help them claim that the war on cancer was being won. According to Ralph Moss, "Relative survival rates take into account the 'expected mortality figures.' Put simply, this means that if a person hadn't died of cancer he might have been run over by a truck, and that must be factored into the equation."[8]

These *adjusted* rates are used in a very misleading way because they are presented to the public as representative of mainstream medicine's ability to help a cancer patient recover from their life-threatening cancer. The only way this sort of adjustment could be used *correctly* is if the resultant statistics were presented with full knowledge of what they reflect. In other words, the American Cancer Society, or your doctor, would have to clearly say, "These figures represent your chances of living past five years with your cancer, given that you are using conventional medical treatments *and given that you might be run over by a truck, suffer a heart attack or stroke, or might be shot by a gun.* In truth, the relative survival rate adjustment is just one more way that cancer cure-rate statistics are manipulated to make conventional treatments look better than they really are.

The above six major fudging tactics are the real *back story* behind the "official" cancer cure-rate claims currently being advertised to the public. It is only by using extreme statistical manipulations and a totally misleading definition of "cure" that the cancer industry can make bogus statements like *40 to 50 percent of all cancers are curable.* It takes very little research to see that these statistics are *not real*, and that conventional medicine has failed in the arena of cancer treatment.

Because these tactics are not institutionally ingrained in mainstream cancer treatment and research, the conventional data available start out distorted from the get-go. Therefore, the real data needed to figure out the "true" conventional cure-rate statistics for cancer just aren't available. However, we don't need those data to know that we are in the midst of a very serious problem. All we need to know is that in just one year (1996), more people in the United States died of cancer than the number of U.S. soldiers who died in all of World War II, the Korean War, and the entire Vietnam War combined![9] This is quite a sobering thought. Another is that Americans are dying of cancer at a rate approximately equivalent to 10 September 11 terrorist attacks every month!

So, in the bigger picture, the first basic truth is "conventional cancer treatments have failed."

Second Basic Truth — Successful Alternative Treatments Abound

How many times have we heard television commercials that imply the pharmaceutical companies are working very hard to find a cure for cancer? Yet, you will discover in the following pages that many successful treatments for cancer have *already* been developed. They just don't get any publicity since they are labeled "alternative." To put it briefly, the cancer treatments that have been relegated to the alternative world have generally involved natural forms of treatment that could not be patented or otherwise controlled by the big multi-billion-dollar cancer industry. This huge cancer industry is run by powerful pharmaceutical companies and even bigger corporate cartels. Its big profits are threatened by any natural or individually owned treatment that can't be patented or controlled by big business for profit.

The truth is that there have been many highly successful cancer treatments developed over the past century that *should have been incorporated into mainstream medicine.* Most of them were developed and pioneered by highly respectable physicians or scientists — not quacks or con artists. The best of the alternative, non-toxic treatments for cancer have had blatantly higher success rates than conventional treatments, and these success rates reflect "real" cures, not phony redefined cures! But these successful cancer treatments have been *suppressed* to one degree or another, and many misconceptions about alternative cancer treatments have flourished.

One misconception is that, in order for treatments to be suppressed, there must be some kind of centrally located, well-planned "conspiracy" going on with little evil men in dark clothes wringing their hands and tittering "hee-hee" while eagerly anticipating peoples' deaths. This is not at all how it works. The suppression has been carried out in many different ways by many different organizations and is simply the result of business economics and common unethical tactics that tend to occur when large money interests are involved in any field.

Surgery, chemotherapy, and radiation involve billions of dollars of profit for the industries that supply them. Moreover, the current system for new drug development and full acceptance by the FDA is set up such that the cost of developing and bringing a new cancer drug to market is close to a billion dollars. (Common costs are 700 to 800 million dollars in the United States.) Without a patent, this type of cost investment is not economically feasible for a pharmaceutical company. This means that, since any treatment made up of natural ingredients is not patentable, a natural form of treating cancer will never be pursued by a drug company! Unfortunately for the public, the most successful treatments for cancer either involve natural substances or are privately owned and patented by creative individuals who were willing to think "out of the box" to develop something totally new. What they have to offer is always going to be an economic threat to the multi-billion-dollar cancer industry that is largely in control.

Thus, to say that there is a "conspiracy" to suppress alternative cancer treatments is like referring to industries that pollute the environment as joining in a "conspiracy" to sacrifice the well-being of our natural ecology. That would be ludicrous and would show a total lack of understanding that the way big businesses get where they are is by being profit-motivated. When it comes to the environment, it is true that some of the tactics used by industries to circumvent environmental protection laws or public safety may seem conspiratorial, especially if they involve falsifying paperwork, paying off Congress, or illegally dumping waste under the cover of darkness. But that does *not* mean there is a broad conspiracy by big business to pollute the environment. In the same way, there is no broad conspiracy by big business to suppress alternative cancer treatments. In both cases, *big businesses are just doing what they do best—protecting their profits.*

Another misconception about alternative treatments for cancer in general is that they simply involve going to the nearest health food store and buying everyday types of supplements. If you find it hard to believe that doing this would be a successful way to overcome such a powerful health challenge as cancer, your instincts are right. This is *rarely* how it is done. Most of the successful alternative approaches involve much more powerful treatments than that, and often revolve around very innovative methods that require the help of an experienced alternative practitioner or a knowledgeable support group to be done properly.

There is actually an *amazing* human story going on in the world of alternative cancer treatment these days. With conventional medicine failing most cancer patients, more and more people are turning to alternative medicine every year to save themselves. And large numbers of them are winning! They are beating their cancer even though conventional medical experts are claiming that what they are doing cannot be done. They are beating their cancer even though the big insurance companies are not recognizing or paying for the treatments they are using. They are beating their cancer because they are "outsmarting" their cancer with alternative, non-toxic treatments that work. Thus, the second basic truth of the cancer reality today is that "successful alternative treatments abound."

Third Basic Truth — The "Disbelief Factor" Is Alive and Well

Another widely held misconception about alternative cancer approaches is that, if they really worked better than the current conventional approaches, then cancer doctors and clinics everywhere would be using them. This misconception is at the heart of what I call the "disbelief factor." The disbelief factor is a dynamic that occurs in people's minds when they say, "If there really *are* natural, non-toxic treatments for cancer that can bring about real, long-term cures, even in cases of late-stage metastasized cancers, then why aren't all doctors using these treatments?"

Finding it hard to understand why all doctors are not using the most effective and least toxic treatments for cancer is not the problem. The real problem arises when a person finds this so hard to believe that he or she simply can't accept the possibility that there could be alternative approaches out there that really work. And when they are told there *are*, they often don't listen at all because it is just too preposterous to believe. This is the disbelief factor at work.

For those people with cancer who let the disbelief factor win, it is a tragic situation. Their disbelief keeps them from doing any further research on their own. They trust their doctors, not knowing that their doctors have only been taught the mainstream treatments and usually know nothing of the alternative ones. What these people don't realize is that most doctors are just people who *also* have a hard time believing in alternative treatments, and who ask, "If these treatments really work, why wasn't I taught them in medical school?"

And patients often do not realize that, even if their doctor did think an alternative treatment for cancer would help them, in most states that doctor is *not* legally allowed to prescribe or even recommend anything other than the big three of surgery, chemotherapy, and radiation. That is why cancer patients who are doing alternative treatments will so often hear from their conventional doctor monitoring them, "Just keep doing whatever it is you are doing!" These oncologists often don't even want to know what the patient is doing that is working because they know they can't prescribe it anyway. Unfortunately, the legal straightjacket that conventional oncologists are in only contributes to the prevalence of the "disbelief factor." The fact that "the disbelief factor is alive and well" is the third basic truth of the cancer reality today.

As you can see, the "bigger picture" of cancer treatment in modern countries such as the United States puts cancer patients at a disadvantage. The almost total separation between conventional and alternative therapies requires patients to do their own homework if they are to make a fully informed decision about their treatment. The good news, however, is that there *are* excellent alternative approaches available. But before we delve into those approaches, there are two basic questions to answer first: "Why so much cancer?" and "What causes it?"

Resources:

Book

Ralph W. Moss, Ph.D. *The Cancer Industry*. New York: Equinox Press, 1999. (ISBN 1-881025-09-8)

Video

Lorraine Day, M.D. *Cancer Doesn't Scare Me Anymore*. To order, call (800) 574-2437, or visit Dr. Day's website: www.drday.com.

CHAPTER 2

Why So Much Cancer and What Causes It?

More and more people who have never smoked, who do not drink heavily, and who have exercised and been health conscious all their lives are being diagnosed with cancer. And they are wondering how this could have happened to them. It is common for a person's first question after diagnosis to be, "Why me?" When they find out that they are far from alone, then the questions become, "Why so much cancer?" and "What causes it?"

It seems that if we listen to doctors, pharmaceutical companies, or advertisements on television about cancer clinics and treatments, we come away with the idea that cancer is some sort of *mysterious affliction* that no one completely understands. Other than knowing that too much sun exposure can cause skin cancer, smoking too much can cause lung cancer, and drinking too much can cause liver or kidney cancer, we somehow get the idea that, for just about any other case, the medical profession is "stumped" as to what causes cancer. What the public does not know, however, is that it is only the conventional medical world that is stumped. Researchers and practitioners who have been relegated to the alternative no man's land have been putting important pieces of the cancer puzzle together for decades and have already proven a number of key causes. Understanding these causes is important for the cancer patient because it moves cancer out of the realm of "something I can't fight" into the realm of "something I have control over."

Is Cancer Genetically Caused?

What about cancer being *genetically* caused? We hear so much about modern cancer research focusing on genes and how certain people are "predisposed" to cancer because of their family history. In

17

fact, looking at cancer as a genetically inherited disease has become so common that some women who have never been diagnosed with cancer are actually considering have both of their breasts surgically removed because they have a family history of breast cancer. This incredibly extreme preventive measure exhibits a powerful belief that cancer is genetic!

Although it is certainly possible that "a predisposition" to a few cancers may be genetically inherited, I will go out on a limb here and say that *most* cancers are *not* a result of genetic inheritance. In her video, *Cancer Doesn't Scare Me Anymore* (mentioned in Chapter 1), Dr. Lorraine Day presents two compelling reasons why we must assume that most cancers are *not* genetically inherited. Her first reason is based on the incredible rate at which cancer incidence has risen over the past century. As an example, she refers to how the incidence of breast cancer has risen dramatically since the early 1900s. Yet, those were the days of our grandmothers. Since the women of today are so closely linked genetically with their grandmothers, if breast cancer were a genetically inherited disease, then the grandmothers would have about the same basic rate of incidence as their granddaughters. But the grandmothers of today's women had a much *lower* incidence of breast cancer than today's women. For instance, as recently as the 1960s, about 1 in every 20 American women developed breast cancer. Now, just 40 years later, about 1 in every 8 American women develop breast cancer. If breast cancer were a genetically inherited disease, there would be no way of explaining this dramatic increase in incidence over just 40 years, and between one generation of mothers to the next generation of their own daughters.

There are many other examples of dramatic rises in cancer rates as well. For instance, Dr. Stoff and Dr. Clouatre wrote in their book, *The Prostate Miracle*, that between 1985 and 1996, prostate cancer diagnoses in this country rose from about 85,000 cases per year to over 317,000 cases per year.[1] This huge increase was over a mere 11-year period! And the incidence rate of non-Hodgkin's lymphoma has nearly *doubled* since the early 1970s. Both breast cancer and prostate cancer have been strongly linked to pesticide exposure, and non-Hodgkin's lymphoma has been strongly linked to herbicide exposure. Thus, it would seem much more likely that pesticides and herbicides are bigger contributors to these types of cancers than genetic inheritance. Moreover, *all* cancer incidence rates have risen over just a few generations. This sort of rise in all types of cancer would *not* be happening if cancer were primarily genetically caused.

Dr. Day's second reason to not assume that cancer is primarily an inherited disease is based on the reality that different groups of people
around the world show different incidences of various types of cancers
depending on what lifestyle or diet they are engaged in. In countries
where certain types of cancer are particularly low, the incidence of these
cancers increases when people from those countries adopt a Western
diet. But attributing cancer to dietary factors alone is misleading. As you
will see, there are many environmental and common lifestyle factors
that can contribute to the development of cancer. For example, cigarette
smoking may be the single *biggest* causal factor to cancer in our modern
world today. It has been estimated that a whopping 30 percent of all cancer deaths in the United States are attributable to tobacco smoke. This
means that if everyone were to suddenly stop smoking, deaths from cancer would reduce by about one-third!

The confusing issue is that cancer does, to a certain extent, involve
the genes in cells. But that does not mean it is an *inherited* condition.
For instance, genes in cells can mutate as a result of being hit by radiation or because of damage caused by some sort of toxin. Nutritional deficiencies can also contribute to gene damage. Robert Barefoot and Carl
Reich, M.D., make the point in their book *The Calcium Factor* that
chronic calcium deficiency in a person's diet can precipitate a condition
around cells whereby carcinogens are more able to penetrate the cell
walls and thereby gain access to and cause mutations of genes.

Moreover, researchers have proven that there are certain genes that
can promote the growth of cancer (oncogenes) and certain genes that
can inhibit the growth of cancer (tumor suppressor genes), and that *the
activity of these oncogenes and tumor suppressor genes can be turned on or
off by various physiological factors.* This is critical for people to understand. There are many things in our *inner* physiological environment
that can either promote or suppress the actions of certain genes within
cells. So, yes, cancer does involve the genes within cells, but that does
not mean that cancer is genetically inherited. When it comes to cancer,
gene activity more often reflects the *dynamic* state of genes in their interrelationship with the body's inner environment.

This is not to say that a predisposition to cancer is *never* inherited.
There may be a small percentage of cases involving some inherited factor. But very little has been proven about this to date, and what the evidence proves much more powerfully is that genetic inheritance is *not*
the primary cause of cancer. When cancer appears to run in families, it
is more likely that there are other factors, such as diet, lifestyle, ways of

dealing with emotional stress, and so forth, these family members have in common that are contributing to the development of cancer.

In general, the approach in modern medical science today is to look for just "one thing" that causes every illness. This may be partly why the search for an inherited genetic cause of cancer is so popular. However, a great deal of evidence points to cancer as a "multi-factorial" disease. This means that many factors usually go into the development of cancer for any particular person. I have come to look at these multiple factors as falling into two general categories: (1) "triggers," and (2) "deficient control mechanisms."

Triggers and Deficient Control Mechanisms

To understand how triggers and deficient control mechanisms contribute to the development of cancer, I'd like to use the analogy of a forest fire: What if someone were to ask the question: "What causes forest fires?" Looking for just one answer would be silly. We all know there are *many* things that can "trigger" a forest fire—a commuter throwing a lit cigarette out the car window into roadside brush; a camper allowing embers from a camp fire to blow up into the limbs of an overhanging tree; a bolt of lightning during a storm that hits a tree and causes it to ignite; or sunlight shining through a discarded piece of glass just the right way, causing some pine needles to ignite. These are all examples of factors that can trigger a forest fire.

But does a forest fire occur *every* time one of these triggers happens? No. This is because there are *also* many factors that will determine whether or not the initial spark will turn into a raging forest fire or not. I refer to these factors as "control mechanisms."

Some of the control mechanisms in the forest fire analogy may involve humans actively putting the fire out before it becomes big enough to be classified as a forest fire. But many of the control factors can happen without human involvement at all, and these would be factors in the "environment" around where the initial trigger, or spark of fire, occurred. For instance, environmental control mechanisms for the above examples might be: not enough brush and wind occurs along the roadside to fan a fire, so the commuter's cigarette spark is short-lived and burns itself out; the embers from the camper's fire have blown into the tree leaves of a very healthy, moist tree, so the fire never gets started in the first place; the bolt of lightning during the storm starts a tree blazing, but the accompanying rain drenches the tree and puts the fire out; or the sunlight shining through the glass starts a wisp of smoke in some pine needles, but the area is damp and surrounded by large rocks so the small fire has no where to spread and dies out quickly.

In this way, we can see that there are many "triggers" that can cause a spark that could result in a forest fire, but there are also many environmental "control mechanisms" that could stop that spark from turning into something that rages out of control and causes great destruction. *So too with cancer.* There are many common triggers, such as random errors in cell replication, or too much exposure to ultraviolet radiation, radioactive fallout, pesticides, and other environmental toxins. But there are also many natural control mechanisms within our bodies to keep these sparks from turning into raging forest fires of cancer.

Most medical practitioners and researchers agree that, in fact, we all probably have cancer cells developing in each of us all the time, but our bodies are able to dispose of them before they rage out of control. In other words, a healthy body can normally defend itself quite well against the development of cancer because it knows how to deal with these natural occurrences.

But life in the "modern world" has *skewed the balance between triggers and control mechanisms for cancer.* On the one hand, modern industrialized societies have introduced countless potent carcinogens and other toxins into our air, food and water, so that our bodies now have to deal with many more triggers to cancer than ever before. And on the other hand, modern industrialized societies have created highly processed, less than optimum foods and, through advertising, have promoted eating habits that result in poor nutritional support to our bodies. This lack of vital nutritional support can cause our own natural control mechanisms to become compromised and deficient.

The sad reality is that there are many more triggers to the development of cancer in humans than ever before in history, and peoples' control mechanisms are generally more deficient than ever before. There is just no getting around it. When we ask the question—"Why so much cancer and what causes it?"—the simplest answer is *modern living.*

A Disease of Modern Living

"Modern living" is obviously a broad reference, but it can be easily broken down into the categories of diet, environment, and lifestyle. For each of these categories, there are numerous factors that can contribute to cancer. Some are cancer-causing triggers, others are deficient control mechanisms. Briefly listed, some of the most important cancer-contributing factors of modern living are the following:

Modern Diet

- Not enough fresh fruits and vegetables
- Too many cooked and processed foods
- Foods grown in depleted soils
- Not enough essential fatty acids
- Too much refined sugar and refined flour
- Artificial sweeteners
- Excessive soda, coffee, or tea consumption
- Chronic dehydration (not enough water)

Modern Environment

- Pesticides
- Herbicides
- Chlorine byproducts (from chlorinated water and other sources)
- Fluoride
- Asbestos
- Fiberglass
- Nuclear radiation (from nuclear tests done decades ago)

Modern Lifestyle Choices and Treatments

- Cigarette smoking
- Birth control pills
- Hormone replacement therapy for menopause
- Common medical and dental X-rays
- Toxic teeth (from dangerous dental practices)
- Childhood vaccines
- Chronic stress

This is *not* a comprehensive list by any means, but it is enough to give you an idea of the types of factors today that can contribute to cancer. Now, let's look in a little more detail at these factors. (Each item above is listed in **bold** where it first appears in the following text.)

Diet

One of the biggest problems with the modern American diet today is that it typically involves a huge **deficiency of fresh fruits and vegetables.** Our modern diet has unfortunately developed around speed, ease, and the profitability of the foods being sold. People living fast and on-the-go lifestyles don't generally have a chance to carry fresh fruits and vegetables around wherever they go, so they must rely on **cooked and processed foods,** which are easier to carry around or prepare quickly. Cooking destroys important natural enzymes that aid the body in assimilating nutrients, and highly processed foods are practically devoid of much-needed vitamins, minerals, fiber, and phytochecmials. Fresh fruits and vegetables, on the other hand, provide us with many different nutrients that help our bodies defend against the development of cancer.

When we, in modern industrialized countries, *do* eat fresh fruits and vegetables, we are often eating produce that was grown in **depleted soils.** The more and more commonly occurring soil depletion results from over-cropping and the use of chemical fertilizers that do not maintain a proper balance of minerals in the soil. This means that even our fruits and vegetables may be deficient and imbalanced in their mineral content.

Essential fatty acids are another nutritional category critical to the healthy functioning of the body yet very deficient in the common modern diet. Two of the most important are the omega-3 and omega-6 fatty acids. These are called "essential" because the human body cannot biosynthesize them; therefore, they must be obtained through diet. The omega-6 fatty acids are primarily found in nuts and seeds, and the omega-3 fatty acids are primarily found in fish. When you think about it, seeds, nuts, and fish have been common dietary staples for humans for eons. Yet they are not abundant in the modern Western diet.

When we don't get enough vital nutrients, the cancer control mechanisms in our bodies cannot function optimally. But problems with the modern diet are not only defined by deficiencies. For instance, there is an *over*abundance of certain foods such as refined sugar. **Refined sugars and refined flours** (which are metabolized like sugar in the body) are hundreds of times more prevalent in the common modern diet than in the natural diets humans thrived on for millennia. This overabundance of refined sugars and flours contributes to all kinds of physical problems. One problem is that, if cancer does get started, lots of sugar in the diet may help the cancer to thrive because *cancer loves sugar.*

If a person tries to reduce his or her sugar intake, however, he or she often does this by replacing white sugar with **artificial sweeteners** such as aspartame (the sweetener used in NutraSweet, Equal, and Spoonful). Aspartame is one of the most common artificial sweeteners used today, and yet it was found to *definitively* cause various types of primary brain tumors in rats when studies were done in the 1970s. Even though these studies were conclusive, the FDA approved its use as a tabletop sweetener in July 1981. Two years later, in July 1983, aspartame was approved for widespread use in diet beverages as well. One year after that, the number of human brain tumors in the United States suddenly increased by 10 percent! There are currently more than 5,000 aspartame-containing products on the food market today, and it is estimated that over 200 million people in the United States consume it.

The way aspartame can trigger brain cancer is partly related to what happens to aspartame when it exceeds 86 degrees Fahrenheit, as it often does while being shipped in hot trucks or stored in hot warehouses. At higher than 86 degrees Fahrenheit, the methanol (wood alcohol) in aspartame converts to formaldehyde and then to formic acid. Both formaldehyde and formic acid are potent carcinogens. In fact, formaldehyde is categorized in the same class of deadly poisons as cyanide and arsenic. On the other hand, when methanol occurs naturally, as it does in fruits, it is always in the presence of ethanol. Ethanol keeps methanol stable and prevents it from breaking down into formaldehyde and formic acid. But the methanol in aspartame is "free" methanol, and thus unstable.

Aspartame comprises 10 percent methanol, 40 percent aspartic acid, and 50 percent phenylalanine. Methanol has been proven to cause damage to the optic nerve and can cause blindness. Aspartic acid has been proven to cause holes in the brains of mice. Phenylalanine breaks down into diketopiperazine (DKP), a tumor-causing agent. Thus, not only does the methanol break down into carcinogenic agents, but the ingredient found in largest quantity—phenylalanine—breaks down into a direct tumor-initiating substance. Some neurosurgeons have even reportedly found high levels of aspartame in brain tumors after the tumors were surgically removed and examined!

Moreover, brain cancer is not the only type of cancer aspartame has been linked to. Animal tests performed between 1971 and 1974 proved that aspartame caused mammary tumors (breast cancer) in rats. Nutritionist Janet Starr Hull, Ph.D., wrote a revealing book on the dangers of aspartame called *Sweet Poison*. On page 170, she lists the names of researchers and their universities who have published studies on aspartame. According to Dr. Hull, testicular cancer and endometrial (uterine) cancer have also been associated with aspartame.

Besides cancer, aspartame causes over 90 different documented adverse side effects. These side effects include debilitating MS type symptoms, seizures, coma, blindness, birth defects, and death. Some experts also believe that aspartame was the primary cause of the "Gulf War Syndrome" suffered by so many American troops. This is because thousands of pallets of diet drinks were shipped to Desert Storm troops where they were left to sit for weeks at a time in 120-degree Fahrenheit heat. Dr. Hull states that out of 90 *independently*-funded studies, 83 of them found one or more problems caused by aspartame. But out of the 74 studies funded by the aspartame industry (e.g., Monsanto, G.D. Searle, and ILSI), every single one of them claimed that no problems were found.

Sodas are now one of the most common beverage alternatives to water. But they are either high in sugar or high in aspartame or some other artificial sweetener. They are also high in phosphorus, which can disrupt the mineral balance of the body. And many sodas contain caffeine, which is a diuretic. All caffeinated drinks, whether they are sodas or **coffee or tea,** can actually contribute to **chronic dehydration.** Good, clean water is much more important to drink than many people realize. None of the cells of the body works at optimum functioning levels if they are chronically dehydrated, and some experts believe chronic dehydration can contribute to cancer by causing cell damage.

So, the common modern way of eating and drinking is full of nutritional deficiencies and, at the same time, complicated with an overabundance of harmful substances. This type of diet contributes to "deficient control mechanisms." And when an overload of toxins barrage the body on a daily basis for year after year, there are going to be problems. Unfortunately, most of these toxins come from our environment, which includes our air, water, and foods we eat. And more of these toxins are directly carcinogenic than most people realize.

Environment

This category of cancer-causing factors is probably the worst offender. In our modern world, we are surrounded by toxins in our air, water, and soil. We eat, drink, and breathe them on a regular basis. For instance, we breathe in countless petrochemical molecules every day from smog if we live in a normal industrialized city. But some of the worst chemicals, and *most* carcinogenic, are often the ones we don't ever see, feel, or taste.

One primary source of these invisible chemicals is **pesticides.** Pesticides are amply sprayed onto our food crops and are also used for household or garden insect control. I, like many others, used to have the misconception that pesticides can be removed from our produce once we get the produce home from the grocery store and thoroughly wash it. This is not true. The pesticides sprayed onto crops get *into* our foods.

These dangerous substances cannot be completely removed by washing the fruit or vegetable before eating it because they are *absorbed into* the fruit or vegetable as it grows. This happens in large part as a result of the pesticides being washed into the soil around the crops and then being absorbed by the plants along with water and other nutrients from the soil.

Thus, no matter how much we wash our fruits and vegetables, we will be eating pesticides unless we buy only "organic" produce from reputable sources. But even those people who are conscientious about buying only organic foods will probably also be ingesting at least some pesticides. This is because, through rain and irrigation runoff, pesticides have contaminated virtually all of our surface and ground water supplies so we are commonly drinking them.

Pesticides are similar to artificial sweeteners in that small exposures to them may be considered harmless, but daily exposure over many years is a very different story. Many of the carcinogenic compounds in pesticides do not easily break down over time, and tend to build up in the body, where they are stored in the fat cells. This can cause a *cumulative* buildup over the years. Many pesticides produce potent estrogenic effects, which means they mimic estrogen in our bodies. (More details on their relationship to cancer are covered in Chapter 19, What Women *Must* Know.) Because so many of the pesticide chemicals have estrogenic properties, they can be a *big* factor in numerous cancers of the body where sex hormones play a role—such as cancers of the breast, uterus, ovaries, and prostate.

In 1978, Israel enacted a strict ban of certain pesticides that had been linked to breast cancer. Previous to this, the occurrence of breast cancer in Israel had been steadily rising. Over the next 10 years, after banning these pesticides, breast cancer incidence in Israeli women dropped sharply. (There was an 8 percent overall decline, and a 30 percent drop in breast cancer deaths for women under age 44.)[2] And this decline in breast cancer incidence and mortality occurred while these same rates in the rest of the world were climbing, and while other negative factors in Israel, such as alcohol consumption, fat intake, and insufficient dietary amounts of fruits and vegetables, were increasing.

The 1976 Israeli study that had identified these pesticides found them to occur at much higher concentrations in the malignant tissues of women with breast cancer when compared to normal breast tissues. Over the years following the ban, there was a corresponding noticeable drop of these same pesticides in Israeli cow's milk and *Israeli women's breast milk*. Thus, these carcinogenic pesticide chemicals were clearly associated with breast cancer. The fact that these chemicals have been found in mother's milk also indicates they can be passed on to infants through breast feeding. This scary possibility may be one explanation of why so many young children these days are developing cancer.

One of the pesticide chemicals that Israel banned in 1978 was DDT, which has been linked to breast cancer by many different studies since the 1970s. Most people don't know, however, that DDT is still showing up in our environment here in the United States. For instance, in 1996, 80,000 tons of dirt containing DDT were dredged from Richmond Harbor in the San Francisco Bay at a site that had previously been a pesticide packaging plant.[3] The plant had conveniently dumped much of its residue into the bay. After dredging up this massive amount of dirt, the U.S. government decided to get rid of it by having it moved and buried in a landfill in Arizona. At some point in the future, the DDT in this landfill is probably going to leach into the surrounding Arizona groundwater and become a toxic contaminant to humans and animals once again.

But the use of pesticides on crops is not the only way we are exposed to pesticide carcinogens. A recent *Science News* article highlighted a study that showed a link between "household" pesticide use and childhood leukemia. According to the article, written by J. Pickrell, a team of researchers from the University of California at Berkeley interviewed families in Northern California over a four-year period (1995–1999). Among these families were 324 children age 14 years or younger. Half of these children were already diagnosed with leukemia (mostly acute lymphoblastic leukemia), and the other half were free of cancer. What these researchers found was that[4]:

- Families of the children who had developed leukemia were about *three times as likely* to have employed the use of a professional exterminator in their home than the families who did not have a child with cancer.

- The highest risk to children appeared to occur when a professional exterminator was employed while the child was two years old.

- Whenever a mother was exposed during pregnancy to any kind of household pesticide, the risk of her unborn child later developing leukemia was *twice* as high as for mothers who were *not* exposed to household pesticide use during pregnancy.

Thus, regularly spraying our homes for cockroaches, ants, fleas, or other pests may put us in danger of developing cancer in a similar way that large-scale spraying of food crops can.

Herbicides that are sprayed on lawns and crops to kill weeds also can contribute to cancer. For example, one of the most widely used herbicides in the world, a chemical called "2,4-D" is currently under scrutiny as a contributor to cancer in humans. Used in lawn products since 1944, 2,4-D is particularly good at killing dandelion weeds, which plague parks, residential lawns, and golf courses, but it has also been heavily used on commercial crops.

A revealing newspaper article in the June 1, 2002, *Los Angeles Times*, written by Emily Green, stated that Kansas crop workers who had been working with 2,4-D had a higher than normal rate of non-Hodgkin's lymphoma. This article also reported that the overall incidence of non-Hodgkin's lymphoma had increased in farm workers by 75 percent over the previous 20 years and that some statisticians have now linked heavy wheat growing regions of the United States (which are notable for their use of 2,4-D) to higher incidences of cancers of the esophagus, stomach, rectum, throat, pancreas, larynx, prostate, kidney, and brain.

According to the *Times* article, one reason the carcinogenic effect of this herbicide may have gone unnoticed for about 50 years is that the effect only surfaces as a result of "combining" different ingredients together. In other words, by itself, 2,4-D is virtually biologically inert, but when it is *mixed* with other common ingredients in weed killer products it can combine with other chemicals to become deadly. Yet, this weed killer is still commonly sold for residential lawns and gardens and used by many people who have no idea how cancer-causing it may be.

Smog, pesticides, and herbicides are all sources of environmental toxins that most of us are aware of to at least a certain extent. But some of the most carcinogenic environmental pollutants we are exposed to on a daily basis may be ones that most of us *are not at all aware of*. The biggest, invisible culprits may be chlorine byproducts, fluoride, asbestos, fiberglass, and nuclear radiation. In the following paragraphs, these carcinogens will be introduced briefly. But since they are such important and complicated issues, they will be discussed in more detail in the Appendix of this book.

Chlorine byproducts, also called "organochlorines," are unnatural compounds that are created as a result of the chemical interaction between chlorine and organic material. They occur largely as a result of chlorinating public water supplies, but they also occur in our daily lives from other chlorine sources. According to a joint study conducted by

Harvard University and the Medical College of Wisconsin, the simple act of drinking chlorinated water accounts for about 15 percent of all rectal cancers and about 9 percent of all bladder cancers. These add up to about 10,700 cases of cancer every year in the United States that are suspected to be due to drinking chlorinated water.[5]

More details about chlorination are discussed in the Appendix, but it is worth noting here that one category of chlorine byproduct, called "dioxins," has been referred to by scientific experts as *the single most carcinogenic type of manmade chemical known to science*. Read the Appendix to see how you may be ingesting dioxins every time you eat beef or dairy products, or even every time you drink a cup of coffee.

Fluoride is currently a controversial issue. But it appears to be controversial only on the *political* level, not the scientific level. To researchers who have studied it, there is no doubt that fluoride is an extremely hazardous substance to everyone's health in many ways.

Besides many other serious health problems, fluoride has now been linked to human cancers of the bone, bladder, liver, mouth, and lung, and it may contribute to other cancers as well. Dean Burk, Ph.D., former chief chemist of the National Cancer Institute, has been quoted in many sources as saying, "In point of fact, fluoride causes more human cancer deaths, and causes it faster, than any other chemical." Even Proctor and Gamble(the makers of Crest toothpaste) presented studies to the U.S. Public Health Service that showed fluoride to be a cancer-causing agent *at the lowest concentrations used*.

The public was fooled into accepting water fluoridation because the original tooth-decay prevention tests were done using calcium fluoride, or CaF_2. Calcium fluoride is the type of fluoride found naturally in water and plants. Yet, the type of fluoride that got added to public water supplies and toothpaste was *sodium fluoride*, or NaF. As opposed to calcium fluoride, sodium fluoride is highly toxic, but it is still the type of fluoride added to many public water sources and common dental products!

Unfortunately, even if you *don't* drink fluoridated water or use fluoridated toothpaste, that does not mean you are not being exposed to toxic fluoride. Through water sources, it has now contaminated many of our foods and numerous commercial beverages such as sodas, juices, teas, beer, and wine. Exposure to fluoride contamination in modern countries is just about inescapable. (See the Appendix for more information on the history of fluoridation and studies that link it to cancer.)

Another environmental cancer-triggering substance most people rarely think about is **asbestos**. We have heard bad things about it and have also heard that it has been largely banned and regulated. However, what we don't know is that a great deal of asbestos is *still* in our environment. Countless buildings all over the United States still contain asbestos insulation that releases microscopic fibers into the air the people in those buildings breathe. This includes countless modern skyscrapers and tens of thousands of children's schools. The microscopically small fibers from asbestos get into the air we breathe and take an incredibly long time to settle out of the air. They are also virtually indestructible. Once breathed into the body or ingested into the intestinal tract, these fibers can irritate cells and eventually cause cancer.

Virtually every man, woman, and child in industrialized countries has now been exposed to asbestos-contaminated air, no matter where they live or work. It has been estimated that in the 20th century asbestos killed somewhere around 300,000 asbestos workers, and countless other people whose cancers and other illnesses are suspected to have been asbestos related. According to cancer researcher Ralph W. Moss, some officials of our government have estimated that possibly 10 to 15 percent of all cancer deaths in this country are due to asbestos! (For more details on asbestos and cancer, please refer to the Appendix.)

It took many years before the use of asbestos was regulated in the United States, but as it was phased out, many manufacturers turned to the use of **fiberglass** instead. Fiberglass has not been studied as much as asbestos, but many researchers believe it may be *just as cancer-causing*. This is a controversial subject as well, but if fiberglass *is* this cancer-causing, then we are in very big trouble because something like 90 percent of all the homes in America use fiberglass insulation. Air circulating through air condition and heating vents can pick up and circulate microscopic pieces of this material from the insulation packing. It is as yet unknown as to how much fiberglass pollution is in the air we breathe.

Last but not least, in our look at major environmental cancer-causing factors we rarely think about, we come to **nuclear radiation.** Back in 1954, a Hollywood movie called *The Conqueror* was filmed on sand dunes outside of St. George, Utah. This location was about 150 miles downwind from atomic bomb testing sites. For three months, crew members and stars including John Wayne, Susan Hayward, Agnes Moorehead, and producer Dick Powell breathed in dust that was laced with radioactive fallout. Of the total 220 people involved with that film's production, 91 had contracted cancer by 1980 and half of them died of the disease. Those who died of cancer included John Wayne, Susan Hayward, Agnes Moorehead, and Dick Powell.[6]

We cannot be sure that radiation from nuclear fallout was the only cause of these actors' deaths, but the rates of cancer incidence in some areas of Utah have been so high that, in 1990, Congress officially apologized to the citizens of Utah and other areas downwind from nuclear testing. (See the Appendix for more details.)

Of course, you may be thinking, "Why would nuclear radiation be a factor in cancer today? After all, we're not testing nuclear bombs anymore, and we're not in a war involving nuclear weapons." The answer is that, during the 1950s and 1960s about a thousand nuclear devices were test-detonated in the Nevada desert as well as in a few other places around the United States, and the nuclear fallout from those tests is still affecting us today. Many of the detonations were carried out underground, but 184 were atmospheric, above-ground.[7] Radioactive nuclear fallout from these tests was then wind-blown over just about every part of the United States. Moreover, the tests in the United States were not the only sources of nuclear fallout exposure. It is probable that Americans were also exposed to fallout blown over the Pacific from the World War II detonations at Hiroshima and Nagasaki, test detonations carried out in the Pacific, test detonations carried out in the Soviet Union, and from nuclear power plant disasters such as Chernobyl and Three-Mile Island.

This wind-blown fallout from domestic tests, as well as from sources abroad, resulted in a great deal of "direct" radiation exposure to many people who later developed cancer. But it also settled onto our crops and into our soil and water. Since many of the damaging radioactive substances that settled into our water and soil have a very long half-life, they are still affecting us today. We still breathe them into our bodies when dust blows through the air, and we still ingest them in our crops and drink them in our water.

The important thing to remember about nuclear fallout is that some of the radioactive substances take only about 30 years to deteriorate—but other radioactive substances take *thousands* of years to deteriorate. This means that they keep on emitting radioactivity for a very long time. In other words, the fact that test detonations have stopped does *not* mean radiation exposure has stopped.

Once ingested, these radioactive compounds can get stored in various places in our bodies and keep on radiating. That is why nuclear fallout is capable of causing so many different types of cancers over a very long period of time. Even the National Cancer Institute finally admitted in a government report in 1997 that fallout from bomb tests carried out in the 1950s could have caused up to 75,000 cases of cancer. And since the NCI was only looking at the effects of *one* of the many radioactive isotopes generated, nuclear fallout has probably caused more like hundreds of thousands of cancers in humans.

Modern Lifestyle Choices and Treatments

This is a very important category of modern living because it involves cancer-causing factors we have *control* over. It is also a very disturbing category, since it highlights some big cancer-causing triggers that we may unwittingly *choose* to subject ourselves to without realizing that we are greatly increasing our chances of developing cancer by doing so.

Without a doubt, the first of these factors to look at is **cigarette smoking.** The director of the Harvard Center for Cancer Prevention has estimated that *tobacco smoke alone accounts for about 30 percent of all cancer deaths in the United States.*[8] Only about one-third of these cancer deaths involve tobacco-related lung cancer. This is because cigarette smoking has also been linked to cancers of the head, neck, mouth, throat, vocal cords, bladder, kidney, stomach, cervix, pancreas, and even to leukemia. Of the lung cancer cases that *are* tobacco-related, an estimated 20 percent of them are due to "passive" exposure. In other words, about 3,000 lung cancer deaths occur each year in the United States among *non-smokers* who have been passively exposed to tobacco smoke.[9]

According to W. John Diamond, M.D., and his co-authors of the book *An Alternative Medicine Definitive Guide to Cancer*, the cancer-causing ability of cigarette smoking was known to the tobacco industry back around 1950. Among a number of studies linking cigarette smoke to cancer incidence, in December 1953, researchers at the Sloan-Kettering Institute in New York published the alarming results of one scientific study involving laboratory animals. This study showed that when cigarette smoke "condensate" was simply painted onto the skin of mice, 44 percent of the mice developed cancer.[10]

It is a sobering thought that the number of cancer deaths in the United States could be cut by one-third if people just stopped smoking cigarettes.

One of the *next* biggest cancer-triggering modern lifestyle choices has to do with the use of synthetic hormones by women. Many modern women have chosen to use **birth control pills** or take synthetic hormones for relief from menopause symptoms. Whether or not long-term use of birth control pills can contribute to cancer is still a controversial subject, but there is a great deal of research indicating it *can* be a contributor—at least for young women who start their use of "the pill" before age 20. On the other hand, the cancer-causing ability of synthetic **hormone replacement therapy** (HRT) for women dealing with menopause has been well established. The following is a quote from Dr. Walter Willett, M.D., chairman of the Department of Public Health at Harvard Medical School. He refers to the current common HRT prescription of "Premarin" and "Provera" in the following statements:

> The downplaying of the risk of using animal-derived and synthetic HRT is even more despicable. The spin doctors calmly stated that for every 10,000 women on HRT during one year, only eight more will have invasive breast cancer, only seven more will have a heart attack, only eight more will have a stroke, and only 18 more will have blood clots. Sounds benign, doesn't it? It does, until you do the math.
>
> There are 8 to10 million women currently using HRT. Using conservative numbers, that adds up to 6,400 cases of invasive breast cancer, 5,600 heart attacks, 6,400 strokes, and 14,400 cases of blood clots to organs such as the lungs. That adds up to 32,800 cases of drug-induced morbidity *each year!*[11]

And the above quote only refers to conservative estimates for HRT-induced breast cancers, though HRT-induced uterine cancer has *also* been well-established. (This will be discussed in more detail in Chapter 19.)

Another "choice" common to modern living is the use of X-rays. It has been estimated that approximately 78,000 people every year develop cancer as a direct result of having been given **medical and dental X-rays.** Some researchers believe that a majority of breast cancer occurrences may be caused by medical X-rays given for diagnosing chest and lung problems, or spinal-related back and neck problems.

One of the most insidious sources of contributing factors to cancer, unfortunately, may be the field of modern dental practices. The subject of **toxic teeth** is still controversial, but the evidence linking certain cancers with dangerous dental practices is there. The most common dental practices that have been linked to cancer are: (1) silver/mercury fillings, (2) nickel-alloyed stainless steel used in certain types of crowns, and (3) root canal procedures. Many alternative practitioners who specialize in treating cancer agree that it can be important to deal with one's toxic teeth for a better chance of recovery from cancer. Not everyone has toxic teeth, but those who do may not know it. This is because toxic teeth don't always display clear warning signs, such as pain in the mouth or abnormal shading on X-rays. (Chapter 20 presents more details on toxic teeth and what you can do about them.)

Possibly one of the saddest realities today is that the common practice of administering **childhood vaccines** may be introducing carcinogenic substances into millions of children and contributing to pediatric cancers. This subject is also very controversial, but some researchers have come up with information that is quite alarming.

One couple whose two-year-old son was diagnosed with the most common type of pediatric brain cancer—medulloblastoma—did their own informal research, which they posted on the Internet at www.ouralexander.org/burton.htm. These parents went through agony when their small son was diagnosed and suffered through two brain operations and then chemotherapy. After their little boy Alexander died, these parents tried to figure out why he might have gotten cancer. He had been a strong child, and no one in his family, going back three generations on both his parents' sides, had ever developed cancer.

Alexander's parents researched how long medulloblastoma tumors generally take to grow, then looked into what had happened in the months just before that time. From their son's medical files, Alexander's parents discovered that just before this tumor had most likely started growing, Alexander had gotten numerous pediatric vaccines. Then his parents researched the available material on these vaccines, particularly on the DPT, IPV, OPV, and Hepatitis B vaccines. What they found out was horrifying.

Taken from www.ouralexander.org/burton.htm, here are some of the facts Alexander's parents discovered:

- There are six ways that vaccinations may cause cancer, directly or indirectly.

- Standard medicine really doesn't know if vaccines are carcinogenic or not, because no official studies have ever been done on this. In fact, according to Alexander's parents, "*None* of the vaccines injected into children has ever been tested for their carcinogenic (cancer causing), mutagenic (mutation causing), or teratogenic (developmental malformation causing) potential."

- Most vaccines contain carcinogenic chemicals in them, usually in the form of mercury derivatives, aluminum, and/or formaldehyde. If a parent were found injecting any of these substances into a child, they would be charged with child abuse. Yet these potent carcinogens are in most childhood vaccines.

- Vaccines also can contain viruses, or bacteria that contain viruses, and some viruses have been associated with certain cancers. Also, vaccinations for one type of virus can carry *unexpected* viruses in them that may come from the animals used to create the vaccine. For example, the polio vaccine of the 1950s and 1960s, that was injected into millions of children, was found to carry an unexpected virus from the monkey kidney cells that were used to cultivate the polio vaccine. This monkey virus, called SV40, was found to *definitively* cause cancer. In fact, in studies with young hamsters that were injected with SV40, 80 percent of them developed brain cancer! When this was discovered, polio vaccine manufacturers switched to a different type of monkey to avoid the SV40 virus, but in the meantime, millions of young people had already been injected with it. In 1995, the authors of one study on human brain tumors who published their results in the *Journal of the National Cancer Institute*, stated, ". . . we found SV40 DNA sequences in five of six choroid plexus papillomas, eight of eleven ependymomas, three of seven astrocytomas . . . None of the 13 normal brain tissues were positive for SV40 DNA."[12]

The possibility that many children may be developing cancer as a result of vaccines given to them to avoid illnesses that are less critical than cancer is simply horrifying and is an issue that desperately needs to be more prevalent in the public's awareness.

Last, but not least, modern life is full of stress. **Chronic stress** is probably the most common type of modern stress, as opposed to the type of stress generated by a single, temporary crisis. Chronic stress can result from a lifestyle that creates daily situations where a person is *constantly* feeling as though he or she is racing against the clock or on the edge of a crisis. Mothers and fathers who try to juggle full-time jobs while raising children and dealing with extracurricular school activities, busy freeways, and so forth, are prime targets of chronic stress.

But even *without* fast-paced lifestyles, certain personality traits alone can sometimes generate chronic stress. These tend to be the personality traits, or learned behavioral patterns, involving how we communicate with other people and deal with our emotions. People who chronically stuff their anger, frustration, or fear and don't know how to get their emotional needs met are often suffering on a physiological level from chronic stress.

High levels of chronic stress can negatively affect the body's defenses in many ways. It can cause higher than optimum stress hormones to be produced by the body on a daily basis, which can create an imbalance in other hormones. Chronic stress can even deplete the body's stores of vitamin C, because this vitamin is used up to create some of the stress hormones that the body generates. Along with other weakening effects of environmental triggers and deficient control mechanisms in the body, many cancer researchers believe that chronic stress can actually be a powerful factor in contributing to the development of cancer.

It is clear that, although cancer has been around for thousands of years, and occurs naturally in humans, other animals, and plants, the *frequency* of it today among humans has put cancer into the category of a disease of "modern living." After reading about all the possible cancer-promoting factors in the modern world, it is no wonder that many people who have eaten well, exercised, and otherwise lived conscientiously healthy lives are getting cancer.

How Different Are Different Cancers?

Is lung cancer a whole different disease from liver cancer or uterine cancer or prostate cancer? Are leukemias, bone cancers, and lymphomas different diseases from kidney cancer or bladder cancer? How different are all of these? The simple answer is that conventional medicine tends to look at cancers in different parts of the body as different diseases—but in the alternative cancer treatment world, cancer is cancer no matter where it is.

What you will discover in the following pages is that, once cancer develops in the body, it basically involves the same mechanics and cell functioning *wherever* it occurs. Although there are some *minor* differences among differently diagnosed cancers, these differences are minimal compared to the similarities, or commonalities, all cancers share. And the differences that *do* show up appear to result more from the fact that different types of body cells and body locations are involved in different types of cancer. Thus, rather than say there are different "types" of cancer, it would probably be more accurate to say there are different "manifestations" of cancer.

One minor difference the location of cancer can cause is the *speed* at which the cancer cells grow. This difference is linked to the type of cell involved in that particular system of the body. For instance, cancers of the blood, such as leukemia, replicate faster than many other cancers, simply because blood cells *normally* have the characteristic of replicating more quickly than other cells. Another minor difference is that cancers in sexual organs are generally much more affected by the sex hormones of the body than other cancers are. This is for the obvious reason that normal cells of sexual organs tend to have more receptor sites for those types of hormones, so when those cells become cancerous, they still have receptor sites.

And yet another minor difference that may be caused by the location of cancer in the body is the circulatory system that is involved. For instance, cancers of the lymph system and brain are in areas of the body that have unique circulatory characteristics and this may affect how well, or how quickly, medicines or nutrients from the blood can get to these types of cancer.

However, if we look at the most important characteristics of cancer on the basic level of cellular structure and functioning, different types of cancer are not significantly different. In other words, all malignant cancer cells share important common characteristics. Understanding these common characteristics can help to take the mystery out of cancer and can greatly help to reduce the fear that goes along with a cancer diagnosis. But more importantly, understanding the common characteristics and mechanics of *all* cancer cells, no matter where they occur in your body, provides the keys to understanding how to "outsmart" your cancer!

Common Characteristics of All Cancer Cells

The common characteristics of all cancer cells (no matter what type of cancer is diagnosed) are best explained by five scientific theories. However, to call each of these a "theory" is truly inadequate. As you will see in the upcoming treatment chapters, many years of putting these theories into practice have already proven their validity.

The Trophoblast Theory of Cancer

The trophoblast theory was first put forth in 1902 by John Beard, Ph.D., a Scottish embryologist. Dr. Beard presented evidence that cancer cells are virtually indistinguishable from certain pre-embryonic cells. These cells of early pregnancy are called "trophoblast" cells. During the early stages of every human pregnancy, trophoblast cells are those cells that grow very quickly to produce the umbilical cord and placenta.

One of the characteristics common to both cancer cells and early fetal trophoblast cells is that both types of cells produce a detectable hormone known as CGH, or chorionic gonadotrophic hormone. Luckily, CGH can be readily detected in urine. What is so fascinating is that no other cells in the human body produce CGH other than cancer cells and trophoblast cells of early pregnancy. This means that anyone who takes a CGH urine test and gets a *positive* result, is either a woman who is pregnant, or a man or woman with cancer.

Manuel Navarro, M.D., working at a university in Manilla in the 1960s and 1970s, actually *proved* this particular urine test to be 95 percent effective at detecting cancer of all types. And it turned out that the 5 percent assumed to be inaccurate test results were always false positives, as opposed to false negatives. In other words, the 5 percent supposedly inaccurate test results were only with people who didn't *appear* to have cancer, but after time went by, hindsight revealed that many of those people did in fact later develop cancer. Thus, the CGH test accuracy was very probably much better than 95 percent, and the test could detect cancer even before the disease was otherwise diagnosable. (Unfortunately, this test does not appear to be used for early detection of cancer today.)

Trophoblast cells of early fetal development are vital to the life of all humans. They are the cells that quickly produce a protective environment (placenta) and source of nourishment (umbilical cord) to the developing fetus. Since trophoblast cells perform such an important job during early fetal development, nature has provided them with a brilliant way to remain unaffected by the mother's immune system, which would normally attack them as foreign. This effective defense mechanism turns out to be a special protein coating that surrounds every trophoblast cell. The protective coating carries a negative electrostatic charge that allows the trophoblast cell to resist attack by the mother's immune system because all of the attacking white blood cells *also* happen to carry a negative electrostatic charge. Since "like polarities" repel each other, trophoblast cells are able to *electrostatically repel* any white blood cells that would normally attack them.

An example of this type of repelling process that has been observed by most of us in everyday life occurs when we notice static electricity causing our hair to stand up on our arms or head. What is really going on when this happens is that, for a short period of time, all of the hairs and the skin on a person's body happen to contain a predominance of the same polarity of electrostatic charge. Thus, since like polarities repel each other, each hair is electrostatically repelled away from the skin and at the same time is repelled away from the other hairs around it. This is the same mechanism by which trophoblast cells repel white blood cells of the immune system.

Cancer cells *also* carry this particular type of protective protein coating with a negative electrostatic charge. This protein coating does *not* occur around normal healthy cells of the body. Therefore, cancer cells and trophoblast cells of early pregnancy have the same built-in protection from white blood cells, and this is one reason cancer can be so difficult for a person's immune system to get rid of.

During early pregnancy, trophoblast cells create the umbilical cord and placenta, and they do this very quickly by rapid cell division and invasive growth into the uterine wall of the mother. This rapid invasive growth pattern is very much like the pattern of invasive cancer. The obvious advantage of the rapid growth is that the protective environment and food supply mechanism for the fetus are rapidly formed. So, why do trophoblast cells and cancer cells have so much in common? Dr. Beard of Scotland published a detailed explanation in 1911 in his book, *The Enzyme Treatment of Cancer and its Scientific Basis.* But to explain the trophoblast/cancer connection in a simpler way here, I will present ideas from cancer treatment pioneer William Donald Kelley, D.D.S., Kathy P. Fairbanks, Ph.D. (www.drkelley.info/articles/archive.php?artid=283), as well as other investigators.

In very early pregnancy, within the first five days after fertilization, human embryonic cells divide into two basic types: (1) embryoblasts, which develop into the embryo, and (2) trophoblasts, which form the placenta and umbilical cord. While the trophoblast cells are doing their job to create the placenta and umbilical cord, the embryoblasts are differentiating into the three primary germ layers (ectoderm, endoderm and mesoderm). The ectoderm cells develop into the skin, brain, and nerves of the fetus. The endoderm cells develop into the linings of the lungs, intestines, liver, pancreas, and other areas. The mesoderm cells develop into the muscles, blood, bone, and reproductive organs.

According to Drs. Kelley and Fairbanks, the mesoderm cells develop into the vast majority of cells in the body and eventually make up almost all the different cell types. Because the mesoderm cells can potentially develop into so many different types of body cells, they are referred to as "pleuripotent." Many different complicated factors go into the designation of what type of body cell a mesoderm germ cell will become, and some of the cues come from the germ cell's immediate surroundings and local tissue that it has migrated into. Drs. Kelley and Fairbanks claim that it is normal for every human adult to have a certain number of these mesoderm pleuripotent germ cells still scattered throughout the body in a "sleeping" sort of state. These sleeping germ cells have not yet differentiated and are still very similar to the trophoblast cells of early pregnancy. Under certain conditions, they can turn into malignant cancer cells.[13]

One recent confirmation of this concept is reported by cancer researcher, Ralph W. Moss, Ph.D. According to Dr. Moss, modern-day scientists have now confirmed a "stem cell"-cancer link. He writes:

> In 1998, mainstream scientists made a huge leap in understanding cancer when they discovered (and patented) embryonic stem cells (ESC). They did not reference Beard in their paper, but they used the term "totipotent" that had often been applied to describe germ cells, meaning that they were capable of developing into any other tissue.[14]

Author G. Edward Griffin claims in his outstanding book *World Without Cancer* that there is a normal and healthy function for these trophoblast-like germ cells in the adult body. He says these cells may get triggered into action wherever *healing* in the body needs to occur. They are the perfect cells to do the job because they are trophoblast-like, therefore fast-growing, and they are also able to develop into almost any type of body cell. The body naturally triggers them into action at any site that requires healing, and this is done with the help of certain hormones, such as estrogen and other steroid hormones. These hormones occur in both men and women and are well known to be found in high concentrations around areas of tissue damage.

Thus, according to Griffin and the trophoblast theory, cancer is the result of a completely normal process in the human body (i.e., the healing process) that has *not* been effectively kept under control. It might be said that it is *only when the healing process gets out of control* that detectable cancer can occur.

One-time damage to cells that is temporary, like a laceration, deep bruise, or broken bone, will generate trophoblast activity at the site of the wound that will usually be controllable. In other words, once the healing process is complete, the trophoblast-like healing activity is turned off. But where this healing process can get out of control is with cell damage that is of the "chronic" type. A common example of this would be when a person's cells in his or her lungs are damaged *chronically* through smoke inhalation from cigarettes day in and day out. In this type of situation, there is a constant activation of trophoblast healing activity.

Chronic cell damage can occur from many sources, including exposure to certain chemicals, toxins, radiation, or even as a result of poor diet that does not supply cells of the body with the building blocks they need. The bottom line is that chronic cell damage constantly triggers trophoblast-like germ cells for healing, and these cells multiply very fast and have a way of protecting themselves from the immune system. Under *normal* circumstances, there are natural control mechanisms in the human body that are designed to keep the trophoblast-like cells from multiplying too much, just as there are during early pregnancy and fetal development. So what are these natural control mechanisms?

The discovery of the primary control mechanism first came to light when researchers studied embryonic development. They discovered that the trophoblast cells of early pregnancy multiplied rapidly to form the placenta and umbilical cord *up until the eighth week of pregnancy*. But then the trophoblast cell proliferation stopped abruptly. For a long time, no one understood how or why this happened.

The answer came when researchers realized that it is during the eighth week of fetal development that the baby's pancreas first begins to function. One of the main jobs of the pancreas is to create a variety of pancreatic enzymes. Many of these enzymes go into the digestive tract and help us digest our foods. Breaking down proteins and other nutritional compounds is what they're good at. But others circulate via the bloodstream throughout all parts of the body. When certain pancreatic enzymes come across a trophoblast-like cell, they break down (or digest) the negatively charged protein coating. Once this coating is broken down, white blood cells of the immune system are no longer electrostatically repelled and are then able to attack and destroy the trophoblast cell. Thus, in the case of pregnancy, the fetus' pancreatic development is perfectly timed to occur just when the placenta and umbilical cord development should be stopped.

Critical for understanding cancer is the concept that pancreatic enzymes *continue* throughout our lifetime to attack and destroy the negatively charged protective coating around trophoblast-like cells that are triggered for healing purposes. If a person's supply of pancreatic enzymes is low or chronically stressed and depleted for some reason, and if other factors in the immune system are also stressed, then trophoblast cell growth *can* get out of control during healing processes and possibly turn into cancer. Of the various pancreatic enzymes that are able to break down the cancer cell's protective protein coating, "trypsin" and "chymotrypsin" are two of the most important. (Dr. Beard actually used injections of trypsin to help some patients overcome their cancer.) "Amylase" is another important pancreatic enzyme that has been found in the blood plasma of normal healthy adults, and can be found in particularly high concentrations in the plasma of pregnant women.

It is interesting to note that cancer is almost *never* found in the first segment of the small intestine, or duodenum. This is the area of the intestine that the pancreas transfers its enzymes into first. The duodenum is therefore literally "bathed" in pancreatic enzymes, and cancer of the remaining intestinal tract increases in frequency in direct proportion to the distance from this area.[15]

You might well ask at this point, "If pancreatic enzymes unmask cancer cells, then why does cancer of the pancreas occur?" The answer is that, in the pancreas itself, pancreatic enzymes are in an *inactive* state. They are converted to an *active* state only after they reach the small intestine, and they are circulated into the bloodstream from the intestinal tract after that.

A damaged or underperforming pancreas may not produce optimum levels of enzymes and can thereby contribute to cancer as a deficient control mechanism. (This brings up another interesting observation, which is that people who are diabetic and have a malfunctioning pancreas are actually three times more likely to develop cancer than non-diabetics.[16]) You will read in Chapter 7 how Dr. William Donald Kelley helped thousands of people to successfully "outsmart their cancer" with the use of high doses of specially formulated pancreatic enzymes in conjunction with special enzyme activators and other supportive techniques.

One last point about trophoblast cells is warranted here and has to do with "malignant" versus "benign" tumor cells. In *World Without Cancer*, G. Edward Griffin makes the point that when cancer is in its very early stages, the body sometimes tries to "seal off" the cancer by surrounding it with non-cancerous cells of that area of the body. This can then result in a benign lump or polyp. Griffin explains:

> Under microscopic examination, many of these tumors are found to resemble a mixture or hybrid of both trophoblast and surrounding cells; a fact which has led some researchers to the premature conclusion that there are many different types of cancer. But the degree to which tumors appear to be different is the same degree to which they are benign; which means that it is the degree to which there are *non-cancerous* cells within it.
>
> The greater the malignancy, the more these tumors begin to resemble each other, and the more clearly they begin to take on the classic

characteristics of pregnancy trophoblast. And the most malignant of all cancers—the chorionepitheliomas—are almost indistinguishable from trophoblast cells.[17]

The trophoblast theory describes cancer as a condition that develops after cell damage has triggered a natural healing process. This healing process involves trophoblast-like cells that carry a protein coating to protect them from the immune system long enough to do their job. If a person's body is forced to undergo too much chronic cell damage, or does not produce adequate levels of pancreatic enzymes to break down that protein coating and keep these cells under control, then the healing process may get out of control and become malignant cancer. The trophoblast theory also points out three things that *all* malignant cancer cells have in common:

1. All cancer cells carry a protective protein coating that helps them resist the immune system's white blood cells.

2. All cancer cells secrete the hormone CGH.

3. A sufficient production of pancreatic enzymes in the body is one of our most important control mechanisms for stopping the development of all types of cancer.

The Nutritional Deficiency Theory of Cancer

The trophoblast theory is just one source of information we have for understanding the common characteristics of all cancers. Another source is the nutritional deficiency theory of cancer that surfaced in the 1950s. It was the first theory about cancer development to focus on a specific dietary nutritional deficiency. The specific nutrient was considered to be vitamin B_{17}, a natural component of hundreds of foods commonly eaten by humans. These foods include lima beans, bean sprouts, most berries, yams, many seeds, cashews, macadamia nuts, millet, and buckwheat, to name just a few. In its natural state, vitamin B_{17} is also known as "amygdalin" and is part of a family of natural compounds called "nitrilosides." Almost all wild fruits and most seeds have some form of nitriloside in them.

The connection between vitamin B_{17} deficiency and cancer was first discovered by Dr. Ernst T. Krebs, Sr., a prominent physician and medical researcher. Dr. Krebs took an early interest in cancer. Soon, his son

Dr. Ernst T. Krebs, Jr., who had specialized as a biochemist, joined his father in this research. By 1952, the father and son team had discovered a definite connection between vitamin B_{17} and cancer, and had developed the theory that cancer was, at least in part, a result of nutritional deficiency. They also put forth the idea that the trophoblast theory and the nutritional deficiency theory of cancer are closely connected. The way they are connected is that the body's pancreatic enzymes are the "first line of defense" against cancer. Then, once the protein coating of the cancer cell is broken down by these enzymes, vitamin B_{17} from dietary sources joins forces with the body's white blood cells as a "second line of defense" and attacks the cancer cells directly.

This unusual vitamin actually works like a tiny "smart bomb." On a molecular level, the vitamin B_{17} is composed of four units: two units of glucose, one unit of benzaldehyde, and one unit of cyanide. The cyanide unit is tightly locked together with the other three units so that its toxic characteristics are completely inert under most circumstances. What the two doctors discovered is that there is only one situation in the human body that can cause the cyanide in vitamin B_{17} to be *unlocked* and released as a toxic substance. That situation occurs when the B_{17} molecule comes in contact with an enzyme called "beta-glucosidase." If this happens, then the unit of cyanide is released and is toxic, and the unit of benzaldehyde in the B_{17} is also released and is toxic. Moreover, these two substances working together are about a hundred times more toxic than either one is by itself!

Amazingly, it just so happens that the cyanide-unlocking enzyme, beta-glucosidase, *only* occurs to any significant degree in just one place in the body. It is only significantly present in cancer cells. Thus the toxic cyanide and benzaldehyde are released from vitamin B_{17} in the body *only when the vitamin comes in contact with cancer cells*. After the pancreatic enzymes, nature has provided us with an ingenious second line of defense against cancer—and it is a common dietary nutrient!

But that's not all. Nature even provided normal cells with a back-up *protecting* enzyme called "rhodanese." Rhodanese has the ability to neutralize cyanide on contact. In fact, rhodanese actually converts cyanide into other components that are beneficial to the body. By now, it should be no surprise to learn that the enzyme rhodanese is prevalent in great quantities throughout the body *except where there is cancer*. Thus, if any amount of cyanide from B_{17} does get unlocked near normal cells, the enzyme rhodanese will immediately detoxify the cyanide and convert it into good components. It sure sounds like there is a good plan here.

Vitamin B_{17} is an all-natural, smart chemical bomb that fights cancer. And it is found in so many food sources that all we have to do is eat a varied healthy diet consisting primarily of fruits, vegetables, grains, nuts, and seeds to get plenty of it. G. Edward Griffin points out that the groups of people around the world who regularly ingest high amounts of B_{17} from their diets are the same groups that show extremely low incidences of cancer.

One of these groups of people are the "Hunzakuts," or "Hunza," people of the Himalayas. The Hunza people have become very famous over the years because they are some of the longest-lived people in the world. It is quite common for a Hunzakut to live to be over 100 years old, and not too uncommon for them to live to the age of 120. And this longevity goes along with a very high quality of health and vitality. Cancer, in particular, was unknown to the Hunzakuts before they were introduced to modern civilization. Because of their unusual good health and long life, scientists from around the world have studied their habits and diet in great detail.

There are many healthy aspects of the Hunzakut lifestyle and diet, including clean glacial water, fresh air, fresh vegetables and fruits, and so forth, so it would be wrong to attribute their good health *solely* to just one thing. However, a very interesting fact is that the Hunzakut diet is has historically been high in vitamin B_{17}—possibly the highest in B_{17} of any human diet in the world. This is because apricot trees have always been the Hunza's main crop, and traditionally, the wealth of a Hunzakut man was measured by how many apricot trees he had. And the *most* prized food of all in their culture is the soft inner pit, or seed, of the apricot, which they dry in the sun and eat as an important part of their diet. It just so happens that dried apricot seeds are one of the highest sources of B_{17} found on earth.

Apricot seeds are like little almonds, and though quite bitter, it would be common, Griffin says, for a Hunzakut to eat 30 to 50 of them daily as a mid-afternoon snack. It has been estimated that, largely because of their apricot seed ingestion, the traditional Hunza diet may have had at least 200 times the amount of B_{17} as the average American diet. Thus, it is no wonder they never experienced cancer.

Evidence that the Hunzakuts are not just genetically wired to resist cancer has been shown by the fact that many Hunzakuts who partake in the lifestyles and eating habits of Western industrialized countries often fall prey to degenerative diseases, including cancer.

Another group of people found to be traditionally free from cancer are the Eskimos. At first reflection, this seems unlikely since one would think that an Eskimo's diet would be very poor in fresh vegetables, fruits, or seeds. The secret lies in the fact that the traditional Eskimo diet is very high in meat from caribou, reindeer, and other grazing animals. Grasses around the world are typically very good sources of B_{17}, and the fresh arctic tundra grasses are even higher than most grasses in their B_{17} content. This means that the meat from the arctic grazing animals is itself very high in vitamin B_{17}. There are also certain berries in the arctic summertime that are rich in B_{17}, which the Eskimos would eat large amounts of during the spring and summer. Thus the Eskimo diet has traditionally been *extremely* rich in vitamin B_{17}. And like the Hunzas, whenever Eskimos take on modern diets, they too succumb to degenerative diseases, including cancer.

Researchers over the years have shown similar correlations between diets high in B_{17} and a low incidence of cancer among other native populations of the world as well. These include many of the native North American tribes and native peoples of South America and Africa. One very rich source of B_{17} in the tropics, for instance, is the native fruit called "cassava." Cassava is such a staple of many southern indigenous diets that it has been called the "bread of the tropics," and thus provides protection for these people against cancer.

Philip E. Binzel, M.D., an American physician who specialized in fighting cancer with nutrition, made an interesting point in his book, *Alive and Well*. He stated that millet used to be a common staple grain for humans. Millet is one of the few grains that is very high in vitamin B_{17}. Nowadays, the most common grain people eat is wheat that is generally highly processed, and wheat has very little or no B_{17} content.

Interestingly, Dr. Krebs, Sr., has stated that in the Old Testament of the Bible there is a specification for how to prepare grains to be used in the making of bread. The formula is presented in Ezekiel 4:9 and discusses six ingredients. Five of these ingredients are rich in their nitriloside content and are barley, beans, lentils, millet, and chickpeas (garbanzo beans).[18]

In *Alive and Well*, Dr. Binzel also makes the point that human beings the world over have traditionally eaten meat from animals that grazed on natural grasses, and thus the meat was almost always high in B_{17}. Today, we eat meat from animals that are primarily grain fed. Unfortunately, the type of grain most commonly used has no B_{17} content. Thus, we in modernized countries today are not only eating grains that have no B_{17} content, but we are also eating meat that in the past would have naturally supplied us with B_{17}, but now is virtually devoid of this important cancer-fighting nutrient.

Although B_{17} may be one of the most important single nutrients used by the body to fight cancer, research has shown that the mineral zinc is an important transportation mechanism for B_{17}. In other words, without zinc, dietary B_{17} does not get into the tissues of the body. Dr. Binzel states that research has also proven vitamin C, vitamin A, manganese, magnesium, and selenium to all be important nutritional factors for the health of the immune system in general. Thus, many factors in the total diet of humans can be critically interlinked to support the immune system and the body's natural cancer-fighting "control mechanisms." (For more information on vitamin B_{17}, refer to Chapter 6.)

Otto Warburg and the Anaerobic Cancer Cell

So far, we have seen that all malignant cancer cells are similar to each other in that they have a protective protein coating that makes it hard for the immune system to attack them, and that pancreatic enzymes, naturally produced by the body, are nature's most important way of disabling this protective coating. We have also seen that all cancer cells are vulnerable to destruction by the important nutrient, vitamin B_{17}. Now, we will look at another important common characteristic of cancer cells. This characteristic is that *all* cancer cells are primarily "anaerobic."

The discovery that cancer cells are primarily anaerobic was made in the first half of the 20th century by Otto Warburg, a highly accomplished German biochemist and professor. A brilliant thinker and researcher, Warburg was awarded the Nobel Prize in medicine in 1931 for his discovery of oxygen-transferring enzymes involved in cell respiration. Warburg was intensely interested in the physiology of cancer cells and was the first scientific expert to put forth the idea that cancer cells *do not* use oxygen as their primary source of energy. This characteristic makes them very different from normal, healthy cells of the body, because all healthy cells *do* use oxygen as their primary source of energy.

Simply put, an aerobic cell meets its energy needs through the use of oxygen, and an anaerobic cell does not. Warburg discovered that cancer cells are normal cells that have given up their need for oxygen and have become anaerobic. He showed that, instead of using oxygen for energy, cancer cells are able to thrive in low-oxygen environments and meet their energy needs in large part through the fermentation of sugar, or "glycolysis." (It is worth noting here that researchers have shown that cancer cells may still use some small amount of oxygen in their respiration process, but they primarily use glucose fermentation, as opposed to healthy body cells that primarily use oxygen.)

Warburg adamantly believed that the "prime cause" of cancer was the switching of cells from their normal respiration process, in which they use oxygen for energy, to the very different respiration process in which they use the fermentation of glucose for energy. In other words, according to Warburg, cancer starts when normal cells transform from aerobic to anaerobic functioning.

We may not yet know all the reasons *why* a normal cell switches to anaerobic functioning, but there are some sensible theories that have been proposed. One of these theories suggests that when people with nutritionally inadequate diets develop inner bodily environments that are overly acidic, they are setting up a cancer-prone environment in themselves. We will talk more about the body's acid/alkaline balance in Chapter 18, but the basic concept is that minerals and other co-factors from the foods we eat help our bodies to maintain an optimum acid/alkaline balance.

If a person does not eat a diet sufficiently high and sufficiently balanced in minerals, the extracellular environment of their tissues can become too acidic. Stress, prescription medicines, soda beverages, and other factors can also contribute to an overly acidic body. *On a cellular level, overly acidic environments are low-oxygen environments.* Thus, it is possible that cancer may result partly because normal cells are forced to revert to a more "primitive" *anaerobic* state in order to survive in an unhealthy environment—an environment that is low in oxygen.

The fact that all cancer cells are primarily anaerobic is an important common characteristic to know about. This one characteristic plays a role in many different alternative approaches to treating cancer. In Chapters 9 through 12, you will read how directly targeting the anaerobic cells of the body with the effective formula "Protocel" has helped countless people to completely recover from their cancer. And you will also read in Chapter 17 about "cesium high pH therapy," the most alkalizing approach to outsmarting cancer.

Johanna Budwig's Essential Fatty Acid Deficiency Theory

Dr. Johanna Budwig, a German biochemist, was able to identify yet one more piece of the puzzle called cancer. And her discovery may actually provide us with a big key as to why normal, healthy cells turn anaerobic in the first place.

In the 1950s, Dr. Budwig discovered that cancer (as well as heart disease and some other degenerative diseases) was largely a result of a deficiency of essential fatty acids in our diets. She found that modern humans tend to be particularly low in omega-3 and omega-6 fatty acids, and that this deficiency is disastrous to the integrity of all of our body's cell walls. In Chapter 14, we will look more closely at how this type of deficiency contributes to the transformation of cells from aerobic to anaerobic functioning.

The reason Dr. Budwig's ideas are not more commonly known about today is because she had the misfortune to enter into a battle with the powerful margarine-producing industry that did not want her theory to become well known. This was because Dr. Budwig claimed that our diets are not only deficient in essential fatty acids in their natural form, but that we also eat an *overabundance* of highly processed fats, such as hydrogenated oils and trans-fatty acids. These highly processed fats, or oils, are the result of modern processing techniques developed to make profitable food products easier to market and distribute.

According to Dr. Budwig, this overabundance of "altered" fats in our diet is causing all kinds of diseases, and even killing us. This is because these "pseudo-fats," as she calls them, are being used by our bodies to form faulty cell walls. (Chapter 14 discusses just how these faulty cell walls can contribute to cancer development.) Dr. Budwig went on to prove her point by developing a specific diet that revolved around eating flaxseed oil and cottage cheese to replenish the body's intake of essential fatty acids. Clinical results of her dietary approach showed over and over that she was able to actually reverse cancer and bring about complete recoveries for many cancer patients.

The Microbial Theory of Cancer

There is one last important theory about cancer that needs to be mentioned here, and this one may be the *most* controversial. It is the concept that various microbes may contribute to the development of cancer. These could be bacteria, viruses, or other yet to be identified forms of microbes. Although cancer has never appeared to be an "infectious" disease caused by one particular external microbe, it may be that microbes commonly found in all of us are indeed involved in the development of cancer. These are certain types of microbes that remain in a benign form when the body is in a healthy state. But once the body has become seriously out of balance or unhealthy because of poor nutrition and other reasons, these microbes transform into a different form that is cancer-causing. Several researchers, including Royal Rife, Virginia Livingston, and Gaston Naessens, have produced clear evidence of this type of microbe-cancer link. Rife and Naessens even developed their own extremely powerful microscopes in order to observe these cancer microbes.

What is interesting is that all of the evidence linking microbes to cancer also indicates a "pleomorphic" quality to the microbes. "Pleomorphism" was an idea supported by the 19th-century French scientists, Claude Bernard and Antoine Bechamp (Pierre Jacques Antoine Bechamp). Bechamp and Louis Pasteur waged a huge battle of ideas regarding the characteristics of microbes. Pasteur believed that microbes were distinct organisms with distinct characteristics. In other words each microbe is either a particular form of bacteria, or a particular form of virus, yeast or fungi throughout its life cycle, and there is no crossover between forms. Pasteur's theory of microbes is referred to as "monomorphism."

Bechamp, on the other hand, argued that micro-organisms may not necessarily be limited to one distinct form. He argued the theory of "pleomorphism," which stated that micro-organisms are capable of having more than one form in a given life cycle. This means that the *shape* of a microbe can drastically change (i.e., a rod-shaped bacteria could turn into a spheroid-shaped bacteria), and the *size* of a microbe can also drastically change in response to the state of health of the organism the microbe is living in. Bechamp believed that certain bacteria could actually "devolve" into much smaller forms which he called "microzymia."[19] The theory of pleomorphism even includes the possibility that bacteria could turn into viruses in some situations as a direct response to their environment!

Pasteur's ideas ended up winning out and forming the basis of today's modern views on microbiology. However, if Bechamp's ideas had won out, modern medicine today might be looking at bacteria and viruses quite differently. And we might be looking at cancer development quite differently, too.

The main thing to remember about microbial theories of cancer is that they do *not* refer to cancer as an infectious disease caused by some form of exposure to an outer microbe. Rather, these theories of cancer refer to an inner change in certain microbes already existing in each of us, and that this change is a result of an unhealthy bodily environment and/or trauma to the body. In other words, poor nutrition, metabolic imbalance, toxins, radiation, or other damaging factors may cause common microbes that we each carry within us to pleomorphically change into what could be called a "cancer virus." Some forms of the pleomorphic microbes can also look like yeasts or fungi, and this may explain, in part, why many researchers have also found yeasts or fungi to be frequently associated with cancer.

Thus, microbial theories of cancer actually *support* the concept that the initial cancer-prone state of a person may start with nutritional deficiency or imbalance. Even when the microbial theory of cancer is used, cancer is still referred to as a "chronic metabolic disease," not as an infectious disease. (For more details on pleomorphism and the microbial theories of cancer, refer to Chapters 15 and 16, which discuss the Rife Machine and 714X.)

In summary, cancer is not so much a genetic disease as it is a disease of modern living. There are many contributing factors to cancer and many control mechanisms, as in my analogy of forest fires. These factors include countless known pollutants and toxins that are directly carcinogenic, nutritionally deficient modern diets, and other modern lifestyle habits. Yet, once cancer gets started, *all* cancers share common characteristics no matter where they are found in the body. These common characteristics of all cancer cells, which conventional medicine has disregarded, provide the main keys to how alternative non-toxic treatments work. The final key is provided by the fact that non-toxic treatments can safely be administered over long periods of time, 24 hours a day and 7 days a week. In this way, cancer cells are *never* given the chance to grow back.

Different non-toxic approaches may target different characteristics of cancer, but the outcome is always the same. In other words, they "outsmart" and defeat the cancer by either naturally blocking some aspect of the cancer cell's ability to function, by naturally strengthening the body's own ability to overcome the cancer, or both. If you are currently dealing with a cancer diagnosis, there *is* hope in the world of alternative, non-toxic treatments. In the next section, you will read the details of many different strategies that others have used to "outsmart" their cancer!

Section II

Alternative
Non-Toxic Treatments

CHAPTER 3

The Hoxsey Therapy

We begin our in-depth look at alternative, non-toxic cancer treatments with a completely *herbal* approach called "the Hoxsey therapy." Herbal approaches were not mentioned in the previous chapter as applying to any particular theory of cancer because they tend to work in a variety, or combination, of ways. Also, in some cases, we still don't know fully how they *do* work. Nevertheless, herbal treatments are documented as the oldest type of treatment for cancer and have been used with success for thousands of years by indigenous people all around the world.

In recent years, modern science has proven that many herbs do, in fact, have cancer-fighting properties. They have been shown to support the body's immune system, improve blood circulation, strengthen the functioning of major organs, and enhance the efficient elimination of toxins, among other things. They can act very much like a potent drug, as well. For instance, some herbs have direct cytotoxic effects on the cancer cells themselves, while not harming other cells of the body. Other herbs have been shown to inhibit a tumor's ability to produce new blood vessels to feed itself, thereby strangling the tumor's system of nourishment. And still other herbs have anti-microbial properties. Thus, herbs are often referred to as "nature's medicine" and the Hoxsey therapy for cancer is a wonderful example of this.

The Hoxsey therapy was the first widely used alternative non-toxic treatment for cancer in the modern United States. Still obtainable today, it is an herbal treatment consisting of a topical salve, a topical powder, and an internal herbal tonic. Though many people have never heard of it, this treatment approach was very successful and was actually used by tens of thousands of Americans in the early to mid-1900s. Around 1953, at the height of the Hoxsey therapy, the main Hoxsey clinic in Dallas, Texas had 12,000 patients and was the largest private cancer center in the world. There were also subsidiary clinics in 17 other states.

History

The history of the Hoxsey therapy is a colorful one. Harry Hoxsey, an American man born in 1901, was the person responsible for the widespread use of the Hoxsey therapy for cancer. But the herbal remedy had started farther back in time, and had been passed down to Harry by his great-grandfather, John Hoxsey. It was John Hoxsey, a horse breeder in Illinois, who developed the herbal remedy in the mid-1800s. According to the story as Harry told it, in 1840 his great-grandfather John had a stallion that was expected to die as a result of having developed a cancerous lesion on its leg. This horse had been one of John's favorites, so when the horse had to be put out to pasture, he kept an eye on it. He noticed that the horse exhibited atypical behavior by grazing primarily on one clump of shrubs and flowering plants. He also noticed that the horse's cancer completely healed after a number of months and the stallion made a full recovery.

Curious about his horse's amazing return to health, John picked samples from the plants on which the stallion had been grazing. Through experimentation, he developed an herbal tonic, salve, and powder from them. Some think John Hoxsey may have also gotten input from some of the local Native Americans about the use of these plants, but no one knows for sure. He then started using these remedies to treat other horses suffering from external cancers or other types of lesions. John's herbal mixture proved to be quite successful, and word spread quickly until horse breeders were bringing their horses to him from as far away as Indiana and Kentucky.

John Hoxsey's herbal mixtures were eventually passed down to Harry's father, a veterinarian. Harry's father also used the herbal remedies to treat animals with cancer and other conditions. But he started to quietly use the herbal treatments to help humans with cancer as well.

When Harry was eight years old, he began assisting his father in administering these treatments to some of the local people. These were generally people who had no other hope for recovery, and the Hoxsey remedies were having success . Just before his father's death, Harry, the youngest in a family of 12 children, was entrusted with the secrets of how to prepare the remedies and was given the responsibility to carry on the family's healing tradition.

Harry wanted to do this and enjoyed helping people. He decided to become trained as a doctor so he could legally administer the remedies to cancer patients. But coming from a poor coal-mining family, he had to work very hard to start saving money for medical school. Kenny Ausubel wrote the most in-depth and well-documented book about the history of the Hoxsey therapy, titled *When Healing Becomes a Crime: The Amazing Story of the Hoxsey Cancer Clinics and the Return of Alternative Therapies*. According to Ausubel, Harry did *not* want to treat any person with cancer until he had obtained his medical license. But while Harry was saving up for his medical training, people with life-threatening cancer who had heard about the success of his father's remedies kept coming to him and *begging* him to treat them. He tried to avoid doing this, but eventually treated some of them out of the goodness of his heart.

Unfortunately, Harry later discovered that his efforts to get a medical license would never be successful because, as a result of treating some of these desperate cancer patients without a license, Harry was blackballed from entry into medical schools.

Finally, one physician convinced Harry that he could legally administer his remedies to cancer patients as long as he was working as a medical technician under the supervision of a licensed physician. Since he couldn't get a medical license, Harry agreed to do this and began helping people with cancer under the official supervision of various different doctors. He was just in his early twenties, but he was a bright and energetic young man. The Hoxsey remedies were very successful, which brought more and more cancer sufferers to his door. Then, in 1924, when Harry was only 23 years old, he opened the first official Hoxsey Cancer Clinic in Dallas. It was operational into the 1950s and eventually became the biggest private cancer center in the world.

The Hoxsey therapy was mostly known for its success with external tumors on the surface of the body. People with external cancers were treated with an herbal paste applied directly onto the tumor and given a liquid herbal tonic to drink as well. People with internal cancer that showed no external signs were just given the tonic. Certain dietary changes were also recommended to patients in general, along with a few nutritional supplements. The ingredients of Hoxsey's internal tonic are well known, with most sources saying it was made up of potassium iodide, licorice, red clover, burdock root, stillingia root, berberis root, pokeroot, cascara, prickly ash bark, and buckthorn bark. Though it was not proven at the time, botanists have since found all of the herbs in the

Hoxsey tonic to have various anti-cancer properties. And the external salve contains bloodroot, which has been used by Native Americans to treat cancer for centuries.

But Harry Hoxsey was a renegade self-taught healer, and because he was *not* a doctor of medicine, he was constantly being arrested for practicing medicine without a license. Technically, he ran his treatment facilities legally because he always maintained a supervising physician with a valid license. But despite this fact, and maybe because established doctors felt threatened by him, Harry Hoxsey is said to have been arrested more times than any other person in medical history!

According to Ausubel and others, the *biggest* reason that Harry Hoxsey kept getting arrested was because the powerful head of the American Medical Association, Morris Fishbein, was out to get him. They claim that Fishbein wanted to buy Hoxsey's remedies from him, but Hoxsey refused. Thereafter, it is well documented that the ruthless Fishbein conducted a personal vendetta against Hoxsey.

Unfortunately for Hoxsey, the American Medical Association was just coming into its own as a powerful organization, and Morris Fishbein was not only the head of this organization, but also editor of the *Journal of the American Medical Association (JAMA)*. This journal was becoming a powerful force, and Fishbein used it as his primary vehicle for discrediting the Hoxsey therapy. In numerous articles over many years, Fishbein pronounced Hoxsey's cancer treatment as nothing but quackery. Journal articles also ridiculed and discredited any physician who chose to endorse Hoxsey's therapy. In this way, it soon became political suicide for a doctor or other medical expert to even consider using the Hoxsey treatment. The AMA's adamant disapproval of Hoxsey also seemed to be what prompted many of his arrests for practicing medicine without a license even though Harry always worked legally under the supervision of a licensed physician.

What kept saving Hoxsey was the success of his treatment—as well as his own tenacious character. Virtually every time Harry was arrested, groups of his cancer patients would gather outside the jail as a show of support. The crowds got bigger and bigger, and people brought Hoxsey homemade food and sang hymns outside the jailhouse all day long. Eventually, the wardens would release him.

The success of Hoxsey's cancer treatment was also what kept getting him acquitted in the many court trials he had to go through. According to Ausubel, in one case, a local deputy sheriff refused to serve Hoxsey with a subpoena, even though he was ordered to do so, because the deputy sheriff himself was undergoing treatment for cancer with Hoxsey.

In another case, Hoxsey was acquitted in a trial because 12 of the jury members were either former patients of Hoxsey's or had relatives or friends who had been helped by him. In yet another court battle, the trial ended favorably for Hoxsey because the presiding judge had been raised by a relative Hoxsey's father had cured of cancer.[1] Even several senators endorsed Hoxsey's cancer therapy. And over the many years he was charged with practicing medicine without a license, not a single cancer patient ever testified against him.

One of Harry Hoxsey's vehement opponents in Texas was Al Templeton, assistant district attorney. Over a two-year period, Templeton had Harry arrested more than 100 times. But in an ironic twist of fate, the district attorney's younger brother, Mike Templeton, came down with cancer of the intestine. He went through conventional treatment and a colostomy. But when his cancer was still there and began growing again after the surgery, Mike's conventional doctors told him there was nothing more they could do for him. At this point, Mike secretly went to the Hoxsey clinic for treatment and ended up completely recovering from his cancer. Upon hearing of his younger brother's unexpected cure, ADA Templeton reversed his attitude toward Harry. After years of continually arresting him, Templeton became Harry Hoxsey's lawyer and began legally defending him in court instead!

A Texas nurse named Mildred Nelson also believed Harry Hoxsey to be a quack at first. Mildred was trained in conventional medicine and tried to talk her own mother out of receiving the Hoxsey therapy for cancer in 1946. Mildred's mother, Della Mae, was in a desperate situation. According to Ausubel,

> Ranch wife Della Mae Nelson had uterine cancer that had been extensively treated with twenty units of X-ray and thirty-six hours of radium. She was so badly burned from the radiation that she couldn't even pull a sheet over her body for a year after. Wasted to eighty-six pounds, she was bleeding internally, so severely impaired that she had to learn to walk all over again. Then the cancer recurred.[2]

When Della Mae's cancer recurred, her conventional doctors told the family there was nothing more they could do for her. Against her daughter's wishes, Della Mae then sought treatment at the Hoxsey clinic in Dallas. She, too, completely recovered from her cancer as a result of the Hoxsey therapy. (Della Mae Nelson died about 50 years later, in 1997, at the age of ninety-nine. She had outlived most of the conventional doctors and nurses that had treated her). Needless to say, Mildred was finally convinced that Hoxsey's herbal treatment was effective and went to work for Hoxsey's Dallas clinic as a nurse. Mildred's father was subsequently also treated for cancer by Hoxsey, and he completely recovered as well.

Mildred found Harry Hoxsey to be a compassionate, admirable man with many talents. She recalled that he had a photographic memory and never forgot a patient's name or face. She also said, "He had a sixth sense if somebody was sick. He seemed to have almost a psychic thing of what would work for this particular person."[3] Hoxsey claimed to achieve about an 85 percent success rate for cancers that were external and about an 80 percent cure rate for patients with internal cancer that had *not* been already treated with prior surgery or radiation.[4] Many of the bus and taxi drivers in the local area were so used to transporting and talking to people who were getting well at the Hoxsey clinic, they claimed it was where they would go if they got cancer.

During the time that Hoxsey's treatment was showing great success, however, conventional treatments for cancer were beginning to become a very big business. By the 1950s, conventional cancer treatment had already become focused on surgery, radiation, and the fast-growing field of chemotherapy. Some people believe that Morris Fishbein was not the only obstacle to Hoxsey's Therapy, but that the inexpensive and unpatentable Hoxsey therapy threatened the emerging cancer industry's big profits and stimulated opposition from many sources. The favorite approach from the conventional medical establishment was to label Hoxsey a "quack" or a "hoaxer." These statements went completely against the facts, which unequivocally showed that Hoxsey's treatment really worked for a wide variety of cancer cases.

Since most quacks are in it for the money, if Hoxsey *was* a quack, he wasn't a very good one. All of the Hoxsey clinics admitted and treated any cancer patient who came to them, even *those that could not pay*. Ausubel's book documents numerous times when Hoxsey exhibited generosity to his patients above and beyond the call of duty, including fully treating people who had used up their last dime on bus fare to get to the clinic. Many times Hoxsey then drove them to a local place where they could stay. In reality, Hoxsey was following the advice his father had given him when he handed the responsibility of the family remedies over. His father said:

> Now you have the power to heal the sick and save lives. What I've managed to do in a tiny part of this state, you can do all over the coun-

try, all over the world. I've cured hundreds of people. You can cure thousands, tens of thousands.

But it's not only a gift, son; it's a trust and a great responsibility. Abe Lincoln once said God must have loved the common people because he made so many of them. We're common, ordinary people. You must never refuse to treat anybody because he can't pay. Promise me that![5]

In 1954, an independent group of 10 doctors from various parts of the United States made a point of investigating Hoxsey's clinic in Dallas. After the two-day inspection, which included examining hundreds of case histories and talking to patients and ex-patients, this independent group of physicians made a stunning public conclusion. They reported that the Hoxsey clinic

> . . . is successfully treating pathologically proven cases of cancer, both internal and external, without the use of surgery, radium or x-ray.
>
> Accepting the standard yardstick of cases that have remained symptom-free in excess of five to six years after treatment, established by medical authorities, we have seen sufficient cases to warrant such a conclusion. Some of those presented before us have been free of symptoms as long as twenty-four years, and the physical evidence indicates that they are all enjoying exceptional health at this time.
>
> We as a Committee feel that the Hoxsey treatment is superior to such conventional methods of treatment as x-ray, radium, and surgery. We are willing to assist this Clinic in any way possible in bringing this treatment to the American public.[6]

Here, finally, was the type of official medical endorsement that Hoxsey had been looking for to help him spread the treatment to more and more people. Unfortunately, this was not to be. The report of the 10 independent doctors was ignored by all influential parties.

Thus, Hoxsey was not only powerfully opposed by Morris Fishbein but also by others in the cancer industry. The higher-ups in the AMA may have been his most vehement opponents, but other organizations such as the NCI and FDA also helped to suppress any fair assessment of the Hoxsey therapy. Even though Hoxsey repeatedly pleaded with these groups to conduct scientific studies on his formulas, and even though thousands of patients were recovering from cancer as a result of Hoxsey's herbal mixtures, the official cancer industry's response was not to study it. In fact, unbelievably, official representatives from the FDA would actually "go to patients' houses, intimidate them, tell them they were being duped by a quack, and take away their Hoxsey medicines."[7]

Morris Fishbein eventually delivered a powerful blow by officially claiming Hoxsey as a hoaxer in a segment that was published, not in the AMA journal, but in a Sunday newspaper segment that was read by about 20 million people. Hoxsey sued Fishbein and the Hearst newspaper for libel and slander, and 50 of his cancer patients testified on his behalf in court. Fortunately, Harry Hoxsey won the lawsuit, although he was only awarded 2 dollars by the court.

The following excerpt from Richard Walters's book, *Options*, lays to rest any doubts that suppression of good, non-toxic cancer treatments has truly happened. Referring to Dr. Morris Fishbein after the Hoxsey lawsuit, Walters writes:

> The leader of America's "quack attack" was now on the defensive. Critics charged the AMA with being a doctor's trade union, setting national medical policy to further its own selfish interests. The United States Supreme Court agreed that the AMA had conspired in restraint of trade. Dr. Fishbein was forced to resign.
>
> In 1953, the Fitzgerald Report, commissioned by a United States Senate committee, concluded that organized medicine had "conspired" to suppress the Hoxsey therapy and at least a dozen other promising cancer treatments.[8]

But despite his legal victory over Fishbein, Harry Hoxsey's opponents eventually proved too powerful and all his cancer treatment centers were forced to shut down. The Hoxsey clinic in Dallas closed its doors in 1960, and its long-time chief nurse, Mildred Nelson, ended up moving the operation to Mexico where she faithfully administered the treatment for many more years. Thus, the Hoxsey therapy was finally pushed out of the country and effectively denied from the American public at large.

After a lifetime of fighting conventional medicine, Harry Hoxsey died in 1974. He had developed cancer of the prostate, and some sources refer to how ironic it was that he couldn't cure himself of cancer. However, Ausubel, who researched Harry's history more meticulously than anyone else, says that he *did* cure himself of his cancer using his own remedy and in fact died of other causes. Paul Peters, M.D., Harry's last doctor of record, adamantly claimed that Harry died of liver trouble and a weak heart. He vehemently said that before his death Harry was free of cancer. But Dr. Peters was out of town when Harry died, and another physician was required to sign the death certificate. This physician, not knowing the true cause of death, merely looked at Harry's medical records, saw that he had had prostate cancer, and wrote that down as the cause on his death certificate.[9]

Current Hoxsey Therapy

Effective cancer treatments don't die easily, however, and Mildred Nelson's Bio-Medical Center in Tijuana continues to operate and administer the Hoxsey therapy. She ran the center for 25 years after Harry's death and provided cures for many people until her own death from a stroke in 1999. The Bio-Medical Center is now being run by Mildred's sister, and information below indicates how to contact this treatment center. The Hoxsey therapy has been known to work successfully for many different types of cancer, and the center in Tijuana is currently claiming that the best responders to the treatment are those diagnosed with lymphoma, melanoma, or other types of external skin cancers. Some people find traveling into Mexico for treatment a bit daunting, but the comparatively low price of this treatment makes up for that difficulty for many.

People with cancer who go to the Bio-Medical Center today do not stay there as in-patients but make day visits over the border. These people are difficult to follow up on because they tend to go back home to other countries, so it is not easy to assess whether the treatment still has the same efficacy as it did when it was under Harry Hoxsey's administration. Hopefully, the United States will pass more freedom of medical choice legislation, and this amazing herbal treatment will someday be able to return to its U.S. homeland and be developed and studied further.

Resources:

Bio-Medical Center   Phone: (011) (52) 66-84-9011
P.O. Box 727
615 General Ferreira
Colonial Juarez
Tijuana, Mexico 22000

Treatment at Bio-Medical Center: As of this printing, the total cost of treatment is under $4,000. Patients pay a set "lifetime" rate that is the same for everyone and covers as many times as treatment is needed. Patients are asked to arrive by 9 A.M., Monday through Friday, and will be done by 4 P.M. No appointments are necessary.

For a consultation with the Bio-Medical Center: Consultations are extremely inexpensive. Bring any X-rays, blood test results, and so forth, that are less than one-month old. If you don't have these with you, you may be charged to have them done there.

Video

Hoxsey: How Healing Becomes a Crime can be ordered by calling (505) 989-8575.

Books

Kenny Ausubel. *When Healing Becomes a Crime: The Amazing Story of the Hoxsey Cancer Clinics and the Return of Alternative Therapies.* Rochester, Vermont: Healing Arts Press, 2000. (ISBN 0-89281-925-1)

Richard Walters. *Options: The Alternative Cancer Therapy Book.* New York: Avery Penguin Putnam, 1993. (ISBN 0-89529-510-5)

CHAPTER 4

Essiac

No book on alternative cancer treatments would be complete without a discussion of the herbal tea treatment called "Essiac." Like the Hoxsey therapy, Essiac has been around since the early 1900s and also has a colorful history. One of the Essiac herbs, "burdock root," is also part of the Hoxsey herbal therapy. While the Hoxsey herbal formula came to America from a horse rancher, the Essiac herbal tea came to Canada as a gift from Native America.

The history of Essiac begins in the late 1800s with a Canadian woman who was suffering from advanced breast cancer. She happened to meet an Ojibwa Indian medicine man, who told her he could cure her of her illness. She didn't want to have the surgery her doctors recommended, so she decided to accept the medicine man's offer instead. He showed the woman four herbs that grew naturally in her area and told her how to pick them and brew them into a tea. He instructed her to drink the tea every day. The Canadian woman did as she was told and subsequently completely recovered from her advanced breast cancer.

Thirty years later, in 1922, this same woman was a patient in a Canadian hospital in northern Ontario. Rene Caisse, the head nurse, was bathing the now elderly woman one day and noticed a great deal of scar tissue on the woman's breast. When she inquired about it, the woman told her about how she had been dying from breast cancer 30 years earlier and was cured by an Indian herbal formula. Caisse was extremely interested, especially since the elderly woman had not had a recurrence of her cancer in 30 years. According to one account, Caisse wrote down the names of the herbs from her patient in the hospital. According to another account, she visited the medicine man herself and was given the herbal remedy directly.

According to legend, Nurse Caisse found that the four herbs were sheep sorrel, burdock root, slippery elm bark, and turkey rhubarb root.

There may have been other herbs she was originally told about, too, but these are the four she supposedly ended up using. Nurse Caisse was told that when blended and brewed together in a certain way, these herbs had more curative power than any of the four herbs individually had.

About a year after receiving the herbal formula, Rene Caisse's aunt was diagnosed with stomach cancer that had metastasized to her liver. The doctors had given up on her aunt, so Caisse brewed the herbal tea and administered it to her. The tea worked and her aunt lived another 21 years.

Caisse then started collecting the wild herbs on a regular basis and preparing larger and larger portions of the remedy in her kitchen. She got permission from one doctor to administer the remedy to some terminally ill cancer patients the medical profession had no cure for. Soon, she was treating more and more cancer patients. When she wanted to pick a name for her concoction, Caisse decided to spell the letters of her last name backwards. That is how she came to name the herbal tea "Essiac."

With the supervision of some doctors who supported her work, she was able to leave the hospital and start up her own cancer clinic in Bracebridge, Canada. She was 33 years old at the time. From 1934 to 1942, Rene Caisse treated thousands of cancer patients who had no other hope. Though she never claimed her treatment was a cure, it turned out to be just that for many people. Caisse's own mother developed liver cancer at one point and Rene put her on Essiac. Her mother recovered and went on to live another 18 years.

Most people who tried Essiac came to it as a last resort. Because so many of these people were in very late stages or had already sustained damage to their vital organs, not everyone was able to fully recover. For many, Essiac was only able to "control" the cancer, and for still others it was successful only at alleviating pain. But literally thousands of people reported complete cures from their cancer. Nurse Caisse never required payment for administration of her cancer therapy. She did, however, accept donations from anyone who could afford to give them, and her clinic was supported by these donations alone.

According to Dr. Gary Glum, an expert on Essiac who wrote the book *Calling of an Angel*, the Royal Cancer Commission of Canada held hearings in 1937 and came to the conclusion that Essiac *was* a cure for cancer.[1] Finally, the Canadian Ministry of Health and Welfare and the Canadian Parliament became involved. Around 1938, grateful former patients and friends of Rene Caisse petitioned the Parliament to give Caisse the legal right to administer her remedy to anyone who asked for it. The petition was submitted to the Parliament of Ontario with an incredible 55,000 *signatures* on it. This action initiated a bill in the Ontario Parliament. If passed, the bill would allow Rene Caisse to legally treat cancer patients without the constant threat of arrest. If passed, the bill would also give credibility to Essiac as a recognized treatment for terminally ill cancer patients. Unfortunately, this unprecedented measure fell just three votes short of being passed.

Charles A. Brusch, M.D., was a well-known and highly esteemed doctor in the United States who had been the personal physician to John F. Kennedy. Dr. Brusch heard about Essiac and became very interested in it. Between 1959 and 1962, Dr. Brusch worked closely with Rene Caisse and together they treated thousands of cancer patients out of Brusch's clinic in Massachusetts. Dr. Brusch spent about 10 years studying Essiac in depth and using it clinically. After these 10 years, he concluded that "Essiac is a cure for cancer, period. All studies done at laboratories in the United States and Canada support this conclusion."[2] He even developed cancer himself and used Essiac to bring about his own complete recovery.

According to Dr. Glum, the Memorial Sloan-Kettering Cancer Center in New York also studied Essiac. However, some sources state that Rene Caisse was very protective of her formula and would not reveal all of the ingredients or methods of preparing it. These sources state that Caisse only allowed Memorial Sloan-Kettering to study one of the herbal ingredients—the sheep's sorrel. Dr. Glum states that Dr. Chester Stock at MSK did the research and discovered that the sheep's sorrel did have powerful anti-cancer properties. Glum also claims that this information was *withheld* from the American public, but was given to the Canadian Ministry of Health and Welfare. After receiving this information, rather than supporting the use of Essiac for cancer, the Canadian government immediately *banned* the sale and distribution of the sheep sorrel herb.[3] (It is *not* banned in the United States or other countries, however.) One can only guess at their reasons for doing this.

During the 1960s and 1970s, Rene Caisse tried to get various pharmaceutical companies interested in producing her formula for widespread use. The only stipulation she gave them was "that Essiac be put to immediate use with cancer patients."[4] But Caisse would not give her formula to the pharmaceutical companies for testing unless they signed the agreement she requested, and without being able to test the formula first, the pharmaceutical companies would not sign the agreement.

Finally, in 1977, just before her death, Rene Caisse sold her formula to the Resperin Corporation of Toronto for a dollar. She also reportedly gave her formula to two of her friends, Mary Macpherson and Gilbert Blondin.

Rene Caisse had treated cancer patients with Essiac for almost 60 years before she died in 1978 at the age of 90. Immediately after her death, the Canadian Ministry of Health and Welfare went to her house and destroyed all of her paperwork on the Essiac formula. They burned it in 55-gallon drums behind her house. Again, one can only guess at their reasons for doing this.

The Resperin Corporation took years to run tests on Essiac, and people in Canada could then only obtain Essiac by having a doctor's note saying they had terminal cancer and needed Essiac on an emergency basis. Eventually, however, Resperin Corporation produced the Essiac formula for widespread use. This version of it is now sold commercially out of many health food stores as well as from many sites on the Internet. Resperin's Essiac comes in dry powdered form in a box with instructions on how to brew it up as a tea at home.

But because of the delay by Resperin Corporation to market Caisse's herbal tea, another form of Essiac began to develop for commercial sale in the 1980s. This version of Essiac was backed by Dr. Brusch and was based on his clinical work with Caisse and her herbal remedy. It came to be called "Flor-Essence."

The development of Flor-Essence started out with a radio talk show host and producer in Canada named Elaine Alexander. Alexander had become interested in Essiac and had already interviewed many people who testified to her that they had recovered from their cancer using Essiac alone. In 1984, she phoned Dr. Brusch and told him she was interested in doing a series of radio shows about Essiac and told him she would like to interview him "on the air." He agreed to do this and the first radio interview lasted two hours.

In that first radio show, Dr. Brusch told the public in no uncertain terms that Essiac was, indeed, a cure for cancer. The response from the public was unlike anything Alexander had ever seen in her 20 years in radio. All the phone lines into the station were jammed for hours with people calling in. Before the first show was over, several people had even driven to the radio station and were waiting outside in the hopes that they could get their questions answered!

Elaine did more on air interviews with Brusch and had terminal cancer patients who had been cured by Essiac as guests as well. Her radio shows on Essiac became a phenomenon and she was soon overwhelmed with people needing her help as to what they could do and how they could get Essiac. Some cancer patients got her address and began camping out at her house to get advice and help.

For several years, Alexander and Dr. Brusch did their best to help the people with cancer who were coming to them. Finally, in 1988, Alexander proposed to Dr. Brusch that the two of them become partners and produce their own Essiac product. They both agreed at this point that it would be best to circumvent the medical establishment, which up to this point was not responding to Essiac in any helpful way. They decided to drop the Essiac name because it was too closely associated with "a cure for cancer," and thus too controversial, and they decided to simply sell it as an herbal detoxifying tea.

Brusch and Alexander looked for a manufacturing company that could meet the standards required for producing a high-quality herbal preparation, and they settled on a company called Flora in British Columbia, Canada. The herbal tea was produced and sold in bottled liquid form, and named "Flor-Essence." Flor-Essence can be bought today at many health food stores as well as over the Internet.

Currently there are two main versions of the Essiac herbal tea being marketed. One is Essiac from Resperin Corporation, and one is Flor-Essence from the Flora company. Besides these two, there are countless smaller herbal companies and private herbalists that produce and sell Essiac herbs to be brewed into tea at home. They all seem to have curative effects. Although the various forms of Essiac have never been fully accepted as formal cancer treatments, they are still being used by many people to help them recover from cancer. Right now, it is used in some form in every state of the United States, Canada, Mexico, Australia, Europe, Asia, and Africa.

There is still some controversy, however, as to the details of the original formula Rene Caisse used. The Resperin Corporation claims they have the *true* original formula containing just four herbs. Dr. Charles Brusch and Elaine Alexander, however, assert that Brusch was given the *true* original formula from Rene Caisse and that it contained the four herbs Resperin uses, but also contains four additional herbs: blessed thistle, red clover, watercress, and kelp. These herbs are added to their bottled version of Essiac called Flor-Essence.

It seems impossible at this time to know who has the original formula Rene Caisse used on so many thousands of patients. There are so more sources of Essiac on the market today, that it seems impossible to know which one is the most effective. Other sources of Essiac are sometimes referred to as "Ojibwa Tea" or "Ojibwa Tea of Life."

It is difficult to know which form of Essiac tea is best to recommend. I have read about and heard of some people with cancer getting well through the use of pretty much all the versions available. However, I have also heard of people for whom Essiac was not powerful enough to achieve full recovery for them. One experienced herbalist told me that the quality of the herbs used is critical. There may be a big difference between the potency of herbs picked from good "wild" soil as opposed to chemically fertilized soil. And exactly how and when the herbs are picked and brewed is possibly even more important. Many factors seem to contribute to how potent or effective any herbal treatment will be. Also, Rene Caisse *injected* the sheep sorrel into her patients and none of the herbal remedies today use that approach.

There can be no debate that herbal remedies such as the Hoxsey therapy and Essiac have, historically, been extremely powerful anti-cancer treatments. In today's modern world, there are still people getting well from cancer using these herbal treatments. Finding herbal sources today that use good quality herbs and prepare the herbs optimally is the biggest concern. Since it is difficult to be sure of the efficacy of any particular version of Essiac, it might be best to use it *in conjunction* with another recovery approach with which Essiac tea is compatible. The only approach I know of that is definitely *not* compatible with Essiac, is Protocel. But for all other alternative cancer approaches, Essiac tea can be of great supportive value. Many people even claim that the side effects of chemotherapy are greatly reduced when Essiac tea is used at the same time.

Resources:

Books

Richard Thomas. *The Essiac Report*. Los Angeles: ATIN, 1993. (ISBN 0-9639818-0-3)

Dr. Gary L. Glum. *Calling of an Angel*. Los Angeles: Silent Walker Publishing, 1988. (ISBN 0-9620364-0-4)

Sheila Snow and Mali Klein. *Essiac Essentials: The Remarkable Herbal Cancer Fighter*. New York: Kensington Books, 1999. (ISBN 1-57566-563-8)

Cynthia Olsen. *Essiac: A Native Herbal Cancer Remedy*. Pagosa Springs, Colorado: Kali Press, 1996. (ISBN 1-890941-00-X)

James Percival. *The Essiac Handbook*. (ISBN 0-9651484-9-1)

Websites

www.herbalhealer.com (Order 4-Herb Tea)

www.Essiac-resperin.com/en/history.html (Order Resperin's Essiac)

www.Essiacinfo.org

www.grand-strand.com/suebest/boywho.htm

www.cancer-solutions.net/Homepage.html (Order Dr. Glum's book from this site, or read it for free online.)

www.ojibwatea.com (Order Ojibwa Tea)

www.Essiac-info.org/prices (For many different Essiac sources)

CHAPTER 5

The Gerson Method

While the Hoxsey therapy and Essiac are two of the best-known herbal approaches to cancer recovery, the Gerson Method is perhaps the best-known nutrition/diet-oriented approach. Widely used since the 1940s, it is a natural, holistic approach with a long track record. It is also the method that started the trend of avid carrot juicing and coffee enemas so many people have heard about. Over the past 60 years, thousands of cancer patients have benefited from, or completely recovered, using this method. And many cases of other serious health conditions such as tuberculosis, adult-onset diabetes, lupus, and heart disease have been cured as well with the Gerson approach.

History

The founder of this famous approach was Max Gerson, M.D., a German physician of high acclaim who emigrated to the United States in 1936 and set up a medical practice in New York. But the history of his treatment started in Germany. Dr. Gerson had set up his first medical practice in Germany in 1919 and developed an effective dietary method for treating his own migraine headaches that had plagued him for years. In 1920, he began to treat other patients with migraines and, in the process, discovered that his dietary technique was also able to cure the dreaded disease lupus vulgaris. Lupus is a disfiguring type of tuberculosis of the skin that was considered incurable at the time, and Dr. Gerson was the first physician in Europe to bring about total cures for people with this disease.

While still in Germany, Dr. Gerson also successfully treated the famous humanitarian and Nobel Prize-winning physician, Albert Schweitzer, M.D. Dr. Schweitzer had been forced to retire from his beloved work because of adult-onset diabetes. Using a strict dietary regimen, Dr. Gerson was able to get Schweitzer off all insulin in just one month. With his health restored, Dr. Schweitzer was then able to go back to the humanitarian medical work he loved in Africa, which he continued into his eighties. Schweitzer credited his ability to keep working to Dr. Gerson and once said of him, "I see in him one of the most eminent medical geniuses in the history of medicine."[1]

Dr. Gerson then started to treat advanced cancer patients for whom expert cancer treatment of that day was not working. One aspect of his treatment involved having his patients drink hourly glasses of freshly prepared fruit and vegetable juices. His reasoning was that these juices would supply abundant oxidative enzymes and a potassium-rich array of minerals to aid in the re-balancing and rejuvenation of the body. He began seeing success with his dietary protocols, but also began observing that some cancer patients did not have a healthy enough liver to handle the detoxification process required to recover from their cancer. So, he began to prescribe coffee enemas to help stimulate the liver functioning of his patients.

Contrary to what may be popular belief, the main purpose of coffee enemas is *not* to cleanse the colon. Dr. Gerson understood that coffee enemas were actually a way to cleanse and heal the liver. The way the coffee enema detoxifies the liver is that when this type of enema is taken into and held in the intestines for about 15 minutes, the caffeine and other chemicals in the coffee go directly through the intestinal wall and surrounding blood vessels into the liver. These substances then stimulate the clogged bile ducts of the liver and cause them to dilate and release their buildup of toxic material.

There is also evidence that these stimulatory substances affect the gallbladder and cause its bile ducts to dilate and release toxins as well. Cleansing the liver and gallbladder so they can function more efficiently is important to the process of recovering from many conditions, and cancer in particular. Dr. Gerson also found that an unexpected but welcome side effect of coffee enemas was that they were often able to quickly relieve or reduce pain.

Another way Dr. Gerson began stimulating his patients' livers was by giving them liver extract injections, which also seemed to help stimulate better liver functioning. Dr. Gerson theorized that a combination of toxins and nutritional imbalances was at the heart of cancer, and he was the first practitioner to focus on the liver as a key organ in cancer recovery. His innovative work also focused on some very important electrolyte imbalances within the cells such as the potassium-sodium balance. To restore this type of balance, Dr. Gerson required his patients to stay strictly away from *all* table salt or salt added to foods and would also supplement his patients with extra potassium. Added to this regimen were other supplements as well, including vitamin C, digestive enzymes, niacin, a particular type of iodine, and relatively high doses of thyroid extract.

Besides nutritional supplementation, Dr. Gerson required his patients to go through rigorous changes in their diet. As well as staying away from all added salt, his patients had to severely restrict their intake of fat and protein. Gerson felt that low protein intake increased T-lymphocyte activity and promoted the release of sodium from cells. Patients had to eat primarily organic foods and prepare about a dozen fresh juices each day. They were also required to perform numerous coffee enemas every day.

Dr. Gerson was one of the first medical experts to understand, even back in the 1930s, that people's diets were nutritionally deficient and pollutants in the environment were causing toxic buildups in their bodies. He may have been the first to point out that the foods of the day were being grown in soil that has been damaged (e.g., by overcropping and chemical fertilizers) thereby causing imbalances of minerals in the foods themselves. And he pointed out the deleterious effects of commercially refined foods. He was known to have said, "Stay close to nature and its eternal laws will protect you."[2]

Dr. Gerson's focus on unprocessed foods and nutritional balance was virtually unheard of in the 1930s and 1940s since nutritional science had not become fully developed or accepted yet. In 1936, his innovative ideas for treating serious illnesses with nutrition were not enthusiastically received. Although Dr. Gerson began curing desperate cancer patients at an amazing rate in his New York treatment center, he was shunned and ridiculed by America's mainstream medical establishment. This was at a time when the all-powerful American Medical Association was labeling the idea that diet can affect cancer as a "false notion."

Dr. Gerson's ideas were proven to be right, however, by the incredible successes he was able to achieve with advanced diseases. In fact, he soon became known as someone who could cure "incurables," and many desperate people flocked to his clinic in New York. But Dr. Gerson's impeccable credentials as a top-notch physician and incredible record of success with cancer patients was not enough to keep him from being persecuted and harassed for his unorthodox treatment. He was treated as a "quack" and eventually expelled from the New York Medical Society.

In 1958, S. J. Haught, a New York newspaper reporter, received a letter from a woman who had been given two to six months to live by her cancer specialists, but had been later cured of her advanced cancer by

Dr. Gerson. This reporter then decided to look into the doctor who was being called a "quack" by the accepted cancer authorities. Haught was told by the AMA that Dr. Gerson "had failed or refused to acquaint the medical profession with the details of his treatment."[3]

Haught found out through his journalistic research, however, that the AMA's claim was completely untrue. Dr. Gerson had been anything but reluctant to reveal his methods. In fact, Gerson had published 50 medical papers and three books, including the very detailed A Cancer Therapy, in which he described his cancer treatment methods in depth. Haught learned that many of Dr. Gerson's scientific papers had been rejected by leading medical journals for no reason. Thus, his medical discoveries for treating cancer had been actively blocked from exposure to other doctors.

Haught found out that the Medical Society of the County of New York had already investigated Gerson's treatment center five times, where they had examined patients, looked at X-rays, and explored other aspects of Gerson's clinic and cancer treatment. According to Haught, the findings of this Medical Society investigation were never published or otherwise made available to the public. When Haught requested that the Society's findings on Gerson's treatment be released, his request was refused. Even though Dr. Gerson tried to get his treatment officially evaluated, the medical establishment did not want to do this.

Besides having great successes with "incurable" cancer patients, Dr. Gerson was also very outspoken against the tobacco industry. This did not put him in good stead with the AMA when their biggest source of advertising revenue from the Journal of the American Medical Association came from the Philip Morris cigarette company! As we learned with the Hoxsey therapy, the AMA had a very powerful influence in the 1940s and 1950s over what was accepted by the medical community and what was not.

In 1946, Gerson testified in a U.S. Senate hearing in support of a proposed bill to Congress that would authorize the president to "wage war on cancer." [4] It was the first bill of its kind and if passed, would appropriate $100 million to coordinate research and collaboration by the world's top cancer experts to find a way to prevent and/or cure cancer. Senator Claude Pepper was head of the sub-committee for hearings related to this bill. Dr. Gerson was only one of the experts to testify before this sub-committee, which would go down in history as the "Pepper Commission." Dr. Gerson spent three days presenting documented evidence of recoveries he had achieved in patients who were unable to recover from treatments given by leading cancer clinics and hospitals.

Another expert who testified was George Miley, M.D., the medical director of a hospital where Dr. Gerson had treated many patients. Dr. Miley not only strongly supported Gerson's approach and testimony, he also presented a disturbing study to the sub-committee. According to Dr. Miley, a long-term survey by a well-respected physician had shown that cancer patients who received *no* conventional treatment at all actually survived *longer* than patients who were treated with surgery, radiation, or X-ray![5] James P. Carter, M.D., author of *Racketeering in Medicine: The Suppression of Alternatives*, wrote that this senate bill was ultimately defeated by intense congressional lobbying paid for by big business groups that had interests in the multi-million dollar industries of surgery, radiation, and chemotherapy.[6] Tragically, the bill that could have directed unprecedented funding toward research into other than "established" cancer treatments was defeated by only four votes.

It was just a few months after Dr. Gerson's senate testimony that Morris Fishbein began to attack and ridicule Gerson and his cancer treatment approach. Fishbein used the *Journal of the American Medical Association* as his vehicle. In his book, *Racketeering in Medicine*, Dr. Carter explains that Dr. Gerson was subjected at this point to:

> . . . systematic harassment on the part of the New York State Medical Society and the New York State Licensing Board. Dr. Gerson's publications were blacklisted, and none of the reputable journals would accept them. His hospital privileges at Gotham Hospital in New York City were revoked after his impressive demonstration of success before the Pepper Sub-committee in 1946. He ultimately lost his license to practice medicine in the State of New York. The campaign to discredit him was likely coordinated by individuals in the AMA.[7]

But Dr. Gerson did not give up. In the early 1950s, he submitted five case histories of cancer recoveries to the National Cancer Institute and requested that an official investigation into his approach be carried out. The NCI's response was to tell Dr. Gerson it would need 25 case histories instead of just five. Dr. Gerson promptly supplied them with the requested 25 along with complete documentation. Then, after more than a year later, the NCI responded again to Dr. Gerson saying that 25 case histories would not be enough to justify an investigation, and they would need 125.[8] It appears that the NCI believed it had time and power on its side and could afford to play a cat-and-mouse game. The Gerson therapy was never fairly evaluated.

Even though Dr. Gerson was not able to see his effective cancer treatment accepted by mainstream medicine, he moved his cancer clinic to southern California and tirelessly continued to treat patients until his death in 1959. His cancer therapy is still being offered today at a facility in San Diego called the Gerson Institute. This nonprofit organization is run by Gerson's daughter, Charlotte Gerson. Charlotte Gerson is extremely knowledgeable and experienced in her father's treatment approach, and cancer patients flock from different parts of the world to her facility.

An overview of the Gerson method highlights two basic aspects of the treatment: (1) cleansing the body, primarily with coffee enemas, and (2) flooding it with rejuvenating nutrients, primarily from fresh organic juices. But the details of the Gerson therapy are a lot more complex than that and require careful attention in order for the treatment to be successful. A brief description of the approach is listed below, but to understand it fully one should read the books by Max Gerson and Charlotte Gerson. And the Gerson Institute highly recommends that for best results patients start treatment at either the Institute in San Diego or at another licensed treatment center. It is common for patients to spend three weeks at the Gerson Institute to ensure they understand the full extent of the therapy, as well as to receive unique instructions for their own case, before going home and continuing it on their own.

A Brief Overview of the Current Standard Gerson Therapy

- *Thirteen fresh juices a day* from organically grown vegetables and fruits. This is to flood the body with healing nutrients and live enzymes, which help balance, detoxify, and heal all bodily systems.

- *About five coffee enemas each day*. This is primarily to heal the liver.

- *Very strict diet*. This includes, among other restrictions: no salt, no sugar, and little fat or meat.

- *Nutritional supplementation*. This includes, among other things: potassium (liquid compound solution), potassium iodide (Lugol's solution), vitamin C, digestive enzymes, thyroid, flaxseed oil, niacin, liver/B_{12} injections, CoQ_{10}, brewer's yeast, and castor oil (both orally and rectally). The Gerson Institute now also recommends Laetrile supplementation for some cases. (Laetrile will be discussed in the next chapter.)

The Gerson approach is *not* an easy one to do. Some people have had to hire help in order to carry out all aspects of the program required. Juicing fresh fruits and vegetables 13 times a day in itself is a full-time job. In fact, the Gerson therapy might be the most difficult alternative cancer approach available, and even the Gerson Institute does not recommend it to those who do not think they can follow the program carefully and completely. This is one reason attending the Gerson Institute in San Diego as an in-patient first is a good idea. There, patients can learn how to correctly carry out the protocol while 13 juices each day are conveniently made for them. And initial supervision is especially recommended by the Gerson Institute for those who have already been through chemotherapy or have diabetes, brain metastases, severe kidney damage, or foreign bodies such as pacemakers, breast implants, steel plates, or screws.

Dr. Max Gerson had a broad impact on the field of non-toxic cancer treatments. Because he was the first pioneer to create a widely successful nutritional approach, many of Gerson's protocols have been incorporated into other alternative methods over the years, especially the concepts of daily fresh juices, coffee enemas, enzymes, and mineral supplementation. Many people with cancer are still achieving recoveries using his approach. It is a rigorous method to follow, but for those who are able to do it successfully, the reward is great.

Resources:

The Gerson Institute   (888) 4-GERSON (1-888/443-7766)
1572 Second Avenue   www.gerson.org
San Diego, CA 92101

Treatment at the Gerson Institute: Treatment generally involves being an in-house patient for either one week, two weeks, three weeks, or four weeks at the cost of approximately $5,000 per week (as of this printing). For most people, a minimum of three weeks is recommended. The Institute also offers a Gerson Therapy Home Package, which gives you the information needed to undertake the treatment protocol on your own. The Institute can also refer patients to clinics in other locations that are licensed to provide this therapy.

Books

S. J. Haught. *Censured for Curing Cancer: The American Experience of Dr. Max Gerson*. San Diego: The Gerson Institute, 1991. (ISBN 0-88268-109-5)

Max Gerson, M.D. *A Cancer Therapy: Results of Fifty Cases*. San Diego: The Gerson Institute, 1958/1999. (ISBN 0-9611526-2-1)

Charlotte Gerson and Morton Walker, D.P.M. *The Gerson Therapy*. New York: Kensington Publishing, 2001. (ISBN 1-57566-628-6)

Richard Walters. *Options: The Alternative Cancer Therapy Book*. New York: Avery Penguin Putnam, 1993. (ISBN 0-89529-510-5)

James P. Carter, M.D. *Racketeering in Medicine: The Suppression of Alternatives*. Hampton Roads, 1993. (ISBN 1-878901-32-X)

Ross Pelton and Lee Overholser. *Alternatives in Cancer Therapy*. New York: Simon and Schuster, 1994. (ISBN 0-671-79623-2)

CHAPTER 6

Laetrile

With the Gerson therapy being considered the first widely used nutritional approach to cancer, the use of Laetrile should probably be considered the second. Most of us have heard about Laetrile, but unfortunately, the only thing we heard was that it was some kind of "bogus" or "fad" cancer treatment a few decades ago. I was truly surprised, myself, to find the truth about Laetrile to be quite different. In fact, when I found out what Laetrile is and how effective it could be, I was amazed! Laetrile is simply a concentrated, purified version of B_{17}—the vitamin that tends to be high in the diets of those people around the world who rarely get cancer. (Refer to Chapter 2 for an introduction of B_{17} under the "Nutritional Deficiency Theory" of cancer.) In this chapter, you will see how this purified version of B_{17} has been used therapeutically to help people overcome their cancers.

The Two Dr. Krebs

To briefly review, vitamin B_{17} was originally studied by the two prominent scientists: Dr. Ernst T. Krebs, Sr., and his son Dr. Ernst T. Krebs, Jr. By 1952, they had discovered the ability of vitamin B_{17} to destroy cancer cells. They also proved that the cancer cell is the *only* type of cell in the body that carries the enzyme "beta-glucosidase." Beta-glucosidase unlocks the cyanide molecule bound up in vitamin B_{17} from its inert state, freeing the cyanide portion of B_{17} to then kill the cancer cell. The two Dr. Krebs also proved that all *healthy* cells of the body carry the enzyme, "rhodanese," which has the ability to neutralize cyanide on contact. Thus, if there is any cyanide from B_{17} that does get unlocked too close to normal cells, the enzyme rhodanese will immediately detoxify the cyanide and convert it into beneficial components that can be used constructively by the body.

Although vitamin B_{17} occurs naturally in hundreds of common foods, including various seeds, nuts, millet, sprouts, berries, and meat from animals that graze on grasses, the highest concentration of B_{17} in its natural state can be found in the dried bitter seeds of apricots. For their research purposes, however, the Krebs were able to produce a purified, synthesized version of B_{17}, and they called this "Laetrile." Thus, Laetrile is simply a common, but very important, vitamin.

The Krebses were able to get Laetrile introduced into widespread experimentation in numerous laboratories around the country. In the 1950s and 1960s, countless studies on animals showed Laetrile to be a perfectly safe substance *and* effective in treating various forms of cancer. After seeing the promising laboratory results, a number of physicians decided to see if it could help their human cancer patients as well. G. Edward Griffin, author of the definitive book on Laetrile called *World Without Cancer*, states "As early as 1974, there were at least twenty-six published papers written by well-known physicians who had used Laetrile in the treatment of their own patients and who have concluded that Laetrile is both safe and effective in the treatment of cancer."[1]

Drs. Nieper, Navarro, and Contreras

Laetrile for cancer was not just studied in the United States, it was studied and used around the world. Hans Nieper, M.D., of Germany, Ernesto Contreras, M.D., of Mexico, and Manuel Navarro, M.D., of the Philippines were three of the early prominent practitioners and researchers of Laetrile. They were some of the first physicians to pioneer what at that time was called "nutritional therapy" for cancer. Like Dr. Gerson, these practitioners were considered *unconventional* because they looked at cancer tumors as merely the symptom of the disease at a time when conventional doctors were treating tumors with surgery, radiation, and/or chemotherapy as if the tumor *was* the disease itself.

All three of these internationally famous physicians were dedicated to the development of this new type of treatment and to the publication of their findings. And all three achieved *astounding* results, which other physicians began to read about and duplicate as well.

Dr. Binzel

Philip E. Binzel, Jr., M.D., was one of the American physicians who, in 1973, found out about the work done by Nieper, Navarro, and Contreras. He was so impressed that he started practicing nutritional therapy with his own cancer patients. After about 20 years of treating cancer with Laetrile, he wrote a book about his experiences using Laetrile along with other supportive nutritional therapies for cancer. His easy-to-read and inspiring book is called *Alive and Well*, and I highly recommend it to anyone interested in Laetrile. There were also other prominent American physicians who successfully treated cancer with Laetrile, such as John A. Richardson, M.D., of California.

Dr. Binzel states in his book that no Laetrile practitioners ever claimed the use of Laetrile alone was enough to cure cancer. In other words, it was never meant to be used alone like a drug. Although the use of high doses of intravenous Laetrile was key to the nutritional therapy approach to cancer, other nutritional supplements, enzymes and diet changes were also part of the program. Then, after patients were done with the intensive part of their treatment involving intravenous Laetrile, they were instructed to continue at home indefinitely with certain diet restrictions and generally continued taking Laetrile supplements.

With Laetrile, supplements, and diet changes, an uncommon number of cancer patients became cancer-free and remained cancer-free until their death from other causes. And this treatment, like most alternative cancer approaches, *was not* restricted to just certain types of cancer—it was effective for all types. For example, following are three cases from Dr. Binzel's book, *Alive and Well*:

Case No. 1: Polly Todd

This 59-year-old woman was seen by me for the first time on 1/10/75 with the history that she had her left breast removed one month previously because of carcinoma. Three positive nodes had been found. I will let the patient tell you the rest of her history in her own words:

"It was recommended by a prominent physician that I be a part of an experiment in a (then) new chemotherapy program. For a second opinion I went to another city where I had a personal contact with the head of a large hospital. There they told me that my odds of survival were slim, and that I should be treated with strong doses of chemotherapy and radiation. At this point, a friend told me about the Laetrile-nutritional program, which I chose."

The lady was placed on a nutritional program at that time and she has remained on it ever since. She is now 79 years old, in good health, and she has had no recurrence of her disease.

In a recent letter the patient said, "None of the above people on the chemotherapy program lived beyond 1 1/2 years. Friends who scoffed at our choice then have much more respect now because others choosing the conventional treatment are gone, while I survive!"[2]

Case No. 9: Rex Perry

This 42-year-old man that I first saw on 6/27/79 with a history of having malignant lymphoma, which was originally diagnosed in August 1978. He had 8 months of chemotherapy, which he tolerated very well. His doctors felt, however, that there was a significant amount of disease still present. They wanted to do several more months of chemotherapy and follow this with total body radiation. The patient did not want to do this because of his concern about what it would do to his immune system. He chose, instead, to use the nutritional approach.

It has now been almost 15 years since he started his nutritional therapy. The most satisfying part of such a case history is that this patient has had no further problem with his disease. He is well and very active.[3]

Case No. 18: B. W.

This 44-year-old woman was seen for the first time on 2/6/81. She had been found one month prior to have carcinoma of the descending colon with 7 positive lymph nodes. A colostomy was not required. She received no radiation or chemotherapy.

She was started on a nutritional program. Now, some 13 years later, she has had no recurrence of her disease and leads a normal, active life.

What is so unusual about this patient? She had cancer of the colon with metastases. The odds of her surviving 5 years were one in one-thousand. Yet, she lives a normal life with no recurrence of her disease after 13 years.[4]

After many years of working with cancer patients using Laetrile (nutritional therapy), Dr. Binzel analyzed the success of his treatment. He separated all of the patients he had treated into two groups, those with primary cancer, and those with metastatic cancer. In the primary cancer group, there were 180 patients with 30 different types of cancer. After 18 years, 87.3 percent of these patients *did not die* of their cancer. When he subtracted the seven patients who died of unknown causes to conservatively concede they *may* have died from cancer, he still showed an amazing 83.3 percent long-term recovery![5]

According to Dr. Binzel at the time he published the above results, the American Cancer Society was officially claiming that with conventional treatment involving *early detection* and treatment of primary cancer that *had not yet metastasized*, ". . . eighty-five percent of the patients *will die* from their disease within five years."[6] Thus, nutritional therapy using Laetrile was clinically shown to be *by far* more effective than conventional cancer treatments.

Successful treatment of metastatic cancer is always more difficult to achieve because of the damage already done to the body, but even Dr. Binzel's rate of recovery for the metastatic group was impressive when compared to conventional treatment methods. His group of metastasized cancer patients consisted of 108 patients treated with nutritional therapy. After 18 years, 70.4 percent did *not* die from their cancer, and when he conservatively subtracted the 9 patients who had died of unknown causes, he still had a whopping 62.1 percent who did not die from their cancer in 18 years! This is truly incredible when compared to the American Cancer Society's official statistics on modern conventional cancer treatment. Recent ACS statistics show that *only 0.1 percent (or only one person out of every thousand) of patients with metastasized cancer who are treated with conventional treatments will survive five years.*[7]

Thus, Dr. Binzel could keep an average of 62 patients out of every 100 with metastasized cancer alive for a minimum of 18 years, while the conventional doctors could only keep about one in every 1,000 patients with metastasized cancer alive for five years. And Dr. Binzel's treatment success with nutritional therapy was similar to most of the other pioneering physicians using Laetrile, such as Dr. Hans Nieper, Dr. Ernesto Contreras, Dr. Manuel Navarro, and Dr. John A. Richardson. So his was not an isolated record.

But once again, the fight with the established cancer industry was a big one. Despite the fact that prominent physicians and researchers all around the world were showing positive results using Laetrile for cancer, the president of the American Cancer Society of California wrote a condemning article at the end of 1973, claiming that "Laetrile is goddamned quackery!"[8]

The Suppression

Unfortunately, nutritional therapy involving Laetrile was the recipient of one of the worst onslaughts of suppressive tactics ever used by the cancer establishment. These tactics involved outright harassment of physicians who administered it as well as intentional dissemination of disinformation (outright lies to the public as to its effectiveness). *Every* physician in the United States who attempted to help their patients with Laetrile was harassed by various agents of the cancer industry. This included physicians being arrested, hauled into court for no good reason, sometimes thrown in jail, and eventually having their medical licenses taken away. To go into the details of these physicians' ordeals would be beyond the scope of this book, but simply researching the history of any American practitioner of Laetrile will show this to be true.

The disinformation put out about Laetrile was focused around two general issues: (1) that Laetrile is too toxic for people to use because it contains cyanide; and (2) that it is simply not effective in treating cancer. The "toxic" argument is laughable. How can something be called toxic when it is ingested whenever a person eats lima beans, bean sprouts, almost any seed or nut, berries, millet, and other foods; when animals thrive on natural foods high in it; and when the healthiest people on earth eat diets extremely rich in it? Also, if it is so toxic, then why is vitamin B_{12} allowed to be sold as a health supplement? Most people don't know that vitamin B_{12} *also* contains the same type of cyanide molecule that is in vitamin B_{17}.

Moreover, according to Griffin, "aspirin tablets are twenty times more toxic than the equivalent amount of Laetrile."[9] Yet aspirin is a highly touted and promoted product. Of course, when compared to the radiation and chemotherapy treatments that are routinely approved by the FDA, the subject of Laetrile being toxic moves into the realm of the absurd. Unlike most drugs that *may* have toxic side effects, when it comes to chemotherapy and radiation, toxicity *is the goal*. Chemotherapy and radiation treatments routinely involve toxicity that is simply off the scales, and many deaths have been documented as a *direct* result of these treatments. Apparently, the FDA and the cancer industry believe that the side effect of "death" is tolerable, as long as it comes from treatments they endorse!

As to the claim that Laetrile is simply *not effective*, this long ago moved out of the realm of the "absurd" and into the realm of the "criminal." Powerful people at Memorial Sloan-Kettering, the American Medical Association, the American Cancer Society, the National Cancer Institute, and even the FDA *lied* to the public and press about Laetrile. And they did it effectively enough to get Laetrile suppressed almost completely. For the most complete exposé of this, there is no better source than the well-documented book *World Without Cancer* by G. Edward Griffin. Let's look at some of the information presented by Griffin to get an idea of how the public has largely been denied an effective non-toxic cancer treatment.

According to Griffin, one of the first dramas of deception occurred at the Mayo Clinic around 1978. Studies on Laetrile there were *not* conducted according to the correct protocol given by the physicians who had been using it, and there have been serious doubts that the Laetrile used in the Mayo Clinic study was even of good quality or purity. As a result of their improperly done studies, the Mayo Clinic researchers concluded that they found no effectiveness of Laetrile on cancer. Many practitioners who had already witnessed great success using Laetrile on their own cancer patients believed that the Mayo Clinic clinical trials had been deliberately designed to fail.

The next drama, and possibly the most criminal story of deception, occurred at Memorial Sloan-Kettering Cancer Center in New York. Between the years 1972 and 1977, Laetrile had been tested on animals with cancer under the direction of one of the country's most respected scientists, Dr. Kanematsu Sugiura. Dr. Sugiura was Memorial Sloan-Kettering's senior laboratory researcher, and he found Laetrile to be *highly effective* against cancers of all types. Yet most medical professionals never knew about his findings because the higher-ups at Sloan-Kettering found ways to get around his results. According to Griffin,

> Dr. Kanematsu Sugiura . . . reported that, in his experiments with mice, Laetrile was more effective in the control of cancer than any substance he had ever tested. This was not acceptable to his superiors. Instead of being pleased at the possibility of a breakthrough, they brought in other researchers to duplicate Sugiura's experiments and to prove they were faulty. Instead, the follow-up studies confirmed Sugiura's. Undaunted, his superiors called for new experiments over and over again, following procedures designed to make the tests fail. Eventually they did fail, and it was that failure that was announced to the world.[10]

Support for the above facts can be found in Ralph W. Moss's book, *The Cancer Industry*. Ralph Moss was a Ph.D. science writer when he was hired to work at Memorial Sloan-Kettering Cancer Center in 1974, and he went on to become its assistant director of public affairs. He claims he was fired in 1977 for "opposing their coverup of positive data on the drug laetrile."[11] But Moss was not a writer to simply curl up his tail and run. He went on to write several books in which he presented in-depth exposés of the cancer industry's outright opposition to and suppression of non-toxic, alternative treatments.

Even though Memorial Sloan-Kettering claimed Laetrile was ineffective against cancer, other respected laboratories around the world came up with positive results in carefully controlled studies on mice. Some of these were Scind Laboratories of San Francisco in 1968, the Pasteur Institute of Paris in 1971, and the Institute von Ardenne of Dresden, Germany, in 1973.[12] There were also numerous prominent physicians around the world who found Laetrile to be effective with their human cancer patients. One of these physicians, Dr. Shigeaki Sakai of Tokyo, published an article in 1963 in the *Asian Medical Journal,* in which he stated:

> Administered to cancer patients, Laetrile has proven to be quite free from any harmful side effects, and I would say that no anti-cancer drug could make a cancerous patient improve faster than Laetrile. It goes without saying that Laetrile controls cancer and is quite effective wherever it is located.[13]

And in 1972, Dr. Hans Nieper of West Germany told U.S. reporters:

> After more than 20 years of such specialized work, I have found the nontoxic Nitrilosides—that is, Laetrile—far superior to any other known cancer treatment or preventative. In my opinion it is the only existing possibility for the ultimate control of cancer.[14]

One piece of "misinformation" that was publicized in the early 1980s may have been the final straw in breaking down public acceptance of Laetrile. It was widely reported that actor Steve McQueen died as a result of going to Mexico in 1980 for treatments of Laetrile in an attempt to treat his cancer. What the presses around the country *failed* to report was that McQueen actually *was* cured of his cancer over about four months as a result of Laetrile and other alternative treatments. However, a benign, non-cancerous tumor remained in his abdomen, which he chose to have removed for cosmetic reasons. It was because of complications from this surgery that he died, not from the cancer[15].

The Steve McQueen case is just one example of how incorrect media reporting caused millions of Americans to believe that Laetrile was just another hoax.

Current Laetrile Therapy

Like the Hoxsey therapy, the use of Laetrile for cancer was largely pushed out of this country and into Mexico. However, some physicians in the United States still administer it, and one of these is Douglas Brodie, M.D. Dr. Brodie is a well-known alternative cancer practitioner practicing in Reno, Nevada. He refers to his treatment modality as "Complementary and Alternative Medicine," or CAM, and one of the most powerful tools he uses is Laetrile.

Primary to Dr. Brodie's approach is the administration of intensive intravenous treatments. These usually involve each patient spending three to four hours a day in his clinic Monday through Friday for an initial two to three-week period. After that, the patient can usually go home with a diet and supplement plan and return to the clinic at varying intervals for follow-up treatments. Each patient is treated as unique, and each treatment plan is tailored to that patient's situation. The intravenous treatments received include Laetrile, vitamin C in high doses, vitamin A, DMSO, germanium, and other natural cancer-fighting substances.

DMSO is an organic sulpher compound that was largely pioneered by a Houston physician named Dr. Eli Jordan Tucker for the treatment of cancer. His results, along with those of other researchers, showed DMSO to be an effective anti-cancer agent for a variety of reasons. Thousands of articles have discussed the efficacy and safety of DMSO when administered under a doctor's care, and several books have been written about it as a remarkable and persecuted substance. It is unfortunate that, in the mid-1960s, the FDA shut down further investigations of it.

Some other major aspects of Dr. Brodie's protocol involve: thymus gland support, oxygenation therapy, ultraviolet blood irradiation, and darkfield microscopy diagnosis (which is a way to visually analyze the state of the blood as an indicator of immune system functioning). And there are more tools in his integrative approach as well.

I was able to visit Dr. Brodie's clinic and speak with some of the cancer patients undergoing treatment. Here are two impressive stories I was told by the patients themselves.

The first story came to me from an elderly man whom I met in the waiting room. He told me he had been bringing his wife to see Dr. Brodie for the past two years, and that she had been diagnosed with intestinal cancer. She had initially undergone surgery to cut out the cancer, but the doctors were unable to get it all so she was told she had only a short time to live. At that point, she and her husband searched for alternatives and found out about Dr. Brodie. This man said that for about the first year of bringing his wife in for treatment, he was pushing her into the clinic in a wheelchair. She gradually felt better and better under Brodie's care, and two years later, she was living a happy and vibrant life *without* the wheelchair.

The second story I heard was the personal account of a man with lymphocytic leukemia. He also had been receiving treatments from Dr. Brodie for a couple of years and was in for one of his follow-up appointments. This man appeared to be perfectly healthy and attested to the fact that he, like so many others, had been given only a short time to live by the conventional doctors who diagnosed him. When I spoke to him, however, he was living a normal life, symptom-free and as far as anyone could tell was cancer-free as a result of Dr. Brodie's treatments. As with some of his other patients, Dr. Brodie guided this man to receive a combination of alternative and conventional medicine, and this protocol had worked very well for him.

When I asked this man how he had found out about Dr. Brodie, he said that, about five years before, his brother-in-law had been diagnosed with prostate cancer. Amazingly, within a matter of weeks, his brother-in-law's friend of the same age was also diagnosed with prostate cancer. This man told me that his brother-in-law had opted for conventional treatment for his cancer and was now dead. However, his brother-in-law's friend had opted for treatment with Dr. Brodie and was now alive and well. That was apparently enough to convince the man I met to go straight to Dr. Brodie when he was diagnosed with cancer himself.

In the room where Dr. Brodie's patients were getting their intravenous treatments, I observed a positive healing atmosphere. People were talking in friendly ways to each other while they were getting treatment, or reading books while quietly munching on some food or drinking fresh juice. Every once in a while someone would crack a joke and make others laugh. It was a light atmosphere for people who were getting serious treatment, and there was an overall sense of healing and hope in the room.

Recently, Dr. Brodie's clinic has incorporated a new technique into its impressive arsenal: "Insulin-Potentiated Hypoglycemic Therapy," or IPHT. In this technique, insulin is used to briefly lower the blood sugar level in the patient, then a glucose solution is quickly supplied intravenously *along with* various cancer-fighting agents. This method works by taking advantage of the fact that cancer cells thrive on sugar and need it desperately. When they are deprived of it (even momentarily), they get very hungry, so they start to gobble up whatever they can to survive.

According to Dr. Brodie, IPHT

. . . has a remarkable effect on malignant cells . . . . The cancer cells open their membranes in response to a metabolic need for sugar as food by the insulin's producing a drop in blood sugar. Thus, IPHT stimulates each cancer cell to seek greater quantities of sugar. By the IV feeding of glucose solution containing ascorbic acid, potassium, magnesium, selenium, germanium, and laetrile the cancer cell opens itself to greater membrane permeability in order to suck up larger amounts of glucose as a required food substance. The IPHT greatly potentiates IV infusions of healing substances which cancer cells don't like.[16]

With IPHT, the natural, non-toxic cancer-fighting agents such as Laetrile, vitamin C, and so forth, can get to the cancer cells even *more* effectively than with normal intravenous treatment.

According to Dr. Brodie, IPHT can also potentiate the administration of conventional chemotherapy and some doctors who are using it this way are finding they can get the same results with only 10 percent of the dose of chemotherapy normally required. This means that, when using conventional treatment, less toxic material needs to be introduced into the body and less damage to healthy cells is done. Also, the unpleasant side effects of chemotherapy such as nausea and hair loss are greatly reduced.

With so much evidence of Laetrile's effectiveness, not only through laboratory controlled studies, but also through patient use around the world, it is hard to believe that the cancer industry was able to suppress it so effectively in the United States. And it is just as hard to understand why. The only possible answer appears to be "money." According to Griffin,

> The trail of corruption leads all the way to the FDA itself. A study conducted by USA *Today* revealed that more than half of the experts hired to advise the government on the safety and effectiveness of medicine have financial relationships with the pharmaceutical companies that are affected by their advice.[17]

The lengths the cancer industry has gone to in order to make sure that Laetrile does not pose a threat to their profits have been truly amazing. Unbelievably, even *the sale of apricot seeds*, one of the richest natural sources of B_{17}, is greatly restricted. It is almost impossible to find apricot seeds in stores anywhere, including health food stores, and the only way to obtain apricot seeds now is by ordering them from a few sites on the Internet. I was not too surprised to find out that these sites are not allowed, by law, to list any benefits for cancer along with the product, and it appears that even these few sites are getting pressured to shut down.

Many people have been influenced to believe that Laetrile is no more than a "quack treatment," yet this is just the *opposite* of the truth. It is not as easy to find or as readily available as it should be, but it can still be obtained as a cancer treatment. Anyone interested in obtaining intravenous Laetrile treatments can contact Dr. Brodie's clinic, or search the Internet for other practitioners using it. There are still some courageous doctors in the United States who offer it, and there are also clinics in Mexico that anyone can go to for treatment. As with any other type of treatment, be sure to look into the credibility of the doctor or clinic you are considering, and try to talk with some patients who have been successfully treated by that practitioner to make sure the treatment is being administered effectively.

Once cautionary note: Laetrile stands for "*laevo*-rotatory mandelonitrile beta-diglucoside." Laevo refers to a purified form of B_{17} that turns polarized light in a left-turning direction. In his book, *The Cancer Industry*, Ralph Moss states that the original form of Laetrile, patented by the Krebses, was purified to only contain this left-turning form. However, many of the commercial versions of Laetrile in use today are mixed (or racemic), meaning they contain both the left-turning and right-turning forms of B_{17}. According to Moss, Dr. Krebs, Jr., believed that only the left-turning form was effective against cancer and that the commercial racemic versions were much less effective than the pure Laetrile he and his father had patented.[18] Thus, it is a good idea to double-check the purity of the Laetrile in use by any practitioner with whom you are considering working.

Resources:

W. Douglas Brodie, M.D.   (775) 829-1009
6110 Plumas, Suite B   www.drbrodie.com
Reno, Nevada 89509

Treatment with Dr. Brodie: Treatment charges vary according to individual cases. However, the cost for the first three weeks of intensive treatment is generally about $10,000 (as of this printing). Follow-up treatments are often necessary and are not included in this cost.

For Consultation: Consultations with Dr. Brodie are available and reasonably priced. Often a dark-field microscopy blood test will need to be performed, which costs around $75 extra.

Treatment Centers in Mexico

Oasis of Hope   (888) 500-4673
Tijuana, Mexico   www.oasisofhope.com
(Dr. Ernesto Contreras's clinic)

American Biologics Integrative   (800) 227-4473
  Medical Center   www.americanbiologics.com
Tijuana, Mexico
Chula Vista, California Office   (619) 429-8200

Books

G. Edward Griffin. *World Without Cancer: The Story of Vitamin B_{17}, revised edition.* Westlake Village, California: American Media, 1997. (ISBN 0-912986-19-0)

Dr. Philip E. Binzel. *Alive and Well: One Doctor's Experience With Nutrition in the Treatment of Cancer Patients.* Westlake Village, California: American Media, 1994. (ISBN 0-912986-17-4)

W. Douglas Brodie, M.D. *Cancer and Common Sense: Combining Science and Nature to Control Cancer.* White Bear Lake, Minnesota: Winning Publications, 1997. (ISBN 1-884367-03-8)

Ralph W. Moss. *The Cancer Industry.* Equinox Press, New York, 1999. (ISBN 1-881025-09-8)

CHAPTER 7

Dr. Kelley's Enzyme Therapy

E nzyme therapy, or "Metabolic Therapy," is another very impressive natural approach to cancer recovery that was developed by Dr. William Donald Kelley in the 1960s and 1970s. This approach revolves around the primary factor of high-dose supplementation with *pancreatic enzymes*.

History

As mentioned in Chapter 2, the Scottish embryologist, Dr. John Beard, was the first medical expert to propose the trophoblast theory of cancer cell development. After discovering that fetal trophoblast cells and cancer cells both carried the same type of protective protein coating, and that the growth of trophoblast cells during early pregnancy was halted when the fetal pancreas started functioning, he began to look into the effect of pancreatic enzymes on cancer cells as well. In 1906, Dr. Beard surprised the world by proposing that the pancreas supplied the body's *main* defense against cancer by secreting proteolytic enzymes that could circulate throughout the body. (Proteolytic means "breaks proteins into smaller parts.") Dr. Beard published a book as early as 1911 that described his proposed method of treating cancer under the title, *The Enzyme Therapy of Cancer*.

Years later, a retired Yale University professor named Dr. Howard Beard (who was, strangely enough, *not* related to Dr. Beard of Scotland), further advanced the understanding of how pancreatic enzymes affect cancer by discovering that the two most important cancer-controlling enzymes of pancreatin are "trypsin" and "chymotrypsin." But it wasn't until the 1960s that any medical practitioner really put these ideas to the test, and actually began *treating* cancer patients with high doses of pancreatic enzymes. The first pioneering practitioner to do so was Dr.

William Donald Kelley, and his method of treating cancer began with curing himself of his own advanced, metastasized cancer.

A dentist by training, Dr. Kelley was diagnosed in 1963 with cancer of the pancreas, liver, and intestine. Both pancreatic and liver cancer have historically been considered very "deadly" types of cancer, and the survival rates remain dismally low with conventional treatment even today. For localized pancreatic cancer, *caught early*, modern surgery can still only offer a five-year survival rate of about 5 percent. And for *metastasized* pancreatic cancer, the long-term survival rate with current conventional treatment is about zero. Approximately 30,000 Americans are diagnosed with pancreatic cancer each year and most of them die within a year of their diagnosis.

It is no wonder that when Dr. Kelley was diagnosed with *both* pancreatic and liver cancer, as well as intestinal cancer, his doctors only gave him a few weeks to live. Yet, Dr. Kelley found a way to naturally overcome his metastasized, late-stage cancer by developing and following his own personal program. And he has remained cancer-free for about 40 years.

After attaining his own cure, Dr. Kelley went on to help thousands of other people overcome their cancers, attaining one of the highest cure rates of any practitioner. His treatment protocol is estimated to have benefited approximately 33,000 people over a 30-year period, and the cancer patients who diligently stuck to the program had a very high rate of complete recovery.

Dr. Kelley named his form of treatment "Metabolic Therapy." He saw cancer as a result of faulty metabolic functioning and felt it was of key importance to tailor the treatment to each patient and their metabolic type. To this end, he developed a system to classify each of his patients into one of 10 basic metabolic categories. In general, the five basic components of Kelley's metabolic program were:

1.   Supplementation of high doses of pancreatic enzymes (following an on/off cycle) along with other nutritional supplements

2.   Detoxification of the body primarily through coffee enemas

3.   Nutritionally adequate and balanced diet

4.   Neurological stimulation (chiropractic adjustments, physical therapy, craniosacral therapy)

5.   Spiritual attitude

Dr. Kelley incorporated many of Max Gerson's concepts into his treatment approach, such as fresh juices and coffee enemas, but his approach differed in numerous details from Dr. Gerson's as well. Probably the contribution that Dr. Kelley is best known for is his promotion of the understanding that pancreatic enzymes are of *key* importance to natural cancer recovery. He did this by being the first practitioner to prove the role of pancreatic enzymes in cancer recovery over three decades of clinical practice and thousands of patients.

As early as 1969, Dr. Kelley published a book about his method of treating cancer. Called *One Answer to Cancer*, the book soon became very popular in underground nutritional circles. However, like Hoxsey and Gerson, Dr. Kelley was harassed by the establishment. Amazingly, even Dr. Kelley's freedom to write a book about his methods was denied when, in a 1970s federal court trial, he was ordered to never speak or write about cancer again!

Dr. Kelley was repeatedly attacked for not focusing strictly on dental medicine, and in 1976 his dental license was suspended for five years. In 1986, after many years of harassment, Dr. Kelley finally gave up his practice of metabolic counseling and stopped treating cancer altogether. He claims in his recent book, *Cancer: Curing the Incurable Without Surgery, Chemotherapy, or Radiation* (published in 2000), that there were numerous sinister attempts to suppress his innovative cancer therapy. Unfortunately, these attempts were successful enough to keep his treatment approach out of mainstream medicine, even though he had been achieving "unheard-of" successes with metastasized cancer cases the establishment had little hope of curing.

Although Dr. Kelley is no longer treating cancer patients, there are other practitioners around the country who are administering forms of his treatment to cancer patients with success. Two of these practitioners work together in a New York practice: Nicholas Gonzalez, M.D., and Linda Isaacs, M.D.

Dr. Nicholas Gonzalez

Before Dr. Kelley closed down his metabolic counseling practice, Nicholas Gonzalez, a medical student at Cornell University, decided to look into Dr. Kelley's method of treating cancer. When he approached Dr. Kelley about this in 1981, Kelley freely allowed Gonzalez to review the records of more than 10,000 cancer patients he had treated and to contact the patients. Gonzalez was astonished to find that so many accurately diagnosed cases of metastasized cancer had been cured. Many of these people were thriving 10 or 15 years after their diagnosis.

Gonzalez interviewed and evaluated over 500 cases in detail, and also performed a rigorous independent study of Kelley's pancreatic cancer patients. Gonzalez chose pancreatic cancer for his detailed report because of its extremely low cure rate among conventional approaches. He focused on 22 pancreatic cancer cases in Kelley's files, each of which had been diagnosed through biopsy at a major medical institution. The results of his study were extremely impressive:

- Ten of the 22 patients who *never* followed Kelley's protocol lived an average of 67 days.

- Seven of the 22 patients who followed Kelley's protocol *partially* lived an average of 233 days.

- Five of the 22 patients who followed Kelley's protocol *completely* experienced total, long-term recovery.

Because Gonzalez only focused on the 22 cases that rigorously met his high research standards (such as being diagnosed through biopsy at a major medical institution), the results of his study boldly refuted the common myth that most people who recover from cancer using alternative approaches were misdiagnosed and never had cancer in the first place. Yet, even though Gonzalez used rigorous standards for his study and wrote up his results with careful documentation, he was scorned and ridiculed when he tried to publish his findings. Unbelievably, even in the 1980s, the academic medical world could not accept that a nutritionally based treatment approach to cancer could bring about such incredible recoveries in advanced cases.

Current Treatment

Many of the basic aspects of Dr. Kelley's method are continued by Dr. Nicholas Gonzales and Dr. Linda Isaacs in New York City. They currently treat people using their own modified Kelley approach. Although the Gonzalez-Isaacs program is best known for the treatment of pancreatic cancer, they also treat *all* other types of cancer, as well as other debilitating diseases such as multiple sclerosis, chronic fatigue, and lupus.

Typical treatment involves patients taking up to 45 grams of pancreatic enzymes each day (five to seven capsules six times a day). These specially developed enzymes are unique to the Gonzalez-Isaacs program and cannot be purchased commercially elsewhere. Including other supplements, each cancer patient may consume a total of 130 to 160 capsules a day. Also included in the program are digestive aids such as pepsin and hydrochloric acid, and supplemental concentrates (in pill form) of raw beef organs and glands. Patients must generally prepare three fresh juices each day and, for detoxification, most are required to perform two coffee enemas a day. Both the supplementation protocol and the dietary regimen for each patient are individualized according to the patient's metabolic type and disease state.

In an article about the Gonzalez-Isaacs program published in a 1996 issue of *Life Extension* magazine, writer Terri Mitchell sums up Gonzalez's theory about metabolic typing in the following way:

> Dr. Gonzalez believes that the physiology of patients with cancer invariably turns up as either too acid or too alkaline. Patients who have too much acidity have a predominance of sympathetic nervous system activity. Those who are too alkaline lean towards parasympathetic activity. The sympathetic nervous system is the part of the brain involved in 'fight or flight' activity. This primitive survival mechanism gears up the heart and lungs at the expense of other organs such as the pancreas and stomach. People who are born with a propensity towards sympathetic activity have hyper-vigilant stress responses, but low parasympathetic activity such as digestion.
>
> People who lean towards the parasympathetic are the opposite. Their pancreas, intestines and other organs are working overtime, but their stress response organs are asleep. Dr. Gonzalez' goal with these patients is to augment their sympathetic activity. The idea is to balance sympathetic and parasympathetic physiology.[1]

Like Dr. Kelley, Gonzalez believes that personal psychological and spiritual changes also need to be part of a cancer patient's program. He has been quoted as saying, "I've had patients whose cancer didn't get better no matter how perfectly they did my program, until they resolved serious emotional issues in their lives."[2]

Interestingly, Dr. Gonzalez doesn't worry about the *size* of a person's tumor, and actually prefers to see the tumor enlarge during treatment. In his thinking, this means that the body is causing a natural and healing inflammation response. He also does not believe that it is always neces-sary to destroy a tumor in order for a patient to heal. In other words, Gonzalez says that ". . . sometimes the body will wall off a tumor and just keep it there like an old bird's nest."[3] Dr. Gonzalez's concepts are supported by the many long-term recoveries of his patients. He claims to be able to achieve a 70 to 75 percent success rate with those patients who comply with their individualized program.

Case Stories

A number of different journal articles about the Gonzalez-Isaacs pro-gram have been written and published. The following case stories 1 and 2 were published in the October 1996 issue of *Life Extension* magazine and are paraphrased here:

Case Story #1 — Lung Cancer Metastasized to Liver, Pancreas, and Adrenals

In 1991, a 70-year old man named Mort was diagnosed after X-ray and surgery with lung cancer. CT scans then showed that his cancer had already spread to his liver, pancreas and adrenals. His oncologist recom-mended *no treatment*, indicating that there was none available that could help Mort. Within 2 months, Mort's wife found out about Dr. Gonzalez and Mort started on the Gonzalez-Isaacs program. In four months, Mort's tests indicated he was improving. Five years after his di-agnosis, Mort was still alive and doing well.[4]

Case Story #2 — Breast Cancer

A woman named Henri-Etta had gone through traditional treatment for breast cancer, including surgery and six months of chemotherapy. She went into remission, but about four and one-half years later the breast cancer came back. Her oncologist offered chemotherapy again, but this time she refused. Henri-Etta found out about the Gonzalez-Isaacs approach and, after an evaluation, started on that program instead. About nine years after her cancer diagnosis, in 2003, Henri-Etta was still alive and feeling great.[5]

The following story is paraphrased from the October 2000 issue of *Total Health* magazine (vol. 22, no. 5).

Case Story #3 — Metastasized Melanoma

In 1983, a man named Bill began having chronic sinus problems. An ENT specialist prescribed various treatments that didn't help. Finally, surgery was performed and some polyps were removed. Lab reports on the polyps indicated melanoma. A CT scan was performed which revealed a small tumor behind Bill's left eye. In 1984, a lengthy neurosurgery was done to remove the tumor along with a small piece of bone. Bill's oncologist thought they had successfully removed all of the tumor.

But in 1987, Bill started having abdominal pains. Another CT scan showed a large abdominal tumor which a needle biopsy indicated was, once again, melanoma. Surgery was performed at Sloan-Kettering to remove the tumor, but this time all of the cancer could *not* be removed due to risk of damaging some vital organs. At this point, Bill chose to decline follow-up chemotherapy or other conventional treatment. Instead, he searched around for alternatives.

Bill finally started seeing Dr. Gonzalez and Dr. Isaacs in May 1988. By December of that year, his tumor had stabilized. In the summer of 1992, four years later, his tumor began to grow again. After discussing his situation with Dr. Gonzalez, Bill again went to Sloan-Kettering to have the tumor surgically removed. The surgery was very successful and revealed that his tumor was completely encapsulated, and there was no evidence that the cancer had spread anywhere else. Three years later, when his testimony was taken in 1995, Bill was still happily thriving, and still doing the Gonzalez-Isaacs program.[6]

It is evident from these case stories, as well as from the accounts of many other cancer patients, that the Gonzalez-Isaacs approach to treating cancer, based on the approach originally developed by Dr. William Donald Kelley, is effective. Although it is well-known for treating pancreatic cancer, it can also bring about long-term recovery for a variety of other cancers, and includes cases of metastasized or late-stage cancer. Much of the credit for this treatment approach must go to Dr. Kelley who developed it. Dr. Kelley is no longer in practice, but Dr. Gonzalez and Dr. Isaacs in New York are excellent practitioners who can be sought out currently. The following information gives instructions to people wishing to pursue this effective treatment approach as a way to "outsmart their cancer."

Resources:

Nicholas J. Gonzalez, M.D., P.C.   (212) 213-3337
Linda L. Isaacs, M.D.   www.dr-gonzalez.com
36 East 36th Street, Suite 204
New York, NY 10016

[Lecture tapes are available that give a detailed explanation of the program, and can be ordered from the above website.]

For Evaluation and Consultation: If possible, prospective patients should review the requirements for evaluation that are listed on the above website before applying for treatment. Along with one's application, prospective patients should send any relevant biopsy and blood work results along with their CT or MRI written reports. (But don't send the actual film.) Pre-appointment evaluation of this material will be done, then, a two-session "in-person" evaluation meeting in the New York office will be scheduled over two consecutive days.

Treatment: The overall cost of the Gonzalez-Isaacs treatment program will vary with each patient, but generally is about $600 a month, or $5,000 to $6,000 per year (as of this printing). About three-quarters of this cost is for the supplements. Every patient is required to return at certain intervals for a repeat physical exam and assessment of their dietary and nutritional needs, as these may change over the course of treatment. These follow-up evaluations will be an extra charge.

Books

William Donald Kelley, D.D.S., M.S. *Cancer: Curing the Incurable Without Surgery, Chemotherapy, or Radiation.* Baltimore: College of Metabolic Medicine, 2000. (ISBN 09704290-0-2)

Richard Walters. *Options: The Alternative Cancer Therapy Book.* New York: Avery Penquin Putnam Publishing, 1993. (ISBN 0-89529-510-5)

Websites

www.dr-gonzalez.com

www.drkelley.com

www.drkelley.info/articles/archive.php?artid=283

www.drkelleycancerprogram.com

CHAPTER 8

Burzynski's Antineoplastons

Atruly *different* approach to treating cancer came to the United States in 1970 when medical doctor and researcher Stanislaw Burzynski emigrated from Poland. Dr. Burzynski's unique approach is *not* based on healing the body with diet, nutrition, cleansing, or herbs. Yet, his approach is now being heralded by many as one of the most promising cancer treatments of modern day. And, it is non-toxic. For those who can afford it or who qualify for trials, Burzynski's approach is currently being offered at his clinic in Houston, Texas, where patients are treated by a large staff of highly qualified doctors.

History

Like Dr. Gerson, Dr. Burzynski came to this country with an impressive academic medical background. Born in Poland in 1943, he showed remarkable abilities in chemistry at an early age. He studied medicine and, at the age of 24, graduated first in his class of 250 students at his medical academy. One year after obtaining his M.D., he also obtained a Ph.D. in biochemistry. Burzynski gained recognition as one of the youngest people in the history of Poland to receive both an M.D. and Ph.D. diploma.[1]

Growing up in Poland during and after World War II was not easy for the young Stanislaw. His father—a teacher—was imprisoned for two years by the Nazis because he continued to teach Jewish students after the Nazis had segregated Jews into walled ghettos. In the late 1940s, when Poland was overrun and controlled by communist Soviet Union, life became difficult in other ways. The Burzynski family property was taken away from Stanislaw's family, and his brother began to fight in the anti-communist underground, risking his life on a daily basis. Stanislaw's brother was eventually killed in 1948 while fighting in the resistance movement. While still a boy, Stanislaw often had to defend himself in physical fights that were triggered by prejudices during this class-conscious era of Poland. As a result of his own physical fights, and after watching his brother and father stand up to oppression, Burzynski turned into a person who knew the meaning of fighting for what one believed in.

When Burzynski started medical school, he quickly became involved in research. During his years as a medical student, he studied amino acids and peptides and published papers about his work. He first started analyzing amino acids in wild mushrooms to see if he could turn some of the toxic chains of amino acids that were present in the mushrooms into new antibiotics. Then, he moved on to studying other organic fluids, including blood and urine, that contained peptides. (Peptides are short chains of amino acids.) He began finding peptides in human blood and urine that no one had ever known about before. According to Burzynski, "nobody had bothered to identify them. Nobody cared what they were."[2]

Dr. Burzynski decided to see if the unidentified amino acid compounds he was finding might be related to kidney disease, and he prepared his doctoral thesis on this subject. The work of identifying these compounds was difficult and required very modern chromatographic equipment as well as hard-to-get chemicals.

After a while, Dr. Burzynski began to wonder if the peptides he had discovered might be linked, not only to kidney disease, but also to cancer. He suspected this as a possibility because people with primary kidney disease (PKD) appeared to have an overabundance of some of these peptides, and he knew that another researcher in Poland had discovered that people with PKD rarely suffered from cancer. Dr. Burzynski began to wonder if the peptides themselves were able to inhibit cancer in some way.

Just as Dr. Burzynski was beginning to look into this, he began to have problems with the communist regime controlling Poland. Dr. Burzynski had already refused to join the communist party and this had branded him as a dissenter and independent thinker. One way the Polish authorities dealt with free thinkers at that time was to draft them into the army. Thus, in 1970, Dr. Burzynski received orders to report for military duty. If he complied, he would be sent to North Vietnam to fight with the Viet Cong. Because of how the Polish military worked, this could mean it might be decades before he would be able to return to Poland and his scientific research.

Instead of reporting for military duty, Dr. Burzynski quickly obtained a passport and immediately left Poland for New York. When he arrived in the United States, he only had a few dollars in his pocket and his paperwork documenting the 39 peptides he had identified. Soon, Dr. Burzynski received a message from Poland that he would never be allowed to work in any medical school of that country again. He knew then that he would never be able to go back to his home country.

Luckily, shortly after arriving in the United States, Dr. Burzynski got a job at Baylor College of Medicine in Houston. In the university's department of anesthesiology, a scientist named Georges Ungar was studying brain peptides and how those peptides impacted the transmission of memories. Dr. Burzynski's own work on peptides fit right in.

When Stanislaw Burzynski started work at the Baylor College of Medicine in Texas, he had already identified naturally occurring peptides (small chains of amino acids) that could be found in the blood of healthy persons, but not in the blood of people with cancer. Since he thought that the types of peptides he had discovered might have an *inhibitory* effect on cancer, he chose to name them "anti-neoplastons." The term "anti" means opposing, or against, and a common medical term for cancer is "neoplaston." The term neoplaston was derived from the Greek word "neoplasm," which means "new growth."

At Baylor, Dr. Burzynski was able to move forward with his research and to formulate his own theory that certain types of peptides, or antineoplastons, were actually part of a *biochemical communication system* that complimented the rest of the immune system and could actually regulate the out-of-control division of cancer cells and eventually bring them back to a normal state. He also discovered that not *all* the peptides he isolated had an impact on cancer cell cultures. In fact, most of them did *not* show any anti-cancer activity.

As he continued his research, Dr. Burzynski began to identify specific antineoplastons that had anticancer properties against certain types of cancers. Then, he found one special antineoplaston that actually showed anti-cancer activity against a *broad spectrum* of cancer types. This discovery was huge. Dr. Burzynski called the broad spectrum antineoplaston "Antineoplaston A"[3] and began to concentrate his cancer research on it.

Also while doing research at Baylor College, Dr. Burzynski met his future wife Barbara. Barbara was an M.D. and Polish immigrant as well. Barbara Burzynski soon joined Stanislaw in his research, and over the next 15 years or so they worked together, isolating antineoplastons, breaking down Antineoplaston A into smaller fractions, and learning how to produce the most effective antineoplastons synthetically. In 1974, Dr. Burzynski was granted research funding and support from both the NCI and the University of Texas M.D. Anderson Cancer Center.

After a while, the use of antineoplastons in a laboratory setting on cancer cell lines was going so well that it was time to start using them in animal studies. However, what Dr. Burzynski found was that, while the antineoplastons he had isolated could shut down human cancer cell lines, they had very little or no effect on similar cancers in animals. In other words, he discovered that the antineoplastons were "species-specific" in their chemical communication traits.[4]

Since Dr. Burzynski's antineoplastons were ineffective on animal cancers, he decided in 1976 that it was time to go straight to their use on people. He chose to start with terminal cancer patients who were considered untreatable, or for whom all other treatment had failed. Since he had passed the Texas medical licensing exams in 1973, Dr. Burzynski felt he was qualified to do this. But the Baylor College of Medicine would not allow him to perform human clinical trials unless he had an investigational new drug (IND) permit from the FDA. Dr. Burzynski spent months filing paperwork to get the IND, a process that generally only takes a matter of weeks for pharmaceutical companies with promising new drugs. The FDA kept asking for more and more documentation, and Burzynski kept supplying it. Eventually, his IND application comprised thousands of pages—and when stacked on the floor was over 6 feet tall![5]

Dr. Burzynski was never given the IND permit by the FDA. However, he finally got permission by one independent hospital to test his antineoplaston compounds at their facility—as long as he only used his treatment on people for whom all other treatment had failed. These early antineoplaston treatments on humans showed great promise. He began to see people who had been given a short time to live recover and get well. With more and more refinement of his technique, Dr. Burzynski's treatment approach began to show an overall effectiveness that was better than traditional cancer treatment methods.

In 1977, Dr. Burzynski opened up his own private practice in Houston, Texas, which he called the Burzynski Clinic. This became the place where he could legally administer antineoplastons to desperate patients. In the early years, the production of antineoplastons was laborious because the peptides had to be isolated from human urine. Eventually, however, Burzynski perfected a way to synthesize the antineoplaston compounds he needed from chemicals. He developed a large manufacturing plant in Houston and made sure that it met every FDA standard for manufacture of pharmaceuticals. The Burzynski Clinic in Houston is now a large treatment center that employs about 20 physicians and a large staff of other medical personnel.

Over the past 25 years, thousands of patients have been treated at the Burzynski Clinic with antineoplaston therapy for terminal cancer and other types of devastating diseases. Dr. Burzynski has authored and co-authored 184 scientific publications and has presented scientific papers at international conventions. He also holds over 160 patents for his treatments in 35 countries around the world. Antineoplaston therapy is non-toxic and has brought about long-term recovery for countless cancer patients.

Julian Whitaker, M.D., of southern California has looked into Dr. Burzynski's approach in detail. He explains how Burzynski's treatment works against cancer in this excerpt from one of his newsletters:

> Antineoplastons consist of small peptides, components of protein, and peptide metabolites that are given by mouth or intravenously. They work by entering the cell and altering specific functions of the genes: Some activate the tumor suppressor genes that prevent cancer, while others turn off the oncogenes that force the cancer cell to divide uncontrollably. Like rifle shots to the heart of the malignant process, the antineoplastons cause cancerous cells to either revert to normal or die without dividing.[6]

In a 1996 special supplement of his popular monthly newsletter, Dr. Whitaker reported numerous cases of people who had recovered from cancer using antineoplaston therapy, three of which are reported here. Case stories 4 and 5 were testimonials I took from other Burzynski patients.

Case Stories

Case Story #1 — Adult Malignant Brain Tumor

A 35-year-old school psychologist named Pamela began experiencing double vision in 1987 and, after going through tests, was diagnosed with a tumor in her brain stem. It was classified as an "anaplastic astrocytoma, grade 3." She underwent surgery and two months of radiation, but these treatments did not get her cancer under control. The highly malignant tumor in her brain just kept growing. She was offered chemotherapy, but refused it because her doctors told her there wasn't much chance the chemo would do any good anyway.

In April 1988, Pamela had a follow-up MRI which showed that her tumor was about the size of a quarter, about twice as large as when she was first diagnosed. At this point, a resident at the University of California, San Francisco hospital told her to get her affairs in order because she only had 6 weeks to 6 months to live.[7] Luckily for Pamela, she then found out about the Burzynski Clinic. By July 1988, she had started on antineoplaston therapy.

To Pamela's sheer joy, an MRI in September 1988 showed her tumor to have decreased 30 to 40 percent in volume. By the following January, there was no sign of the tumor in her brain at all.[8] She continued on antineoplastons for about two years and her tumor never showed up again. When she was re-checked in 2003, Pamela was still doing fine and had not received any treatment of any kind for 13 years![9]

Case Story #2 — Breast Cancer Metastasized to the Bones

In 1990, a woman named Carol underwent a mastectomy and received chemotherapy for "infiltrative and intraductal cancer of the breast."[10] Four years later, she found out that her cancer was still growing inside her and had now spread to her bones. First discovered in her spine, she soon found out it had also spread to her hip, clavicle, and ribs.

It was at this point that Carol began antineoplaston therapy from the Burzynski Clinic. The antineoplaston treatment first halted the spread of her cancer and then she began to see it reverse. About a year and a half later, the cancer in Carol's clavicle, hips, and ribs was completely gone, and she only had a slight involvement of the lumbar spine which was, in fact, reducing. She also claimed to be feeling better than she had in 10 years.

Case Story #3 — Prostate Cancer Metastasized to the Bones

A 61-year old business man named Ernesto was diagnosed with metastatic prostate cancer in 1995. The diagnosis was confirmed by biopsy. A bone scan showed that his entire skeleton, legs, ribs, spine, and skull were full of cancer as well. At the time of Ernesto's diagnosis, his PSA count was 960. (A normal PSA count would normally be below 4.) He refused most conventional treatment, and only went on a testosterone blocker called Lupron which his doctor hoped would help but did not expect it to stop Ernesto's cancer.

Within just a couple of weeks of his diagnosis, Ernesto started on antineoplastons. After only three weeks of treatment, his bone pain subsided. Six months later, his PSA reading was down to an incredible 1.4! Remarkably, each time he received a scan he could see his cancer receding more and more from his bones.[11] The last anyone heard from him, Ernesto was doing fine and living a normal life.

Case Story #4 — Prostate Cancer

Prostate Cancer appears to respond extremely well to antineoplaston therapy, and here is one more case story from a man I was able to contact personally. His name is John.

In January 1990, when John was 64 years old, he was diagnosed with prostate cancer. His prostate gland was completely encircled with tumors, which when biopsies were taken, were found to be very malignant. (At the time, the Gleason scale and PSA test had not yet been developed for more detailed diagnoses.)

John got an appointment with Dr. Burzynski later that same month. According to John, Dr. Burzynski wanted to be absolutely sure of his diagnosis and sent him to another hospital in Houston for a second opinion. This hospital gave John the same diagnosis as the first one he had gotten. At this point, Dr. Burzynski put John on antineoplastons in capsule form and sent him home with a three-month supply.

In May 1990, after about three months on the capsules, John returned to Houston for an examination. X-rays showed that John's tumors were "healed," but Dr. Burzynski wanted him to continue on the capsules for a few more months. In August 1990, John went back to Houston once again. This time, X-rays showed that John's tumors were all gone.

The PSA test had just become available, so Dr. Burzynski sent John home with a prescription to get this test done. John had several PSA tests performed over the next three to four months. All showed very low readings, so his doctor finally said he didn't need to keep getting them. He now only gets his PSA level checked whenever he goes in for a general health check-up.

John is currently 77 years old and it has been 13 years since he was diagnosed with cancer. He lives a normal, happy life. John has *not* experienced any recurrence of his cancer and his PSA test results have remained completely normal.

Case Story #5 — Non-Hodgkin's Lymphoma

Mary Jo is a woman whose cancer recovery story has been written up in numerous publications. In 1991, when Mary Jo was only 40 years old, she was diagnosed with low grade non-Hodgkin's lymphoma. It was 100 percent follicular lymphoma, and she consulted with physicians at USC, UCLA, Stanford Medical Center in California, and the Dana Farber Cancer Institute in Boston. They all told her that there was no conventional treatment that could cure her cancer. The Dana Farber Institute offered Mary Jo an autologous bone marrow transplant with high-dose radiation as her best chance for recovery. This treatment procedure is extremely risky and can cause serious side effects, including death. Mary Jo decided to turn it down.

Not wanting to give up, Mary Jo and her husband researched other options that might be available and eventually found out about Burzynski's treatment. In 1992, Mary Jo flew to Houston and started on antineoplaston therapy. For about the first two months she took the antineoplastons in capsule form. This involved 60 capsules a day. But the capsule regimen did not seem to be working effectively enough on her cancer, so she then switched to the commonly used "infusion pump." This is the most effective way to administer antineoplaston therapy, and involves carrying around a small pump that is attached to a catheter surgically inserted into the chest. The pump releases a constant slow drip of antineoplastons into the body for about 10 hours a day. Mary Jo says that this pump was not difficult to deal with, and that she could basically do everything she would normally do without any problem. She also says there were no side effects from the treatment.

After 9 months of treatment on the infusion pump, Mary Jo was pronounced in remission by both her oncologist at UCLA and by Dr. Burzynski. She remained in remission for about two years, when two swollen lymph nodes indicated a possible recurrence. It was never determined whether her enlarged nodes were really the cancer recurring or just a reaction to a cold or infection. But just to be safe, Burzynski put her back on treatment immediately. After only three months on capsule treatment, a follow-up CT scan showed Mary Jo in remission again. She has been cancer free ever since, which, at the time of this writing has been for the past 11 years!

Case Story #6—Childhood Brain Tumor

Paul was a five-year-old little boy back in 1986 when he was diagnosed with a large slow-growing tumor in his brain. Doctors told Paul's family that the tumor was inoperable and he would not live to see his tenth birthday. Paul's parents sent his scans to the head of the pediatric neurosurgery department at the Mayo Clinic. At that time, this was Dr. Patrick Kelly. Dr. Kelly reviewed the scans then wrote to Paul's parents:

"I have reviewed the MRI scans on your five-year-old son Paul . . . it is the largest tumor I have ever seen in this area in anybody ever referred to me for surgery. I showed your scans to a number of my colleagues here who feel that it is inoperable . . . .Without surgery, your boy will die."[12]

Because of the serious risks involved in attempting surgery or radiation, Paul's family elected *not* to pursue those treatments. By 1988, they finally found out about and started Paul on Burzynski's antineoplastons. By the time he started antineoplaston therapy, Paul's tumor had grown to the size of an orange. On antineoplastons, the tumor gradually shrank down until it was no longer visible. Today, Paul is a healthy 22-year-old young man.

(*Note:* More personal cancer recovery stories from people who used antineoplaston therapy can be viewed from the website www.burzynskipatientgroup.org. Just click on "Our Stories." These recovery stories include a wide variety of cancer cases.)

Theory and Efficacy

Burzynski and his colleagues at the clinic are now quite specific about how antineoplastons work. They claim that

> . . . antineoplastons work on cancer cells to interrupt the signal transduction in the ras oncogene pathway, which causes cells to divide endlessly. At the same time, antineoplastons activate the p53 tumor suppressor gene, which tell the cells to undergo programmed cell death. Healthy cells remain unaffected under these processes.[13]

Antineoplaston treatment is completely safe and non-toxic to the individual. It is also extremely effective. At one point, Dr. Burzynski presented the FDA with details on 74 clinical trials using antineoplastons to treat cancer. In one of these trials, the antineoplaston therapy was *seven times* more effective than surgery, radiation, and chemotherapy.[14]

By comparison, chemotherapy looks like a barbaric practice from the Middle Ages. It indiscriminately poisons healthy cells along with cancerous ones and is extremely toxic to the body as a whole. Chemotherapy is based on the concept that, though chemotherapy kills all cells in the body indiscriminately, the fast-growing cells of the body are killed the quickest. Cancer cells tend to grow and replicate faster than other cells in the body, and thus are most hard hit by cytotoxic drugs (chemotherapy). Hair cells are also fast-growing compared to most normal cells of the body, and that is why chemo patients often lose their hair.

Chemotherapy is, more or less, a shotgun approach that kills as many of the fast-growing cells of the body as possible in a relatively short period of time.

But chemotherapeutic drugs can rarely be effectively used to kill *all* the cancer cells in a person's body. This is because, to ensure that all the cancer cells are killed, one would probably have to use enough chemotherapy that would also kill the patient. Thus, when a patient is said to be "in remission" as a result of chemotherapy, that does *not* mean the patient is cancer-free. At best, chemotherapy treatment may kill on the order of 90 percent of the cancer cells in the body. This leaves around 10 percent of the cancer cells still surviving, which often is millions of cancer cells. Those cancer cells that are left just begin again doing what they are good at, which is multiplying quickly. And since the cancer patient's immune system has generally been devastatingly weakened by the chemo, these multiplying cancer survivor cells have very little opposition.

On the other hand, because Dr. Burzynski's treatment involves the administration of antineoplastons which specifically turn off the activity of the "oncogenes" of the cancer cells, they interrupt the signal that causes rapid cell division. At the same time, the antineoplastons activate the tumor suppressor genes which stimulate normal cell death. Thus, antineoplastons simply encourage abnormal cancer cells to become normal or die off, and don't adversely affect normal healthy cells at all. Patients can be *deluged* with this treatment for many months until, gradually, all of the cancer cells are controlled. Also, unlike chemotherapy, Burzynski's antineoplastons work on a broad range of cancers. These include brain cancer, lymph cancer, lung cancer, bladder cancer, prostate cancer, and breast cancer, among others.

Brain cancer (which chemotherapy does *not* work well on) responds particularly well to antineoplastons. This is important because the other form of conventional treatment for brain cancer, which is radiation, is also limited in efficacy. In fact, because brain cancer responds so well to antineoplastons and typically so poorly to chemotherapy, a highly respected Seattle oncologist and faculty member of the esteemed University of Washington Medical School carried out his own independent review of 17 of Dr. Burzynski's brain tumor cases. This oncologist, Robert E. Burdick, M.D., carefully examined the 17 patients' medical records and wrote a detailed report. On page 2 of Dr. Burdick's report, he states:

The following is a summary of the 17 cases that I have reviewed. Of the 17 patients there were 7 complete remissions, one patient having had a second complete remission after he discontinued antineoplaston therapy which resulted in his tumor regrowing. There were 9 partial remissions, 2 cases of stable disease and no disqualifications. The average duration of therapy with antineoplastons necessary to obtain a complete remission was 10 months with a range of 2 to 20 months. The average duration of antineoplaston therapy necessary to obtain a partial response was 8 months with a range of 1 to 14 months. The average duration of complete remissions is 16+ months with all 6 complete remissions continuing to remain in remission to the best of my knowledge through January 1, 1997. The duration of complete remissions ranged from 3+ months to 40+ months with the duration of partial remissions averaging 18+ months and ranging from 5 to 78+ months.[15]

In discussing the above results, Dr. Burdick remarks,

The response rate here is an astounding 81 percent, with an equally astounding 35 percent complete remission rate. Such remission rates are far in excess of anything I or anyone else has seen since research work on brain tumors began.[16]

Dr. Burdick also comments,

It is very rare, currently, to ever get a complete remission or cure in a patient who has a malignant brain tumor using our standard modalities of surgery, radiation, and chemotherapy . . . . As a rough estimate, neurosurgeons do well to cure one in every 1,000 brain-cancer patients they operate on. Radiation therapy slows the growth of adult tumors, gaining perhaps one month of life, and again may result in a cure in only one in 500-1,000 patients, those cures being in the pediatric age group. Similarly, chemotherapy research, despite 30 years of clinical trials, has not resulted in the development of a single drug or drug combination that elicits more than an occasional transient response in primary brain tumors.[17]

Dr. Burzynski has tirelessly continued to seek official evaluation and investigation into his antineoplaston therapy. In his book, *The Burzynski Breakthrough*, Thomas D. Elias quotes Burzynski as saying, "I began asking in 1981 for the NCI and the American Cancer Society to review our patient records, but for years, neither would do it."[18] Finally, in 1991, an NCI team of doctors paid a site visit to Houston to investigate Burzynski's treatment. Elias quotes Burzynski commenting on the NCI investigation in the following words:

> I have no idea why, but they spent only one day here. We had prepared 20 brain tumor cases for them, but they had time to examine only seven. They reviewed all the medical records in each case, including MRI and CT scan films and pathology slides. They also inspected our chemical plant. When I asked them to stay longer and look at more cases, they told me that seven would be more than enough to prove the point.[19]

Even though they stayed only one day, the NCI site investigators were able to confirm the anticancer activity of antineoplastons. They also verified five complete remissions of the seven cases they evaluated. Later on, the NCI would minimize Dr. Burzynski's work by implying that he had only presented them with seven of his best cases. In saying this, the NCI was ignoring the 13 other cases Dr. Burzynski had prepared for their evaluation.

In the late 1990s, clinical trials of Dr. Burzynski's antineoplaston therapy produced very positive results in patients with malignant brain tumors and non-Hodgkin's lymphoma. In particular, the trials included 81 patients with astrocytoma brain tumors. Of these brain cancer patients, 73 percent benefited from the treatment; 32 percent achieved either complete remission or more than a 50 percent decrease in tumor size, and 41 percent of the brain cancer patients showed less than 50 percent decrease in tumor size but had no disease progression.[20]

Moreover, researchers in Japan have carried out clinical trials on antineoplaston treatment with very promising results. Japanese doctors treated patients with advanced colon cancer with liver involvement using a combination of antineoplastons and low-dose chemotherapy. Since the dose of chemotherapy was below the threshold of toxicity, they did not identify any significant side effects. In randomized controlled clinical trials they found over five years survival in 91 percent of patients compared to 39 percent in the control group treated with chemotherapy alone! The same center found that antineoplaston AS2-1 capsules given to patients with liver cancer increased time to recurrence after standard treatment to 16 months compared with five months in the control group.[21]

Dr. Burzynski has never claimed that his antineoplaston therapy is a cure for all cancers. However, his clinical practice has proven without a doubt that antineoplaston therapy is able to turn many cancers into manageable diseases with long-term survival and often *does* bring about complete, long-term recoveries.

Attempts at Suppression

Even though antineoplaston therapy has proven to achieve very positive results in clinical trials, Stanislaw Burzynski has been the recipient of repeated attacks from the cancer industry. As early as 1985, agents of the FDA barged into his Houston clinic, accompanied by an armed marshal, and confiscated the medical files of over a thousand cancer patients being treated there. Dr. Burzynski's 11 file cabinets of patient records and other medical documents were never given back to him. Eventually, Dr. Burzynski acquired a court order that allowed him to set up a copy machine in the FDA building 20 miles from his office. Here, he and his staff were permitted to copy medical records as they were needed.[22] This was done, of course, at Burzynski's own expense.

Again, in 1995, the Burzynski Clinic was raided by the FDA and thousands of documents *again* confiscated. Many legal battles ensued with hearings before grand juries. Finally, the FDA indicted Burzynski on 75 counts of mail fraud, contempt, and violation of FDA laws. If convicted, he could face up to 300 years in prison for practicing his proven non-toxic, life-saving techniques. There were a series of congressional hearings, and many of Burzynski's cancer patients testified or wrote letters to Congress in his defense.

In January 1997, Burzynski's court trial began. The FDA had three basic charges against him[23]:

1. Violation of an injunction

2. Mail fraud

3. Selling an unapproved drug in interstate commerce

All of the above charges proved to be bogus, and the FDA could not substantiate their claims that Dr. Burzynski was doing anything illegal. On March 3, 1997, the judge declared a mistrial and dismissed all charges against the doctor. The FDA could not come up with a single patient who would say anything bad about Dr. Burzynski. To the contrary, many of his patients were picketing and chanting outside the courthouse in support of Burzynski throughout the entire trial. Their picket signs read "Save the doctor who saves lives," and "I was cured by Dr. B."[24]

It is interesting to note that the issue of whether antineoplastons *actually work* for cancer patients *was never allowed to be addressed* throughout the trial. Apparently, that was the one issue the FDA wanted to avoid. In fact, when the trial began to look like it was *not* going in the FDA's favor, chief prosecutor Clark complained, "The defense got the best of all worlds. They got to bring in the patients and imply that the stuff works, but we could not bring in experts to question its effects."[25] According to Dr. Julian Whitaker, Congressman Richard M. Burr proclaimed that the government's treatment of Dr. Burzynski was "one of the worst abuses of the criminal justice system [he had] ever witnessed."[26]

Today, Stanislaw Burzynski is still fighting to get antineoplastons accepted by the cancer industry and available to every patient who needs them. He is currently conducting 74 phase II clinical trials at his clinic in Houston where he is using antineoplastons to treat cancer, HIV infection, and other autoimmune diseases. These trials are being overseen by the FDA and have to conform to FDA regulations. Unfortunately, this means that only *certain* patients meet the requirements to qualify for treatment with antineoplastons. In some instances, these requirements involve the stipulation that only patients who have already gone through chemotherapy or radiation with unsuccessful results may be admitted to antineoplaston trials.

Because the Burzynski Clinic is having to comply with FDA regulations for trials, the doctors there are sadly being forced to turn away as many as 90 percent of the cancer patients who come to them for help. The biggest tragedy is that many of the cancer sufferers currently getting turned away are children with brain tumors.

The other tragedy is that, until antineoplaston therapy for cancer is fully approved by the FDA, it is still being considered an experimental treatment and not being covered by health insurance companies. Although Dr. Burzynski's treatment is not as expensive as typical chemotherapy, the difference is that most people can get their insurance companies to pay for chemotherapy. Without insurance coverage, the cost of antineoplaston treatment is too high for many people to afford. Treatment costs vary for different patients, but intravenous antineoplaston therapy for cancer typically runs about $7,000 per month. Antineoplaston therapy via capsules is less expensive.

For those patients who get a consultation but don't qualify for anti-neoplastons, the Burzynski Clinic has other options that have also shown success with cancer. For instance, "sodium phenylbutyrate" is an oral compound that has been found to be transformed by the liver into anti-neoplastons. Sodium phenylbutyrate from the Burzynski Clinic generally costs about $4,500 per month.

The high cost of treatment has been one of the things for which Dr. Burzynski has been criticized. Some critics have accused him of taking advantage of his patients. However, with just the smallest amount of research, anyone can see that just the opposite is true. Both Dr. Burzynski and his wife make much *lower* salaries than the average oncologist in the United States. Also, discussion with some of Dr. Burzynski's patients reveals that there have been many cancer patients who could not ultimately pay all their bills to the clinic who were not pursued. Rather, it appears that the high cost of treatment is a direct result of three factors: (1) Dr. Burzynski must meet the salaries of a large staff of doctors and highly skilled technicians; (2) the expense of running his large plant to manufacture antineoplastons to FDA standards is very high; and (3) he constantly has to pay legal fees to defend his life-saving practice.

It is a shame that people with cancer who carry health insurance can get their medical bills covered if they undergo mutilating surgery, damaging radiation, or toxic chemotherapy, but not if they choose to undergo a treatment that is more efficacious and at the same time is totally safe to their bodies. But for many people with incurable cancer, it has been well worth it to come up with the money they needed for antineoplaston treatment.

To find out whether you or your loved one would qualify for antineoplaston therapy and to find out what the cost would be, call the Burzynski Clinic and set up an in-person consultation immediately. There are many types of malignant cancers being treated at the clinic, and these include:

Brain Cancers—Adult and Childhood:
  Various Gliomas and Astrocytomas
  Glioblastoma Multiforme
  Brain Stem Glioma
  Oligodendroglioma
  Choroid Plexus Neoplasm
  Craniopharyngioma
  Ependymoma
  Germ Cell Tumors

Meningioma,
Neurofibroma
Medulloblastoma
Rhabdoid Tumors
Schwannoma
Breast Cancer
Cervical Cancer
Colon Cancer
Cancer of the Head and Neck
Endometrial Cancer
Esophageal Cancer
Gastrointestinal Tract Cancer
Kidney Cancer (Renal Cell Carcinoma)
Leukemia in Adults
Liver Cancer
Lung Cancers:
   Adenocarcinoma
   Bronchial Alveolar Carcinoma
   Large Cell Carcinoma
   Non-small Cell Carcinoma
   Squamous Cell Carcinoma
   Small Cell Carcinoma
Lymphomas:
   Hodgkin's Lymphoma
   Non-Hodgkin's Lymphoma
   Mantle Zone Lymphoma
   Mycosis Fungoides-Sezary Syndrome
   Primary Central Nervous System Lymphoma
Macroglobulinema of Waldenstrom
Malignant Melanoma
Malignant Fibrous Histiocytoma
Mesothelioma
Multiple Myeloma
Neuroblastoma
Neuroendocrine Tumors
Osteosarcoma
Ovarian Cancer
Pancreatic Cancer
PNET Outside the Central Nervous System
Prostate Cancer
Soft Tissue Sarcoma

Small Intestine Cancer
Stomach Cancer
Unknown Primary Site Cancers
Uterine Cancer
Vulva Cancer
Wilmes Tumor

The treatment protocol and length of treatment varies from patient to patient. Many patients are administered treatment via capsules or tablets and undergo no intravenous treatments. Others receive treatment intravenously via catheter attached to an infusion pump. (The dosage and dosing schedule depend on the type of cancer.) The infusion pump and therapy bags are small and light enough to be carried around by a young child.

Treatment generally requires an initial stay in Houston for one to three weeks. The Burzynski Clinic is an outpatient facility, but daily visits for the first few weeks help to assess how well the patient is responding to treatment and what dosage is optimum for them. After the initial few weeks, patients can then continue their treatment at home with follow-up visits to the clinic about every two months. When patients achieve a complete response of long duration, the intensive therapy may then be discontinued and the patient will continue with less intensive therapy in capsule form for another eight to 12 months.

Recently, to support the growing demand for antineoplastons, two new developments for obtaining antineoplastons have surfaced: (1) A new location outside the United States has just started administering antineoplaston therapy. Called "Sanoviv Medical Institute," this facility lies just over the San Diego, California, border. (You will find their address and phone number listed in the resources section at the end of the chapter.) Sanoviv received the Mexican government's and FDA's permission to use antineoplastons for the treatment of cancer, and is a fully staffed, professional medical center. (2) The second development is that the FDA has recently approved a non-prescription amino acid based food supplement, called "Aminocare A10," that was designed by Stanislaw Burzynski. There are no claims that Aminocare A10 can cure disease, but it does appear to help the overall functioning of the body in many ways, and has reportedly had positive effects on prostate hypertrophy and benign breast tumors.

There may be some insurance companies that will pay for antineoplaston therapy performed in the United States, so if you are interested in this form of treatment, it is worth checking with your insurance group about it. As stated before, many people have found it worthwhile to come up with the cost of this treatment on their own, when their insurance company did not pay for it. This non-toxic form of cancer treatment is simply remarkable in its efficacy and definitely something to look into for anyone with a cancer diagnosis!

Resources:

The Burzynski Clinic   (713) 335-5697
9432 Old Katy Road, Suite 200   www.cancermed.com
Houston, TX 77055

(To request a general information packet through the mail, call the above number or email your request to info@burzynskiclinic.com.)

For Consultation: In-depth consultation appointments at the Burzynski Clinic can be scheduled and generally run two to four hours long.

Cost of Treatment: Treatment costs vary greatly due the treatment protocols being tailored to each patient. A general ball-park figure would be around $4,500 to $7,500 per month (as of this printing). Depending on how many months treatment is required, the total cost could run around $100,000 or more.

Treatment in Mexico

Sanoviv Medical Institute   Phone: (Mexico) (6) 614-9200
Rancho Santini   (California) (800) 726-6848
Playas de Rosarito, B.C. 22712   www.sanoviv.com
Mexico

Aminocare A10 (Health Supplement in Tablets or Capsules)
For information, go to: www.aminocare.com or, call (800) 856-8006

Books

Thomas D. Elias. *The Burzynski Breakthrough.* Nevada City, California: Lexikos, 2001. (ISBN 0-938530-66-6)

Richard Walters. *Options: The Alternative Cancer Therapy Book.* New York: Avery Penguin Putnam, 1993. (ISBN 0-89529-510-5)

Ralph W. Moss. *The Cancer Industry.* Equinox Press, New York, 1999. (ISBN 1-881025-09-8)

Newsletter

Dr. Julian Whitaker's Health and Healing Newsletter, Mid-February 1966 Supplement.

Websites

www.cancermed.com

www.burzynskipatientgroup.org

www.burzynskipatientgroup.org/burdickreport.htm

CHAPTER 9

Protocel
History and Theory

As much as I was amazed by the effectiveness of other alternative non-toxic approaches to cancer, I was stunned by the effectiveness of a brown liquid formula called "Protocel." Because there are few other sources of in-depth information currently published about Protocel, I decided to devote four chapters of this book to the Protocel formula alone.

Protocel is a unique non-herbal formula that was designed to specifically target anaerobic cells of the body, leaving normal healthy cells unharmed. As mentioned in Chapter 2, the brilliant Nobel prize-winner, Dr. Otto Warburg, argued that all cancer cells are primarily anaerobic. Dr. Warburg focused his research on cancer cells, and lectured extensively on his discovery that, in the human body, cancer cells primarily use the fermentation of glucose to obtain most of their energy rather than primarily using oxygen for energy like all normal healthy cells do. He fervently argued that the prime difference between cancer cells and normal healthy cells is that healthy cells are *aerobic* and cancer cells are *anaerobic*.

Protocel targets anaerobic cells by interfering with their cell respiration so they cannot obtain enough energy to function. Since normal healthy cells of the body are aerobic and use a different process to obtain energy via cell respiration, they are not harmed. (More details on this will be presented later.) Since it only debilitates the cell respiration of anaerobic cells, Protocel effectively targets cancer cells and other unhealthy anaerobic cells of the body without harming any of a person's normal healthy cells.

Protocel is currently being sold as a general health-enhancing product. It is marketed as a "cell cleanser" because of its powerful ability to rid the body of non-productive anaerobic cells. Because anaerobic cells are believed to be involved in so many chronic illnesses (such as arthritis, chronic fatigue, high blood pressure, diabetes, multiple sclerosis, viral infections, and others), Protocel can be effective in improving a variety of health problems. It is important to understand that Protocel is *not* currently being sold or advertised as a treatment for cancer and is being marketed with no claims as to its effectiveness for cancer or any other disease.

However, for those people who have cancer and *choose* to use Protocel to help them get rid of their anaerobic cells, it can be extremely effective. And it is one of the cheapest and easiest approaches available. A person can simply order Protocel over the phone and have it delivered to their home in a few days. They don't have to go through the rigors of difficult diet changes, frequent juicing, intravenous treatments, mountains of supplements, or enemas. They merely drink about a quarter teaspoonful of the formula in juice or water four or five times a day. Protocel is non-toxic and costs only about $55 to $75 a month.

human Dose

History

Protocel has an interesting history, particularly regarding how the product was originally conceived. This liquid formula was developed by Jim Sheridan, a chemist. He first called his formula "Entelev," and it was later renamed "Cancell." Today, Protocel is a continuation of Sheridan's original Entelev/Cancell formula. The following is a brief history of how the formula came into being.

Sheridan was born in 1912 in a Pennsylvania mining town. His father and both his grandfathers were coal miners. To help support his family, he had to work side jobs while he was going to high school. Finally, Sheridan was fortunate enough to win a scholarship to Carnegie Tech in Pittsburgh. Sheridan initially had aspirations of being a mining engineer and Carnegie Tech had the best program in the country at the time. In his freshman year, however, he realized he was really destined to be a chemist and switched to chemistry as his field of study instead.

What is important to understand about Jim Sheridan is that, even as a young man, he was a devoutly spiritual person. He knew he had a good mind and in his early teens he would pray to God that he be able to use his intellect to help mankind. Unlike most other boys in high school, he also prayed to be able to help find a cure for cancer. For Sheridan, it wasn't his ego at play here. He truly wanted to be of service to his fellow man.

In late high school, Sheridan started having a series of recurring dreams. They were unusual in that he kept seeing a chemical formula over and over again. This formula meant nothing to him, and he could find no one else who could understand it either. However, after Sheridan started college, he came face to face with the chemical formula of his recurring dreams. It was listed in print in the title of an article he came across by accident. The article was printed in a huge source book, and Sheridan just happened to have opened the book to that page. It was an article related to cancer and known carcinogens.

The next important event that led to the development of Sheridan's unique formula occurred in April 1931, while he was demonstrating some chemistry concepts at a Carnegie Tech open-house meeting. A high school boy asked Sheridan if the bright yellow color of a liquid in one beaker was caused by something called "chromate." Sheridan said that it was, and one of the students then wanted to know how that color could be changed to a different color. To this, Sheridan answered that any change in the oxidation state of the sample would result in a color change. He then went to a shelf and picked an acid at random and proceeded to add the acid to the solution in the beaker to demonstrate. To Sheridan's complete surprise, the liquid in the beaker turned all the colors of the rainbow in perfectly defined layers! He and the high school boys stood there dumbfounded, looking at six layers of color in the beaker in the very order they would occur in a rainbow—red, orange, yellow, green, blue, and violet.

This unusual result even astonished the professors who were there, and everyone gathered around to see the amazing sight. One professor stated that it looked like a case of "rhythmic banding," and if it were, then each band of color would be 2.7 times the width of the band above it. Upon measuring the bands of color in the beaker, they found this was indeed the case, though none of the professors or students understood the significance of this "rhythmic banding" phenomenon.

Shortly after this episode, and unconnected with the incident involving the beaker, Sheridan was given a long-term project by his advisor that involved studying the effects of changes in dielectric constant on reactions between positive and negative ions. This work was related to a recently published theory called the "Debye-Hückel Theory." For several years after the odd incident with the rainbow colors in the beaker, Jim worked on testing the validity of the Debye-Hückel Theory. In order to be competent enough to do this, he had to take two years of physical chemistry. He was also forced by his advisor to take an advanced course called "Theory and Thermodynamics of Solutions" *three times* (despite the fact that he received an "A" each time he took the class).

Once Sheridan started studying the Debye-Hückel Theory, he also realized that the chemical formula he had dreamed about in high school, and then had found by accident after starting college, was in fact associated with the Debye-Hückel Theory! Looking back, it certainly seemed that events were leading Sheridan in a very specific direction.

The final important event in the development of Sheridan's formula occurred on September 6, 1936. It happened in the afternoon while he was taking a nap. During this nap, Sheridan had an unusual dream. He explained it in these words:

> The dream brought together the event of the rainbow in the beaker and the work on the Debye Theory. In the 1936 dream, the layers of the rainbow represented the respiratory enzymes. Each color represented an enzyme at a specific redox level. The electrons from the Debye Theory represented the energy units in the respiration moving from glucose to oxygen via that respiratory system. Somehow, the dream suggested the possibility of controlled altering of the pathway of energy flow and energy production in the respiratory system to: (a) cause a cancer, or (b) cure a cancer.[1]

Jim Sheridan was profoundly affected by the guidance he felt he had received in this dream. As he, himself, wrote:

> When I woke up, I felt that I had received my *marching orders*. Three years later I bought my first mice and I was on my way in my basement lab. The suggested cure was to make the cancer cell even more primitive—to the point where the cancer cell would lyse.[2]

The terms "redox," "lyse" and "respiratory enzymes" will be explained shortly.

Jim Sheridan dedicated himself to pursuing the goal put forth in his afternoon dream of 1936. It took him many years of hard work and trial and error to develop his formula fully. In fact, he actually worked on the formula from the 1930s until the 1990s. Most of that time, Sheridan worked on "the project" (as he called it) at home after hours, or whenever he had some spare time. He made his living by being employed full-time doing other work. At first, Sheridan was employed as a chemist at Dow Chemical Company. While working there, he studied law and passed his bar exam, eventually becoming a patent attorney. In 1946, Sheridan left Dow Chemical to practice law.

At this point, Sheridan was able to fully stock his laboratory at home where he continued to develop his formula, using mice for testing. He never stopped working on his "project." By the early 1950s, he obtained a private grant to work at the Detroit Cancer Institute, where he further improved his formula in a more formal laboratory environment. After a while, Sheridan began getting 70 to 80 percent positive results on the mice cancers he was treating. He kept working on his material and improving it, and by 1983, he felt he finally had a formula that could consistently cure about 80 percent of the mice cancers on which it was used.

Sheridan originally named his product "Entelev," which stems from the classical Greek phrase "Entelechy" (pronounced enteleekee). Sheridan's understanding was that "Entelechy" translated as "that part of man known only to God," and he added the letters "EV" to represent "electro-valence." Thus, he created the name "Entelev" to mean the *electrovalence of man known only to God*. The electrovalence part will be explained in the next section as we look at the theory behind Sheridan's formula.

Theory

To understand the theory behind Sheridan's formula, we start with the concept that all cancer cells are primarily anaerobic. Cancer cells are not the *only* type of anaerobic cell found in the body, however. In other words, we can have *other* types of anaerobic cells in our bodies that are not necessarily cancer cells. But any human cell that is anaerobic is unhealthy, or abnormal, and these unhealthy anaerobic cells tend to be involved in illnesses of various sorts. Sheridan believed that cancer cells form some of these anaerobic cells.

In a nutshell, this is how Protocel works: When a person takes Protocel regularly every day, the formula biochemically lowers the voltage of every cell in the body *just a little bit*. (Actually, for those with technical backgrounds, the more accurate term is "capacitance," but most people understand the term "voltage" better.) This results in a voltage reduction of about 10 to 15 percent, and Protocel accomplishes this by interfering with the production of ATP (adenosine triphosphate). Because anaerobic cells obtain their energy by fermentation of glucose, or "glycolysis," instead of by oxidation like normal cells, they operate on a minimum energy level and sustain a lower voltage than normal cells. The slight reduction in voltage caused by Protocel shifts the cancer cells downward to a point below the minimum that cancer cells need to remain intact. When this happens, the cancer cells (as well as other anaerobic cells of the body) break down, or "lyse," into harmless protein. In other words, they cannot hold themselves together anymore and they simply fall apart!

Normal healthy cells of the body, on the other hand, sustain such a high voltage level that the slight reduction in voltage promoted by Protocel does not hurt them. This is why Protocel is deadly to cancer cells but harmless to the rest of the body. The details of how this happens are somewhat complicated, but the following is a simplified explanation of how Protocel works, using an analogy to car batteries.

One could say that all the cells of the human body are somewhat like little car batteries in the sense that they must manufacture and deliver energy throughout the cell so that the cell can perform its important functions. This process of producing and distributing energy in each cell is called "cell respiration." (Most of us think of respiration as the process of breathing oxygen, but on a cellular level, the term "respiration" refers to the acquiring and distributing of energy for the cell, not to breathing oxygen.) Every cell in the body can only grow, divide and carry out its specific functions as long as the cell can continue to get sufficient energy to support those functions. This could be likened to how the battery in a car can continue to do its job only as long as the engine is kept running to resupply the battery with the energy that continually gets used up. If the supply of energy to the car battery is cut off while the energy from the battery is still outgoing, as when a person turns the engine off but leaves the lights on, then the battery energy reserves will be used up and the car battery will eventually "die."

Although human cells are somewhat like car batteries, they are also infinitely more sophisticated. So, when *more* energy is being used up than is getting supplied to the cell through respiration, the cell doesn't immediately die. Instead, it tries to compensate by transforming itself to need less energy. It does this by making changes in its respiration.

To understand this process, we need to know that, central to the respiratory system of each cell, there is something called the "oxidation reduction system." Scientists often refer to this as the "redox system." Although every cell in the body has a redox system, there are gradations of how advanced, or efficient, this redox system is in various types of cells. These gradations could be looked at as the steps on a ladder. Different types of cells in the body could then be represented as different points on this ladder. In Sheridan's own words,

> The oxidation reduction system can be thought of as a ladder, with a
> different chemical reaction taking place on each step. The respiratory

reaction which takes place on each step of this ladder is the same as on every other step in what it produces (i.e. energy for the cell to do its work), but each step is also different from every other step in the sense of how effective the reaction is.

The bottom steps of the ladder involve relatively simple or 'primitive' respiratory reactions. An example of a primitive reaction would be yeast while it is fermenting. Keep in mind that this is still an amazingly complex reaction. It is only 'simple' or 'primitive' compared to the other reactions in the oxidation-reduction system.

The higher steps involve more complex respiratory reactions. The primitive reactions at the bottom of the ladder take place without oxygen being present. The higher respiratory reactions require the presence of oxygen. Generally, for 'reduction' you are moving down the ladder. For 'oxidation' you are moving up the ladder.

Each 'step' on this ladder has a different 'potential'. 'Potential' means a measurable *electrical voltage*, like a small battery would have. Primitive yeast cells which are fermenting will give off a certain amount of electrical energy, i.e. movement of electrons. (We are talking about very *small* amounts of electrical energy.) As you move up toward the top of the ladder you will get increased potential energy. Thus, the potential electrical energy at the top of the ladder is greater than at the bottom. The top of the ladder has a potential of about +0.4 volts while the bottom is about −0.2 volts.[3]

Thus, a normal, healthy aerobic cell would be represented high on the ladder, and anaerobic and primitive cells would be represented lower on the ladder.

According to Sheridan's theory, a healthy cell will maintain a balance of ingoing and outgoing energy and will remain over time in its same position on the redox ladder hierarchy. Short-term drains of energy on cells are usually no problem, and cells can normally regain their balance without serious difficulty. But just like a car battery, if there is a *long-term*, severe drain on the energy of a cell, then there can be a serious problem. In a chronic energy drain situation, the balance point of the cell's respiration system will eventually be affected to where the point of balance *will be forced to occur at a lower oxidation reduction level for the cell to survive.*

When this energy balance point is forced to go lower, the cell could be said to move down the redox ladder. And it can continue to move down the ladder until it hits what Sheridan called a "critical point." According to his theory, this critical point is the lowest point the cell can go on the redox ladder and still retain its primary similarities to a normal cell. However, at this critical point, the cell is also now on the highest point of the ladder that could be said to apply to primitive cells. In other words, the cell that is forced to move down the redox ladder to survive can get to a point where it is, essentially, straddling the fence between being "normal" and being "primitive."

This is a very interesting point for a cell to be at. At this straddling point, the cell actually becomes quite stable because it is not enough like a normal cell to be differentiated and to function normally, but it is also not enough like a fully primitive cell for the body to know how to get rid of it. It is also at this critical point where the cell may become an anaerobic cancer cell!

Sheridan concluded that it would be difficult to move a cancer cell *back up* the redox ladder and make it normal again. He devised his formula to work by taking advantage of the fact that the cancer cell sits on the critical point of the ladder, or right on the dividing line between normal cells and primitive cells. By reducing the voltage (or potential) of every cell in the body just a tiny bit, those cells that are sitting on the fence are the most affected. The reduction of potential caused by Protocel effectively reduces their respiration ability just enough to push them *down* the redox ladder to where they are fully in the primitive zone, or even past it. At this point, the cancer cells are not able to produce enough energy to survive, and they subsequently die off and are disposed of by the body. According to Sheridan, the way his formula affects cell respiration is

> . . . by shunting off 'energy units' of the cell as it is working, so the energy is not going through the respiratory system. (An 'energy unit' is two electrons and a proton). Thus, work is being done by the cell, but not respiration . . . If work is being done, but not respiration, the cell is forced further down the oxidation-reduction ladder. Thus, once respiration is reduced, the cell is forced down completely into the primitive state.
>
> One of the chemicals which reduces respiration is catechol. The natural catechols have many different oxidation-reduction potentials (i.e. the level on the oxidation-reduction ladder where the particular catechol will work or operate.) The trick is to find one that works at the same level as a cancer cell, i.e. at that 'critical point' level.
>
> Entelev/Cancell was developed to act like a catechol, i.e. to inhibit respiration at the critical point.[4]

By following guidance that came to him in a dream, Sheridan was able to develop a truly ingenious way to cause cancer cells, as well as other anaerobic cells of the body, to self-destruct.

Tony Bell, Ph.D., is a chemist who understands on a detailed, technical level how Sheridan's formula works. To put it in simple terms that most of us can understand, Dr. Bell explains that for each cell in the body, the voltage of the cell operates as the cement, or glue, that holds the cell together. Healthy aerobic cells operate on a much higher energy level, or voltage, than do unhealthy anaerobic cells. So, in terms of energy voltage, healthy cells have plenty of energy to spare. But according to Dr. Bell, cancer cells sit right on the edge of the cliff in terms of voltage, and have very little to spare. When the voltage of a cancer cell is reduced by 10 to 15 percent the cell subsequently loses the "cement" that holds it together, and it breaks down into harmless protein that the body can then easily dispose of.

This process of the cancer cells breaking down is called "lysing," and it often results in a clear or somewhat yellowish, egg white-like substance. The body then processes this substance (which is really just "dead cancer cell parts") out through various elimination systems. In other words, when cancer patients use Protocel, this egg white-like material *may* come out of them through any avenue that the body uses to get rid of waste. Thus, people using Protocel for cancer will often see mucousy material in their feces and/or urine, or experience a runny nose or crusty eyes in the morning. Sometimes, people will even cough up mucousy whitish stuff. If any of this happens, it can generally be taken as a good sign that dead cancer cell parts are being ejected out of the body.

Protocel's ingredients are a proprietary blend of Tetrahydroxyquinone, Rhodizonic Acid, Sodium, Potassium, Croconic Acid, Triquinoyl, Pyrocatechol, Leuconic Acid, mineral and trace elements including Copper. These ingredients should not be evaluated individually, however, since putting them together with just the right process produces a unique end result—a powerful formula that acts like a super catechol which is able to inhibit respiration at the critical point in cancer cells. Side benefits of the Protocel formula are that it is less toxic than an aspirin a day, it is an immune system booster, and it is an extremely powerful antioxidant. Testing done at the Brunswick Laboratories in Massachusetts showed Protocel to have an ORAC antioxidant value of approximately 1.4 million (μmole TE/L).

In the next chapter, we will look at some remarkable testimonials from people who have used Jim Sheridan's unique formula to *outsmart* their cancer.

Chapter 10

Protocel

Case Stories

This chapter highlights 16 real-life case stories of people who used Entelev, Cancell, or Protocel for cancer. Each of these testimonials was written by myself after personally interviewing the people involved. Dr. Bell, who was mentioned in the previous chapter, became interested in this formula when one of his own family members came down with cancer, and we'll start with his story first.

Case Story #1 — Lung Cancer Metastasized to Brain

Dr. Tony Bell first became acquainted with Sheridan's formula (then called Cancell) when his brother, Frank, was diagnosed with cancer in 1989. Frank's cancer was non-small cell lung cancer, the type of lung cancer that smokers typically get. His doctors proceeded with treatment by first surgically removing one of his lungs. Then, in 1990, they found out that the cancer was in Frank's other lung as well and had also metastasized to his brain. Frank's doctors administered radiation directed at the brain tumors, but it had little effect and the tumors remained.

Shortly after the radiation treatments, Frank had a heart attack because his lung cancer had seriously stressed his heart. He survived the attack, but was too ill to undergo chemotherapy at this point. Frank's doctors sent him home and gave him about two months to live. They told the family not to worry about the cancer, because at this point it was probably Frank's heart that would kill him.

Frank then heard about Cancell and asked his brother, Dr. Bell, to look into it for him. Dr. Bell looked into it and didn't think it would work, but told his brother he might as well try it because it wouldn't hurt him. After taking Cancell for a while, Frank told Dr. Bell, "I don't know if the Cancell is working on the cancer or not, but it sure is a lot better than morphine because I'm not in any pain anymore!"

After seven months on Cancell, more tests and scans were done and the doctors couldn't find any evidence of cancer in Frank's lungs or brain, or anywhere else in his body. Luckily for Frank, his heart was somehow strong enough for him to play golf on an almost daily basis for six more years, during which time he remained cancer-free. When Frank finally passed away, it was due to heart failure—*not* cancer.

Case Story #2—Kidney Cancer

Another amazing testimonial comes from an 86-year-old man named Gunther. In early 1997, when Gunther was 80, he started feeling lousy. He went in for a general checkup and renal cell cancer was found in his left kidney. Gunther's doctor told him that chemotherapy does not work very well for kidney cancer, and he recommended that Gunther have his kidney entirely removed.

While Gunther was thinking about this, he searched the Internet for more information. Incredibly, he found four other people who had been in a similar situation to him. They all four had renal cell cancer in one kidney, and they all four had had their kidneys removed. Unfortunately, they all four said that the kidney cancer had then metastasized to other parts of their bodies. The good news, however, was that all four of these people had then recovered from their metastasized kidney cancer by using Cancell. Gunther talked with some of these people and decided not to have the surgery. Instead, he found someone who had a few extra bottles of the formula, and in mid-April 1997 Gunther started taking Cancell.

Toward the end of April, Gunther traveled to Germany. Someone there convinced him to seek a second opinion about his kidney cancer. He agreed to do this and had a consultation with a cancer specialist there. The German specialist came to the same conclusion as Gunther's American doctor, and told him he should have his kidney taken out.

At this point, Gunther decided to have his kidney removed and made an appointment with the German doctor for the surgery. But before the surgery was performed, Gunther heard that a doctor back in the United States at the Cleveland Clinic was one of the world's best specialists on kidney cancer. He immediately called from Hamburg to make an appointment at the Cleveland Clinic, cancelled his surgery, and flew back to the United States to consult with this top kidney cancer specialist instead.

In Cleveland, another CT scan was performed and the specialist pronounced again that Gunther had a dangerous renal cell tumor on his left kidney. His right kidney looked fine with just a benign cyst on it. This doctor said the same thing as the other two had. He suggested Gunther have his kidney removed. Gunther finally scheduled the recommended surgery with this specialist and it was set for mid-July 1997.

Three days before surgery, Gunther was back at the Cleveland Clinic to have his pre-surgery exam. But he was by this time feeling so good, his doctor thought it would be all right to postpone the surgery. So Gunther once again cancelled his appointment to have his kidney removed. He just kept taking the Cancell and visiting this doctor for checkups.

In December of that year, Gunther underwent another CT scan. It showed no change in the size of the tumor. But Gunther was still feeling good, so the doctor said, "Let's just continue to watch it." In another six months, another CT scan was performed that also showed no tumor growth. At this point, Gunther got lazy about getting his cancer checked and went a while without another scan. He kept taking the Cancell for about two years (from April 1997 to mid-1999), then stopped the Cancell and didn't worry about it anymore.

In September 2000, however, Gunther became ill and developed a high fever. After hearing about his history of cancer, the doctor did an ultrasound on his kidney and surrounding areas. The result was that the doctor could not find any tumor at all.

Gunther is now almost 87 years old and more active than many people who are a lot younger. He swims laps every morning for 45 minutes, he is still active in business, and he travels around the world quite a lot for pleasure. No one would guess that he'd been diagnosed with kidney cancer six years earlier. And no one would guess that he had never gone through any surgery, chemotherapy, or radiation. The only treatment he ever did was to take Cancell.

Case Story #3 — Pancreatic Cancer

Pancreatic cancer is well known as one of the most deadly types of cancer. So I was truly excited to be able to speak with a man who had recovered from this type of cancer many years ago through the use of Cancell alone. His name is Bill. Bill is now 69 years old, but back in March of 1988 he was diagnosed with pancreatic cancer and his doctor didn't think he would live more than six months. He chose not to do conventional treatment of any kind, and instead immediately started taking Cancell. Bill took Cancell for two-and-one-half years, between 1988 and 1991. After doing so, he was pronounced cancer-free. His doctors were astonished.

Bill didn't take any vitamins, minerals, herbs, enzymes, or supplements of any kind while he was on Cancell. All he did was take 1/4 teaspoonful of Cancell four times a day (every six hours), along with going off sugar and cutting back on his intake of red meat. He has remained healthy and completely free of cancer for about 15 years!

Case Story #4 — Breast Cancer Metastasized to Bones

A story of breast cancer that had metastasized to the bones was told to me by a woman named Roberta. Roberta is now 65 years old, but when she was only 41, she was diagnosed with breast cancer. That was in October 1979. Back in those days, doctors didn't do lumpectomies, they just went straight to mastectomy. So she underwent a mastectomy immediately after her diagnosis and during the surgery five of her lymph nodes were removed to see if the cancer had already metastasized. Unfortunately, it had. After the surgery, Roberta was treated for about six months with chemotherapy and toward the end of that period she also went through a three-week round of radiation.

Roberta went through the full treatment regimen that her doctor had planned for her. But after completing it, she started having some physical problems as a result of the chemotherapy and radiation. One of the problems was that, as a result of the radiation being targeted near her throat, Roberta began having serious difficulty swallowing. The other problem was that she suddenly developed insulin-dependent diabetes. This last development was quite a surprise, since she had never suffered from any sort of diabetes before, nor had she shown signs that she was starting to develop it. Although it can't be said for sure that she wouldn't have developed diabetes at some point, no one in her family had ever had diabetes so she wasn't expected to be genetically predisposed to it.

To be sure that the cancer was all gone, Roberta was given a bone scan. But the results showed that the cancer was not gone and, instead, had metastasized to her bones with spots on her clavicle and in her rib cage. Luckily for Roberta, she had heard about Entelev and had already started taking it. (This was the name of the formula before it was called Cancell.) Her doctor didn't think it would do her any good but didn't discourage her from taking it.

A couple of months after her first bone scan, Roberta was given a second scan. This time, the suspicious spots had reduced in size considerably. For a number of months more, Roberta did nothing in terms of treatment except take Entelev. In those days, there wasn't as much known about the effects of diet or supplements on cancer, and so she didn't take any other nutritional supplements or do anything different with her diet at all. She didn't even reduce her sugar intake. She stayed on the Entelev until all of her scans and blood tests were completely normal, and the doctors couldn't find evidence of any cancer whatsoever. Then she continued to take the formula for a few months more just to be sure.

A little more than a year and a half after Roberta was diagnosed, she finally stopped taking the Entelev. She hasn't had a recurrence of cancer since. She has been monitored regularly by a cancer specialist for the past 23 years, and all her tests have continued to be normal.

Case Story #5 — Central Nervous System Cancer (Glioblastoma Multiforme, Stage IV)

The following case of a woman named Elonna is considered one of the most celebrated of all Cancell recoveries. That is partly because Elonna was diagnosed with a very rare form of nervous system cancer called Glioblastoma Multiforme, stage IV. (According to conventional medicine, malignant glios are virtually always fatal.) Her case is also celebrated because when Elonna was diagnosed with this cancer she had just given birth to quintuplets. One baby unfortunately did not survive, but the other four did. According to Elonna, she was given a CT scan when the four babies were about two-and-one-half weeks old in order to diagnose some severe pain she had been having during and after the pregnancy. They found that the source of the pain was a tumor on her spinal cord in the thoracic area.

An additional MRI and a consultation with a neurosurgeon were done, then Elonna was taken into surgery to have her tumor removed. After the surgery, she was paralyzed from the waist down and told that the tumor was malignant and they were *not* able to remove all of the cancer throughout her spine. She was also told that now there would be free-floating cancer cells in her spinal fluid that would travel to her brain and develop into new tumors. Her doctors said she would not live to see her four babies' first birthday.

Elonna's doctors wanted to put her through either a very aggressive bone marrow chemotherapy treatment, or 30 treatments of radiation at very high calibration. Either treatment choice would cause her body great damage and with either treatment the doctors could still not hope for her to live more than three to six months. Her options were not good. But because of the media attention that Elonna got as a result of giving birth to quintuplets and receiving a rare cancer diagnosis right afterward, many people saw her story on TV or in the newspapers. As a result, she and her husband were barraged with mail containing concerned sugges-tions as to alternatives. One of these suggestions was about Cancell.

Elonna was skeptical about Cancell at first. Her initial words to her husband were, "If there was a cure for cancer, don't you think they would be using it instead of letting thousands of people die?" But she had no other choice and her husband seemed to have faith that Cancell would work. On November 12, 1989, Elonna started taking Cancell. She decided to refuse the conventional treatments of chemotherapy and radiation that had been offered to her since they could promise her no more than six months anyway. She really wanted to be able to take care of her babies and watch them grow up.

At the end of Elonna's second week on Cancell, and into her third week, she was admitted back into a local hospital for eight days because of blood clots and a hemoglobin problem. Luckily her doctor allowed her family to come into the hospital every day and administer the Can-cell to her around the clock. According to Elonna, after several weeks, she began to notice an improvement in her condition, though she still could not walk. However, it was only 18 hours after her first dose that she began to eliminate the cancer waste product. She says, "It literally poured out of me: I threw it up; my bowel movements were extremely loose and stringy and frequent. I lost it in my urine; my nose ran so much I had to keep a tissue with me at all times. I sweated it out pro-fusely; and I had hot and cold flashes and night sweats. When the nurses would give me a sponge bath after a night sweat, the water would be a golden brown color with what they referred to as 'tapioca balls' floating in it."

The lysing symptoms Elonna experienced were worth it. Amazingly, by February 1990, only about three and one-half months after she started on Cancell, new scans of her brain and entire spinal cord came back negative for any signs of cancer.

Elonna stayed on Cancell for a total of two years and three months to be sure all of her cancer was gone and to help repair a great deal of the extensive nerve damage that had been caused by the cancer and surgery. She had to go through agonizing physical therapy to regain her ability to walk again, but she is now walking and living a normal life. Best of all, she has been able to see her children grow up and enjoy them to the fullest, thanks to Cancell. It is now 14 years after Elonna's bout with can-cer, and she continues to be completely cancer-free.

Case Story #6 — Melanoma, Stage IV

Roma is an 80-year-old woman who also has quite a story to share. Back in October 1989, when she was 66 years old, Roma was diagnosed with melanoma. A few months before, she had noticed a dark spot on the big toe of her right foot. She didn't think anything of it, but it came to the attention of a doctor she was seeing about a bone spur problem in her foot. The doctor did not suspect cancer, and he proceeded to cut into the dark spot with a knife and attempted to dig it out with tweezers. This obviously didn't do any good, and the opening he created never healed.

Roma finally went to another doctor, who took some scrapings of the now oozing dark spot for biopsy. The diagnostic results came back: melanoma. Her doctors then debated whether or not to surgically remove the whole foot or just part of it. They settled on removing her right big toe and a great deal of extra tissue going about halfway up her foot. But in just two weeks after the surgery, melanoma spots started showing on her *second* toe, the one next to the big toe that had just been removed.

At this point, Roma decided to try an alternative treatment and went down to a clinic in Mexico where she was instructed to do 13 juices and several coffee enemas each day. She stayed there for one week, which cost her $3,000, then went home and continued the juicing and enema regimen for a full three months. But although the melanoma was not spreading throughout her body, it continued to grow slowly. At this point, her melanoma cancer was now considered to be stage IV.

Then a friend told Roma about Cancell. On May 23, 1990, she started taking Cancell. No longer doing the juicing/enema regimen, she simply took Cancell, and eliminated sugar and cut back on red meat in her diet. Roma says that it wasn't until about the second to third month on Cancell that she noticed the melanoma was getting smaller. Finally, it quit seeping around Christmas 1990. The spots never completely went away, but they eventually changed color to a light brown. In every other way, she felt normal.

After two-and-one-half years on Cancell, Roma's doctors performed another biopsy and could find no indication of cancer at all. At that point, she stopped the Cancell and has not experienced any recurrence of her melanoma since.

Case Story #7 — Intestinal Cancer

Sarah is 83 years old. Back in May 2001, she got very sick and experienced a lot of vomiting and diarrhea. She was finally taken into the hospital and an ultrasound revealed a mass in her intestine which turned out to be a large malignant bowel tumor. Sarah went into surgery where the doctors removed as much as they could of the tumor, but proclaimed that they couldn't get it all. Her cancer had not yet metastasized, but the tumor was shaped like a large comma and the tail end of it, which would have been too risky to remove, still remained in her body after the surgery. Sarah spent three weeks in intensive care, and then her doctors wanted to schedule her for more aggressive treatment with chemotherapy. Sarah did not want to undergo this course of treatment and flatly refused.

Toward the end of the summer, Sarah had still not done any more treatment of any kind since the surgery and was back to feeling very sick every day. But by this time her daughter had heard about Protocel from some people in her church and she was able to convince her mother to try it. In August 2001, Sarah started on Protocel. According to Sarah, after just one week of taking Protocel she started to feel better. Soon, she began to notice mucousy material coming out in her bowel movements.

At one point that summer Sarah's daughter, Elizabeth, was in church and met up with her mother's doctor. The doctor told Elizabeth, "Your mother's *got* to have chemotherapy." Elizabeth knew this doctor personally and liked him very much. But she replied to him, "No, she's going to go the natural route." Upon hearing that, the doctor grabbed Elizabeth's arm and marched her out of the church with him. Once outside, he adamantly said, "Your mother will be dead in a year if she doesn't do chemotherapy!"

But Sarah chose to remain steadfast in her use of Protocel and continued to decline conventional treatments. Over the next few months, Sarah felt better and better, and now, more than two years later, she is feeling great. As of this writing, the latest results of a series of comprehensive lab tests all indicate that she is still in remission—and Sarah says she is still "on Protocel and prayer!"

Case Story #8 — Prostate Cancer

Sarah's husband, Bernard, now 89 years old, also has a Protocel story. Three-and-one-half years ago, Bernard was diagnosed with prostate cancer. His doctors surgically removed a tumor on his prostate and Bernard was scheduled to get some follow-up treatments to make sure the cancer did not recur. But unfortunately, Bernard's doctor suddenly died, and as a result Bernard did not get any more treatment of any kind for eight months. Then he heard about Protocel from his daughter and started taking it at the same time his wife Sarah did. When he started the formula, his PSA count was 19. In about eight months' time, just through using Protocel alone, his PSA was down to 4.

Bernard never did any conventional treatment other than the surgery for his prostate cancer. Thanks to Protocel, he is currently doing fine and is still cancer-free.

Case Story #9—Prostate Cancer

Albert is 73 years old. Five years ago, Albert was diagnosed with prostate cancer. A needle biopsy was performed that included five or six samples, and from these Albert's prostate cancer was given a "Gleason" scale rating of 4.5. (The Gleason scale is a scale from 1 to 10 that indicates how aggressive, or fast-growing, a man's prostate cancer is.) Thus, Albert's cancer was just about in the middle of this scale. His PSA level at the time was 13, and his prostate gland was enlarged.

Luckily for Albert, he already knew about Protocel at the time he was diagnosed and he immediately went on the formula. Albert never underwent surgery, radiation or any other conventional treatment for his cancer. After six months on Protocel, his PSA count went up to 16. But then it started to go down, eventually stabilizing at 9.7. For many men, this would still be a high PSA count. But in Albert's case, a PSA of 9.7 had been his "normal" reading for five to six years prior to his cancer diagnosis. His doctor theorized that Albert has calcification in his prostate gland, which causes irritation and inflammation, and that this raises his PSA level above what is considered normal for most men.

For a few more years, Albert's PSA count remained stable at 9.7. He continued to get tests done over the years (including PSA tests, digital exams, CT and bone scans, blood work-ups, and even an MRI), and his doctors have continued to pronounce him free of cancer. In early 2003, Albert's PSA reading went down to 7.0. This is the lowest PSA reading that Albert has ever had. Albert continues to feel great and to show no sign of cancer.

Case Story #10 — Brain Cancer

Steve is a 41-year-old, happily married man with two sons. On Christmas Day 2000, he suffered a grand mal seizure during a nap. After being unconscious for about 30 minutes, he woke up with blood on his shirt (from biting his tongue) and his family and paramedics staring down at him in horror. A CT scan showed that Steve had an abnormality in the left frontal lobe of his brain. He was given a common anti-convulsant drug called dilantin to keep his seizures under control. A few weeks later after a biopsy, Steve was told that he had a malignant tumor, just under the skull in his speech center, which was about 80 percent the size of a golf ball. It was surgically removed and diagnosed as an "anaplastic astrocytoma, grade III." Steve's prognosis was grim. He was told he had about a 10 percent chance of living five years, but *only* if he did numerous rounds of radiation, likely to be followed by chemotherapy.

At this point, which was 35 days after his surgery, he underwent another MRI. The cancer he was dealing with was apparently *extremely* aggressive (fast-growing) because this MRI showed that the tumor had already grown back! Steve spent an arduous recovery after the surgery and opted for the recommended 35 days of radiation treatments. But he did only three days of treatments and decided he had gathered enough evidence that he believed Protocel was going to take care of his condition without any more conventional treatments.

Steve subsequently refused more radiation and went on Protocel alone. After four weeks on Protocel, another MRI was performed. This time, no change in the size of the tumor had occurred. This was a really good sign, since the cancer was so aggressive and any lack of growth at this point was positive. Steve continued on the Protocel, and two months later another MRI was performed. This time, the result showed that the tumor had greatly reduced in size. Two months more on Protocel and the surgical tumor was even smaller and no longer enhancing! This meant that the MRI no longer showed "active" cancer and the remaining tumor mass could be considered benign.

Steve was told by others who had used the formula that, after about four to five weeks on Protocel, he might go through a period of dizziness and difficulty thinking and talking. Steve was warned that this could occur because the tumor might be lysing enough at that point to cause a certain amount of edema. He was also told not to worry if this happened, because this would mean that the tumor was shrinking. According to Steve, four weeks and four days after he started Protocel, he did experience a period of dizziness and difficulty thinking. But he got through it without much trouble, and then he just started to feel better and better.

Steve continued to feel fine for more than three years after being diagnosed with a very aggressive type of brain cancer, and all his follow-up MRIs continued to show no tumor activity. However, Steve stopped taking Protocel shortly after his tumor stopped enhancing and apparently he stopped too soon. In December 2003, after he started feeling a return of symptoms, an MRI showed new enhancement and tumor growth in his brain. Steve immediately went back on Protocel, and as of this writing in March 2004, he is continuing on Protocel to get rid of his new tumor growth.

(*Note:* In general, tumors anywhere in the body other than the brain will eventually disappear completely over time with the use of Protocel. Small brain tumors will also eventually completely disappear. However, large tumors in the brain will sometimes only shrink to a point, then stop highlighting and stop growing. At this point, some people have chosen to have the benign mass surgically removed, while others have been able to easily live a normal life with the benign mass still in their brain. Steve's experience is an important reminder that when an active tumor has become benign, even though there is no discernable enhancement on an MRI, there could still be some active cancer cells within the mass somewhere. And these active cells could start growing again as soon as Protocel is stopped. Thus, Protocel users agree that it is probably best to stay on Protocel indefinitely as long as there is any mass left in the brain at all.)

Case Story #11—Childhood Leukemia

Sydney is a wonderful seven-year-old girl. In 1999, when she was only two, she was diagnosed with "acute lymphoblastic leukemia." Two-year-old Sydney was given chemotherapy for about a year. At that point, her doctors and family were hoping that she would be able to transition to "maintenance" therapy, but a bone test in October 2000 showed that she still had cancer in her bone marrow. Sydney had relapsed, and her doctors wanted to perform a bone marrow transplant involving aggressive chemotherapy at this point. Her family was told that even *with* the bone marrow transplant, Sydney probably only had a 10 percent chance of survival.

Before making a decision, Sydney's family sought a second opinion from another prominent hospital. The doctors at this hospital told them that Sydney would probably only have a 5 percent chance of survival after the transplant.

In January 2001, Sydney's family chose to decline the bone marrow transplant which offered so little hope. They also declined any further chemotherapy or other conventional treatment. Instead, they started Sydney on Protocel. Sydney showed mild symptoms of lysing which mostly involved loose stools with what looked like lysed material in them. Amazingly, when Sydney went back for her next checkup, which seemed to her mom like after just a matter of weeks, there was no more evidence of leukemia!

Sydney has continued to take Protocel and has also continued to get tested about every three months (including bone marrow tests) for the past four years. All her tests have continued to be negative for cancer. Recently, Sydney's doctor told her family they don't have to bring her in for checkups anymore, but Sydney's mother still feels more comfortable doing the testing once in a while. Sydney's last test was on January 8, 2003, and again showed her to be cancer-free. Little Sydney feels perfectly fine and is currently enjoying attending school.

Case Story #12—Kidney Cancer Metastasized to Both Lungs

Many people whose cancer has already metastasized to other organs have fully recovered through the use of Entelev, Cancell, or Protocel. Like Roberta (case story #4), Kathy was one of these people. In late 1991, Kathy became sick. She was extremely tired and achy and had lost 40 pounds. For a while, the doctors couldn't figure out what was wrong. Finally, in March 1992, they discovered that she was suffering from renal cell carcinoma in her right kidney. Later that month Kathy went into surgery and her right kidney and surrounding lymph nodes were removed. The lymph nodes were clear, but the kidney tumor was big. It measured 7 by 14 centimeters. The surgeons actually had to remove two of her ribs to get it out!

After surgery, Kathy's doctors were going to discuss follow-up chemotherapy or radiation with her, but she didn't want to do either. Kathy had too many nurses in her family who had seen the horrors of these treatments, and her own research indicated that there was no effective conventional treatment for renal cell cancer anyway.

Kathy declined further treatment after the surgery. But in June, she was worried about her lungs and requested a chest X-ray. The X-ray indicated that something was there and the doctors then did a CT scan. The scan showed numerous nodules in both of Kathy's lungs. To diagnose these nodules more specifically, Kathy underwent a two-hour needle biopsy procedure. The biopsy result came back as "metastasized renal cell carcinoma, stage IV." The other result from the biopsy was that the procedure collapsed one of her lungs, and Kathy had to recover in the hospital for five days.

At this point, with metastasized renal cell cancer, Kathy's doctors did *not* recommend follow-up treatment. They did not say specifically, but their attitude suggested that there was no hope and they had nothing to offer her. So she went home. She had already been looking into alternatives and circumstances finally led her to Cancell.

At the end of August 1992, Kathy started taking Cancell. She took only one other supplement, which was Bromelain. Other than the Cancell and Bromelain, Kathy followed a very healthy eating program she created on her own. She stayed completely away from white sugar (though she did use honey and pure maple syrup) and drank a gallon of distilled water every day. She also drank one glass of fresh juice each day (apple, carrot, and spinach) and ate a lot of organic fruits and vegetables. She kept a healthy mix of organic almonds, sunflower seeds, and raisins around at all times for snacking and made vegetable soup with cabbage, potatoes, celery, and V-8 juice. Kathy did not restrict her intake of meat, and freely ate chicken, fish, and beef.

On January 25, 1993, five months after starting on Cancell, Kathy got another scan of her lungs. This time, she only had two nodules left, one in each lung. This was a great improvement since the doctors had initially diagnosed her with "numerous" nodules. Then in March, Kathy went into surgery to have a swollen lymph gland in her collar bone area removed. She was worried that it might be malignant, but the biopsy showed there was no cancer in it. This was good news, but the *really* good news was that the doctors did one more chest X-ray before the lymph node surgery, and this X-ray revealed that the last two nodules in her lungs were both gone. A few months later, in June 1993, Kathy got a total body CT scan, along with a variety of blood tests. All of the results came back the same—no evidence of cancer anywhere.

Kathy's metastasized renal cell cancer was completely gone after 10 months on Cancell! She stayed on the Cancell another eight months to be sure that there would be no return of her cancer, after which she went to a maintenance schedule of taking Cancell just three to six months each year. For the past 11 years she has had no recurrence of cancer.

The year that Kathy was pronounced free of cancer—1993—she organized an informal picnic gathering for Cancell users so that people could share their stories and learn more about it from others. She has continued to organize this picnic every year since then, which is now attended by veteran Cancell users as well as more recent Protocel users. According to Kathy, "I promised the good Lord I would do something to help more people know about this."

Case Story #13 — Stomach Cancer Metastasized to Lymph and Bones

Another remarkable story of recovery from metastasized cancer belongs to Robert. In May 2000, when Robert was 54, he and his wife were vacationing in Las Vegas. One day, Robert suddenly fainted and then began vomiting blood. He was rushed to the hospital, and after scoping his stomach, the doctors told Robert he had stomach cancer, stage IV. The scope had revealed a 5.8 centimeter tumor. Also, the wall of his stomach was about 3 inches thick around the tumor instead of the normal 1-inch thickness. The doctors gave Robert 2 pints of blood to get him back home so that he could be treated by his local doctors.

At home, Robert's doctors performed a cauterization in his stomach to stop the bleeding and administered antibiotics to him. More tests revealed, however, that Robert's stomach cancer had already metastasized. He was soon diagnosed with MALT lymphoma, which is a cancer of the stomach lining, as well as non-Hodgkin's lymphoma. (MALT stands for mycosa-associated lymphoid tissue.) As if that was not enough, a bone scan and bone marrow biopsy then showed he had cancer in his bones as well, and another scan showed two spots on his liver.

Robert's doctors recommended a chemotherapy regimen called "CHOP" along with radiation directed at the stomach tumor. (CHOP stands for four drugs: cyclophosphamide, doxorubicin, vincristine, and prednisone.) They told Robert and his wife that if he did *not* undergo this type of treatment, he would probably live no more than three months.

Robert found out about Protocel in June 2000, and he started taking the formula. He refused all chemotherapy and radiation and just took Protocel every day in distilled water. He also started taking Ellagic 21, enzymes, and aloe vera juice for detoxing and cleansing. After a while, Robert started experiencing a lot of odd stuff coming out of his body in his feces and also saw that his urine was often "bubbly."

Exactly two months after starting Protocel, at the end of August 2000, Robert underwent another stomach scoping. He was thrilled to hear that his tumor had shrunk from 5.8 to 3.5 centimeters in size. They then found out that the two spots on his liver were gone! On his next visit two months later, his stomach tumor was again decreased in size. Finally, on December 22, 2000, after undergoing yet another scoping, a set of scans, and blood tests, Robert was told that all of his cancer was gone. In just six months, his stomach, lymphatic, and bone cancer had disappeared! (The spots on his liver had disappeared as well, but it had never been *definitively* determined that they were cancer. They may have been a pre-cancerous or other sort of condition that also got resolved through the use of Protocel.)

Robert continued to take Protocel for a total of two years from the day he started to make sure that all the cancer in his body was completely gone. He knew that modern diagnostic tests cannot detect all of it. He now plans to take just one bottle of Protocel each year, which is about a two-month supply, as a maintenance program for the rest of his life. Robert's recovery from metastasized cancer is an incredible success story.

What did Robert's doctor think of his recovery? In late December 2000, when Robert was told that all his cancer was gone, his wife asked his main doctor to what he attributed the recovery. The doctor knew all along that Robert was taking Protocel, but for some reason, he couldn't believe it was the Protocel that did it. The doctor's reply was that it was probably the strong antibiotics that had been administered to Robert for his stomach ulcerations early in the summer that brought about his remarkable cure.

Case Story #14—Cervical Cancer, Stage 3B

Janis is another person with an amazing Protocel recovery story. At only 48 years old, she was diagnosed in January 2002 with "small-cell cervical cancer, stage 3B." Prior to the diagnosis, she had been quite sick for more than six months but had been misdiagnosed as having "polymyalgia rheumatica." Her doctor had placed her on a very heavy regimen of prednisone at the amount of 80 milligrams a day for five-and-one-half months. By the time they realized she had cervical cancer, the tumor was very large and had probably been stimulated to grow quickly by the high doses of prednisone, as prednisone suppresses the immune system.

In January 2002, Janis started bleeding profusely. She was rushed to the hospital where she was given seven units of blood. She was told that she nearly died, but as a result of this episode, she was finally diagnosed correctly. Janis was told she had a large tumor on her cervix (about 8 centimeters, or 4 inches, across) that had attached to her pelvic wall. Because her cancer was "small-cell," surgery was out of the question. Janis was told that if surgery were performed on small-cell cervical cancer, the small cancer cells would escape into the bloodstream and quickly spread to her spine and brain.

The very day after her diagnosis, Janis was started on beam radiation treatments. She continued to receive this type of radiation five days out of each week for three months. During that time, she was also treated with two lots of radiation implants. Along with the radiation, on her second week after diagnosis, Janis was started on chemotherapy as well. The chemotherapy continued throughout the entire three months of treatment.

By the end of the three months of aggressive radiation and chemotherapy, however, Janis's cancer had *not* responded to the treatment, and her tumor was even *larger* than before. Moreover, she was so sick at this point she was throwing up every half hour and couldn't even keep a tiny bit of water down. Her bowels had completely seized up and stopped functioning due to the heavy amount of pain medication she had to take. Her weight had plummeted from 240 to 140 pounds, and she was very near death.

At this point, her doctors could no longer successfully rehydrate Janis, and they concluded that one more treatment of chemotherapy would kill her. Her doctor finally arranged for hospice care and told her husband that if Janis was extremely lucky, she might live three months, but realistically, she probably would live only two to four weeks.

The very day Janis was started on hospice, in April 2002, Janis's husband began searching on the Internet for another solution. He found a doctor of naturopathy who knew about and had used Protocel. He advised Ralph to obtain a bottle of it for Janis to start taking immediately, which Ralph did.

At first, it was difficult for Janis to take the formula and keep the liquid down. She was just barely able to manage the small doses throughout the day. Janis and her husband had no idea whether Protocel could help her, but they had no other options.

As Janis tells the story, after two-and-one-half weeks on Protocel she threw up for the very last time. After seven-and-one-half weeks on Protocel, she was finally out of pain and able to stop all her pain medication. This allowed her bowels to start working again as well. Also, at this point, she went back to her doctor for a checkup on her cancer. Her doctor was amazed to see Janis walk into the office. Moreover, examination showed that the tumor had already reduced half in size!

When Janis went back about four months later, her tumor was measured at only 2 centimeters, which was less than one-quarter its original size, and she was back to living normally. Thanks to Protocel, Janis got her life back. She continued to feel better and better, and began spending much of her time helping others to recover from cancer using Protocel.

Unfortunately, Janis felt so well that she stopped using Protocel too soon. (As noted in case story #10, it is imperative that people do *not* stop taking Protocel as soon as they appear to be in remission, but should stay on it much longer to be sure that every last cancer cell has lysed.) Sadly, a number of months after stopping Protocel, Janis suffered a recurrence of her cancer in her liver. By the time it was noticed, it was too late for Protocel to save her. But Janis's husband, Ralph, comments that when she passed, an examination showed the cancer in her cervical area to be completely gone. He is grateful for the extra time his wife had and feels that if she had just continued on Protocel longer, she would *not* have experienced the metastases to the liver.

Case Story #15—Childhood Brain Cancer

Dylan is seven years old. In December 1999, when he was just three, he started to have trouble with his balance that impaired his walking. At this point, Dylan's doctors could not tell that he had brain cancer because he did not have a solid type of tumor mass. Instead, he had a diffused form of cancer that just looked like swelling in the brain. They treated him for encephalitis until April 2000. Dylan did not respond to this treatment and his symptoms were getting worse. So the doctors did a biopsy and discovered that Dylan was suffering from a "glial cell" type of brain cancer. The exact diagnosis is still somewhat uncertain, but Dylan's doctor settled on "ganglioglioma."

In April 2000, when Dylan's diffuse tumor was diagnosed, it was located on the right side of the cerebellum and was about the size of a half dollar. A combination of two chemotherapy agents, called "carboplaten" and "vincristine," were administered to Dylan for the next nine months continuously. But this was not effective and his tumor kept growing. Dylan's symptoms were also getting worse and now he not only had the headaches and trouble with balance, he was also experiencing drooling and some droopiness on the left side of his face. All of these symptoms were tumor-related.

Since the chemotherapy had no positive effect, they finally stopped it after nine months and put Dylan on aggressive radiation treatments to the head and spinal cord. This did not halt the progression of the cancer either, so the doctors (who seemed at this point to be grasping at straws) put Dylan on a different type of chemotherapy, called Temador, which they gave him for three months.

But the Temador had no effect either. Over the first year and a half after Dylan's diagnosis, none of the chemotherapy or radiation treatments administered to him showed any effect on his very aggressive cancer. Dylan's tumor just kept steadily growing. By December 2001, his original cerebellum tumor had become larger, had spread to his brain stem and moved down his spinal cord. An MRI that month showed it had grown all the way down to vertebra T5, which is about at the bottom of Dylan's shoulder blades.

Around this time, because of damage to Dylan's autonomic nervous system, he started having problems swallowing, and he began choking. After five days in the hospital, Dylan complained of a stomach ache, which had probably resulted from not eating anything for five days. But the hospital staff responded by putting Dylan on morphine. Since Dylan's breathing was already very slow due to apnea, the morphine caused him to "code." Fortunately, the doctors were able to get him breathing again by intubating him, and Dylan was kept in the intensive care unit for a while. There, he was given a tracheotomy to help him breathe.

However, things went wrong with the tracheotomy procedure. While trying to get the trach tube in him, the doctors tore Dylan's esophagus twice and severely damaged his lungs. Now, the doctors had to put Dylan into a drug-induced coma so that his esophagus could heal.

Dylan's mother, Sharon, felt that the doctors did not expect Dylan to ever leave the hospital alive. His condition was so critical that, at one point, his parents even started to find out what they would need to do to donate Dylan's organs. However, Dylan opened his eyes and came out of the coma on Christmas Eve 2001. On January 15, 2002, after going through a year and a half of chemotherapy and radiation that didn't work, then almost dying and having to be hospitalized for 48 days, Dylan was sent home to die. The doctors told his parents that he would only live two weeks to two months—at best.

Luckily, however, at this point Dylan's oncologist told his parents of another family that was getting good results with their child's brain tumor using an alternative approach, and he gave them their phone number. The other family turned out to be using Protocel, and Dylan's parents started him on it on January 24, 2002.

In February 2002, Dylan was able to completely be weaned off steroids, which he'd been on continually since December 1999. Then, in March, about six weeks after being on Protocel, Dylan was taken in for another MRI. This time, the tumor had *not* grown since the last MRI, and this was the first time in two years that it had not shown any growth!

Three months later, in June, the next MRI was taken. This time, the tumor in Dylan's spine had *shrunk* the length of two vertebrae, from T5 up to T3. It was the first time in two and one-half years of treatment that his tumor had reduced in size. According to this MRI, the rest of Dylan's cancer in his cerebellum and brain stem had not decreased in size, but those areas were remaining stable. The next MRI was on September 5, and this one also showed stable, with no decrease or increase indicated. But Dylan's condition continued to improve every month he was on Protocel.

According to Dylan's parents, his lysing has been very heavy over the months that he has been taking Protocel. They explain that the lysed material is very obvious to them because they suck all his secretions from his trach tube. Sharon says, "It is definitely an egg-white substance coming out of his lungs but mostly it is post-nasal drip, which causes sore throat or tickle. At night it seeps out his nose and looks like 'whipped egg whites or foam,' and it only drains from his right nostril. (The side his tumor is on.)" Dylan also has excessive dandruff and huge amounts of ear wax, which are known symptoms of lysing as well. "We know some people don't see any evidence of lysing," Sharon says, "while others, like Dylan, seem to have it coming out of every orifice."

An MRI performed January 16, 2003, showed another decrease in tumor width. Although the tumor still showed the same length down Dylan's spinal cord, this MRI showed a reduced diameter to this part of his tumor. All other parts of the tumor still showed no growth and remained stable. However, there is another improvement that showed up. On the contrasted MRI, Dylan's cancer overall was not highlighting as much as before (it appeared darker and more like the color of the rest of his brain), which most likely meant that Dylan's tumor was becoming less dense.

Dylan's next MRI was performed in April 2003, and this one showed another shrinkage in overall size. His tumor shrank from vertebra T3 to T2. Then, true to form, an MRI at then end of July 2003 showed the tumor size to be stable again.

The best news is that Dylan did *not* die two weeks to two months after leaving the hospital, and he is getting better and better all the time. It has now been about two years since he was sent home to die. Amazingly, he has been able to go back to school and is now participating in a regular class because the cancer and chemotherapy and radiation treatments never impaired his mental functioning. Since he is still on a "trach" and a ventilator for breathing, he is currently wheelchair-bound and has to have a nurse with him all day. But Dylan still has the ability to think, talk, and walk (although his walking is currently restricted by the wheelchair he has to be in). With a little more shrinkage of the tumor, Dylan's parents hope he will finally be able to have the trach and ventilator removed. Once that can be done, he will not need the wheelchair and will then be able to build up the strength in his legs to walk and run again. (For more information about Dylan, you can access his personal website at www.caringbridge.org/page/dylansworld.)

Case Story #16 — Childhood Brain Cancer

Nicki is an eight-year-old girl, currently living a completely normal life. But just over three years ago, soon after she turned four in June 2000, Nicki developed a fever and had a grand mal seizure. She was rushed to a hospital emergency room where a CT scan was taken, then transferred to the hospital, where doctors surgically inserted a "shunt" to treat the hydrocephalus condition that had developed. After that, a biopsy was performed on little Nicki, which showed she had a slow-growing tumor in her brain. The biopsy diagnosis came back "low-grade astrocytoma, grade 1 to 2," and was located in the basal ganglia and thalamus regions. The doctors concluded that the tumor had grown to the point where it was pressing on a ventricle in Nicki's brain, and this is what caused the seizure and the hydrocephalus.

Because Nicki's tumor was "octopus-like" and had tentacles infiltrating the rest of her brain, it was considered non-operable. She was also considered too young to undergo radiation. So, after recovering in the hospital for a few weeks, Nicki was started on chemotherapy. Nicki's mom, Vicki, was led to believe by the doctors that they would be giving Nicki some "new" type of chemo that had been achieving great results. The doctors also said that Nicki had a strong likelihood of living five years, which they considered to be a very good prognosis. (This, on the other hand, did not sound so good to Nicki's mom.) The chemotherapy regimen that was prescribed was procarbazine, vincristine, and CCNU.

According to Vicki, administering the chemotherapy to her daughter was a terrible ordeal. The chemo was in capsule form, but the pills were large and very difficult for Nicki to swallow. They had to hold her down and force the pills into her. Forcing these pills down at times caused little Nicki to cough up blood. Vicki hated to do it, but she wanted her daughter to live, so they continued with these pills for about 10 months. Finally, one doctor told Vicki she could open up the capsules and mix the contents into some sweet food for her daughter to eat, but this ended up a disaster. Nicki got red all over and covered with hives. Paramedics had to be called, and they gave her an injection of Benadryl.

After 10 months of chemo, Nicki's tumor was still unaffected. It had not decreased in size, although it had not increased either. After Nicki's bad reaction to the opened-up pill, the doctors decided to switch her to a different chemotherapy regimen. This time, they put her on vincristine and carboplaten. This second protocol was so devastating to Nicki that her mother had them stop it after only three treatments. Nicki's blood counts had dropped severely, she needed a blood transfusion, and her mom felt deep down that the new protocol was killing her little girl.

Vicki just couldn't put her daughter through any more chemotherapy. None of the treatments had caused a reduction in the size of the tumor. The very night Vicki said "enough," and took Nicki home from the hospital, she read about Protocel from her Internet research. She started Nicki on Protocel immediately, which was on September 10, 2001. Nicki was five years old.

Giving Nicki Protocel was easy. Vicki just put a quarter teaspoonful of it into a little bit of juice for Nicki to drink at various intervals throughout the day. After two months of being on Protocel, Nicki went back for another MRI. When she was first diagnosed a year before, Nicki's tumor had been measured at 7 centimeters by 3.5 centimeters by 2.5 centimeters. Now, the tumor measured 6.5 centimeters by 3.0 centimeters. It was the very first time in over a year of chemotherapy that Nicki's tumor had reduced in size!

Nicki's next MRI three months later showed the tumor to be stable again with no visible decrease in size. But another MRI in October 2002 did show another decrease. This time the tumor measured 5.4 centimeters by 3.0 centimeters. When the neurosurgeon came out of the room where he had been looking at Nicki's scans, he said, "Keep doing what you're doing!"

Nicki's life has been perfectly normal since she's been on Protocel. She was fortunate to not suffer any serious neurological damage or noticeable cognitive impairment from the cancer or the chemotherapy. Whether or not Nicki sustained minor neurological damage is still pending, but she does not appear to have any significant problems. Nicki feels well enough to go to school, play, and do everything else eight-year-olds do. She experienced little in terms of visible lysing effects during her recovery. Her MRI in June 2003 showed the tumor to be stable in size, but she doesn't act like she has a tumor at all, and it may be that the tumor is now benign. Nicki has just started second grade and is able to perform on the same level as the other children.

Nicki's mother, Vicki, claims that what the doctors told her when they first prescribed the chemotherapy, was not true. They told her that the chemo they wanted to put Nicki on was "new" and had been achieving very good results. Vicki's subsequent research, however, showed that the chemo they prescribed had actually been around for about 30 years and was *not* achieving great results according to everything she read. Looking back on it now, Vicki can see how much she needed to trust the doctors in the beginning. She says she understands people who hear about Protocel but don't choose to use it. Vicki says, "If I had been told about Protocel when Nicki was first diagnosed, I wouldn't have believed it could work either. I know I wouldn't have put her on it then. I would have still gone along with whatever the doctors said we should do." Now, she just feels grateful that she came across Protocel when she did, and tells others about it who are dealing with cancer.

CHAPTER 11

Protocel

Suppression of the Formula

After reading the Protocel case stories of the previous chapter, the first thing most people wonder is, "Why did this formula *not* become an accepted cancer treatment?" In other words, the obvious question is, "Why aren't all the doctors and cancer treatment centers around the country recommending it?"

Well, the answer is simple. *It was officially suppressed.* As a result of the suppression by the official cancer organizations, Jim Sheridan's Entelev/Cancell formula never got approved by the FDA. And if a medical treatment is not approved by the FDA and endorsed by the leading cancer organizations, doctors generally won't hear anything about it. If a doctor does hear about it, he or she will not have any accepted source to go to and read about the treatment, and in any case probably would not be legally allowed to prescribe it even if he or she wanted to.

How did Jim Sheridan's formula get suppressed? As is commonly the case, it happened over a period of years and as a result of a variety of events. It was not, however, a result of Sheridan's not going through the right channels, or not working with the right organizations. In fact, Sheridan had worked from 1935 to 1937 in the analytical lab at Dow Chemical Company in Michigan, from 1950 to 1953 at the Detroit Institute of Cancer Research (now called the Michigan Cancer Foundation), and from 1961 to 1963 at the Battelle Institute in Columbus Ohio, which commonly tested new chemotherapy agents for the National Cancer Institute.

One of the early suppressive events occurred when Jim Sheridan was working at the Detroit Institute of Cancer Research. At that time, the Pardee Foundation was the source of funding for the research Sheridan was doing. Also at that time, Sheridan's formula was resulting in an 80 percent cure rate of cancer in laboratory mice. According to journal writer Marcello Gallupi, who researched and wrote articles on the Entelev/Cancell story in 1991 and 1992, the Detroit Institute's director decided in late 1953 that it was time to put Sheridan's formula through a clinical program. The director consulted with other experts as well, including the Dean of Medicine at Wayne University, three oncologists from nearby hospitals, and Mr. Grant Clark (a New York representative of the American Tobacco Company). These experts all reviewed the formula's results on laboratory mice and agreed that it was time to move to the next step, which was a clinical program. The Tobacco company representative said that a check for $450,000 had been written for this effort and that any number of millions of dollars would follow, if required.[1]

The only glitch in the plan to start clinical trials occurred when the Detroit Institute's director informed the American Cancer Society of the intended clinical program. The American Cancer Society responded by saying that they did not approve of the program "because Jim Sheridan had not proved that he owned the idea."[2] This was a bizarre twist, with no apparent precedent. However, the American Cancer Society was powerful enough to immediately halt the clinical program on Entelev, and within a few months, Jim Sheridan was suspiciously fired from the Detroit Institute of Cancer Research. Sheridan later heard that all the results of his research at the Institute had been burned.

The next event to block Sheridan's formula from being officially analyzed (and thereby kept out of mainstream medicine) occurred in 1963. He had been working for two years in the Biosciences Division of the Battelle Institute in Columbus, Ohio. At that time, Battelle Institute was a research center where many promising chemotherapeutic agents were being tested for the National Cancer Institute. Sheridan's formula was also being tested there. After 10 months of assessing the formula, which was having very good results with cancer, Dr. Davidson of the Battelle Institute requested permission from the NCI to test Entelev in an NCI laboratory. But Dr. Davidson asked if the test could be executed over a 28-day period, rather than the five-day period chemotherapy tests at NCI were usually given. (Since Jim Sheridan's formula was not a poison like chemotherapy agents, but instead worked on blocking the respiration capabilities of cancer cells until they fell apart, his material took a little longer to work.)

The incredible answer that came back from the NCI was, "No!" In other words, the NCI *refused* to study a cancer treatment that took 28 days rather than five days to work. Because of this stance by the NCI, there was also no more money to continue researching the formula at Battelle, so once again, Sheridan's experiments were forced to cease.

Between 1978 and 1980, Sheridan was finally able to get the National Cancer Institute to run animal tests on his formula. As is commonly the case, the NCI requested from him any information on special requirements it should know about to do the tests on mice. He complied by writing them a letter that stated three requirements. Specifically, Sheridan wrote that the NCI: (1) should not inject the formula into mice, but should administer it orally in water; (2) should make the test period at least 28 days long; and (3) should not test the formula on mice with leukemia, because mice with leukemia *always* die within 18 or 19 days, and it takes longer than that for the formula to work effectively.

After the test was done, Sheridan got a letter back from the NCI stating that his formula had been completely ineffective. But when he looked into how they had done the mice tests, he found that they had *not done any of the three things he specified.* They had injected his formula into mice, instead of administering it orally in water. They had used mice with leukemia, instead of mice with any other type of cancer. And they had completed the whole test in eight days instead of giving it the full 28 days.

So Sheridan called the NCI and asked someone to look into the files and see if his letter was actually there. It was, and the person he spoke to apologized and ordered the test to be done again. After the test was completed a second time, Sheridan received the same type of letter as before, stating once again that his formula was completely ineffective. Upon telephoning the NCI again, he found out that they had completely ignored his instructions a second time and had once more injected it into mice with leukemia over an eight-day period. Either the NCI was not competent at giving specific instructions to their laboratories, or it just didn't want the formula to be tested correctly.

Some people who understand the workings of the National Cancer Institute and the laboratories it farms tests out to, believe that the above failure of the NCI to correctly test Sheridan's formula on mice was not so much "deliberate" as it was the result of an "institutional blind spot." All of the procedures for testing cancer treatments have been set up to test highly toxic drugs like chemotherapy. These procedures have been in place for decades, and certain protocols are ingrained in every step. For highly toxic drugs, injecting the drug into mice with leukemia over no more than eight days works perfectly fine. However, for a non-toxic agent that requires just a little more time, but in the process only gets rid of the cancer and does not harm the rest of the body, the institutionalized process fails.

In other words, the current official methods for testing cancer treatments are based on "fixed assumptions" of how any cancer treatment *should* work. Sheridan believed this type of assumption could make it impossible to find solutions. He argued that an example of this folly would be if the federal government had decided to help fund the building and testing of a flying machine back in 1900, and looking around at things that fly (bugs, birds, and bats), it decided that all flying machines should have wings that flap up and down. Enter the Wright Brothers. Their flying machine would have failed all tests because it had stationary wings, rather than the anticipated wings that flapped up and down.[3]

But Sheridan did not give up. On April 9, 1982, he submitted his Notice of Claimed Investigational Exemption for a New Drug under section 505(1) to the FDA, and on May 20, 1982, the FDA issued him the IND number 20,258.[4] Apparently, the wording and implication of the IND granted to Sheridan indicated that his product was now ready for a clinical program. However, soon after this, Sheridan received word from the FDA stating that the material known as Entelev had been put on "clinical hold" because of lack of data assessing its toxicity. The FDA then informed Jim that he needed to have an "LD-50" test performed on his formula. The LD-50 is a toxicity test using animals that is done in various FDA-approved laboratories around the country to establish the safety level of a product.

Sheridan had already had several "minimum lethal dose" (MLD) tests using animals done on his formula *before* the FDA granted him this IND number. MLD testing is where a technician injects a group of mice with the material being tested in bigger and bigger doses. At the point where 50 percent of the mice die from the material, the minimum lethal dose amount is established. The reason Sheridan had done several of these tests was that every time he changed the formula even the slightest bit, a new toxicity test had to be done.

All of the MLD tests indicated the formula was non-toxic. In fact, it was so non-toxic that the laboratory technicians performing at least one of the tests told Sheridan they finally had to stop injecting larger and larger amounts of his formula into the mice when they got to the point that they felt the mice would literally "blow up" if they injected any more into them. Even with the massive doses they were injecting into the mice, they could *not* get 50 percent of the mice to die.

However, getting the official LD-50 test performed on his formula *after* the IND number had been issued was another matter. Sheridan tried for many years to get this toxicity test done. Three different times he had the process started at three different FDA-approved labs. But all three times, as soon as the lab found out what the material was, it would for some reason refuse to do the test. According to Sheridan, the laboratory would either tell him that they were too busy, or keep delaying the test and never get to it. One time, Sheridan had even gotten to the point of paying the lab in full for the LD-50 test he had requested. But then this lab, too, came up with some reason as to why they could not do the toxicity test and refunded Sheridan his money. Sheridan heard through a friend that one of the labs he was trying to get a toxicity test done at was actually visited by an FDA representative who directly threatened the lab out of doing the test. This was the FDA's way of blocking Sheridan from going to the next step in his attempts to get his cancer formula officially evaluated.

Jim Sheridan witnessed other suppressive events as well. For instance, at one point a doctor he personally knew left his position at Memorial Sloan-Kettering to devote his efforts to researching Cancell. Unfortunately, however, this doctor was from another country and before he could do the research, he found himself being threatened with deportation.

Another way that Sheridan tried to get his formula into mainstream medicine was by attempting to get pharmaceutical companies interested in it. Each time, the pharmaceutical company would be very interested at first. But as soon as they found out that the formula was *not* something they could patent and thereby make exorbitant profits from, the pharmaceutical companies always completely lost interest.

In the early 1980s, another development occurred. However, this time it was a very fortunate one. A metallurgist and engineer named Ed Sopcak got involved with Sheridan's formula. Sopcak was already in business for himself and decided to take on the task of producing Entelev so it could be available at no cost to cancer patients. Sopcak believed that Entelev was a gift from God and should be given away to people. So he used the profits from his already established foundry business to pay for the non-toxic ingredients that went into making the formula and to pay for the postage required to ship it to people. With Jim Sheridan's agreement, Sopcak decided to call the formula "Cancell."

From about 1984 to 1992, Ed Sopcak *gave away* about 20,000 bottles of Cancell to people with cancer. Agents from the FDA visited Sopcak regularly, at the rate of about every six months. But there was nothing they could do to stop his activities since he was simply giving the product away and not selling it.

Incredible testimonies started coming back to Sopcak and Sheridan from people using Cancell. More and more people with cancer, many of whom were in late stages, were getting well. At one point, the two men were invited to speak at a meeting in southern Michigan that would be attended by a number of people who had used Cancell for their cancer recoveries. According to Sopcak, four local TV stations had been invited to film the event and air it on the news. But then none of the TV crews showed up. One station claimed it was too short of staff, and the three others that had been invited claimed that the FDA had threatened to have their licenses revoked if they covered the event. Thus, the media coverage was controlled. (Whatever happened to freedom of the press and fearless journalism?)

Finally, on November 13, 1990, the National Cancer Institute agreed to test the formula once again, this time "in vitro," which meant they would administer it to various cancer cell lines in petri dishes. Even though this was just a 48-hour test *not* using animals, the Cancell formula proved to be highly effective against all the strains of cancer that the NCI tested it on. Jim Sheridan felt renewed hope that it would now be approved. But he was shocked when he received a letter from the NCI stating that it was *not* planning to pursue his formula as a medical treatment.

At this point Jim Sheridan's son, James, was amazed and decided to get involved. James Sheridan is currently, and was also at that time, a district court judge for the State of Michigan. Judge Sheridan called the NCI directly for an explanation and spoke to Dr. Ven Narayanan, who was the head of drug testing for the NCI. When asked why his father's formula was considered a failure, Dr. Narayanan agreed that the tests showed the formula to be effective at killing cancer. But he then went on to tell Judge Sheridan, "I could also obtain these results with chemotherapy, if I wanted to, but anything that would get results *this good* would be too toxic to humans!"[5] Judge Sheridan then suggested to Dr. Narayanan that he, for a moment, hypothetically assume the formula is *not* toxic to humans at therapeutic levels. At that point, Dr. Narayanan made it clear he would not even be willing to consider assuming such a thing. Then, he pointed out to Judge Sheridan that his father (Jim Sheridan) had not yet proved his formula was non-toxic. In other words, he had not had an LD-50 toxicity test run on it yet.

Jim Sheridan and his family were stumped. He was caught in a classic "double bind." The FDA would not pursue his formula without an LD-50 toxicity test that was done after the issuance of the IND number. But the only labs able to do the test would not do it because of pressure from the FDA. And the NCI and FDA both chose to ignore the fact that all the Minimum Lethal Dose tests Jim Sheridan had done before the IND number was issued had all shown the formula to be non-toxic. In fact, it is probable that the NCI knew the formula was non-toxic just by looking at the results of the tests performed on November 13, 1990.

Following are nine graphs produced from the official NCI test results. The first eight graphs show the test results of different dosages of Cancell on eight different types of cancer. The ninth graph shows a superposition of all the eight previous graphs.

A brief explanation of these graphs is warranted. The vertical axis on the left of each graph represents the percentage of growth in the cancer cells tested. On this left axis, 0 means "no growth," 30 means 30 percent growth, -30 means 30 percent death of cells, and -100 means that virtually all the cancer cells in the petri dish are dead at this point.

The horizontal axis on the bottom of each graph represents the dosage of Cancell administered. It presents the dosage of Cancell used in micrograms per milliliter (μg/ml), and in a Log_{10} scale. This means that the "1," "2," "3," and "4" on the bottom horizontal line are powers of 10. (Thus, 1 actually means 10 μg/ml, 2 means 100 μg/ml, 3 means 1,000 μg/ml, and 4 means 10,000 μg/ml.)

The different types of solid, dotted and dashed lines on each graph represent different specific cell lines for each type of cancer tested. These cell lines are defined underneath each graph.

To anyone looking at these graphs, two main characteristics jump out. The first characteristic is that, except for the leukemia cell lines, all other types of cancer tested (non-small cell lung cancer, small cell lung cancer, colon cancer, central nervous system cancer, melanoma, ovarian cancer, and renal cancer) proved to respond with either 100 percent cell death, or very near to 100 percent cell death within a certain dose range. In the case of a devastating disease such as cancer, a substance that can simply bring cancer growth to zero is quite an accomplishment. One that can cause almost 100 percent cell death in a 48-hour period is a *remarkably* good result and definitely worth looking into!

The second characteristic that jumps out is that the optimum dose range on all the graphs was approximately between 100 and 1,000 μg/ml. After that, as the dose amount is increased by factors of ten, the amount of cell death decreases. This means that at much higher doses, the Cancell formula was actually *less* effective at causing cancer cell death. What is evident from this characteristic is that Cancell was *not toxic*. No toxic substance would become *less* able to kill cells at higher concentrations. This characteristic was probably an artifact of the tests being done in petri dishes, rather than in the human body. People using this have found higher doses to cause more cancer cell death—but it is not desirable to kill cancer too fast.

The above official National Cancer Institute testing was done on Cancell over a mere 48-hour time period. If continued over a longer period of time, it is likely that ALL of the graph results would have reached −100, meaning 100 percent cancer cell death. But the NCI's in vitro testing procedure is set at 48 hours because the NCI assumes that it will always be dealing with a toxic material. For toxic materials, it makes sense to limit the duration of the test because the human body can only tolerate a toxic substance for a limited period of time. However, Cancell, being non-toxic, could be taken *indefinitely* without harming the body. At the time of this testing, people who had used Cancell to fully recover from their cancer had used it for much longer periods than 48 hours.

The benefits to using a non-toxic treatment approach for cancer cannot be overstated. Besides the fact that toxic treatments can have extremely serious side effects, such as liver, kidney, and heart damage, to the point that the side effects themselves can be life-threatening, there is also another issue. This is the issue that toxic conventional approaches, such as chemotherapy and radiation, do not allow for continual use. They are so toxic that continual use would kill the patient before the cancer could. So, toxic treatments are always administered with doses spaced out in some way. But cancer's best attribute is its ability to grow new cells fast. This means that, in-between the toxic treatments, the cancer cells grow back. And those cells that grow back the fastest are those cells that have some amount of resistance to the treatment.

In other words, when a cancer patient needs a few days or weeks for their body to recover from the toxic cancer treatment being given them, the cancer cells may also recover during this time. They may even start to grow faster than before due to the body's immune system having also been weakened by the toxic treatment. Eventually, a person's body may not be able to recover anymore because it has been too weakened by the treatment.

With *non-toxic* treatments, however, this vicious cycle is avoided. For instance, Protocel can be safely taken four or five times a day *every single day* for many months. This allows a therapeutic level to be kept in the body continually, which not only *never* gives the cancer cells a chance to grow back but also keeps attacking the cancer cells 24 hours a day, seven days a week. Because it is non-toxic, Protocel can even be taken for years (if a person chooses to) to ensure that the body stays free of cancer.

What was obvious from the 1990 NCI tests on Cancell was that, as a cancer treatment in the initial stages of testing, it passed with flying colors. The only logical conclusions as to why it was never pursued further would have to be that either: (1) the institutionalized procedural bias was too strong, or (2) the NCI just didn't want to pursue it even though they could see that it worked.

The final blow to Cancell occurred on Friday, November 13, 1992, when a federal judge enforced an FDA injunction to stop all distribution of Cancell for the purpose of treating any disease. This injunction legally blocked Ed Sopcak from being able to ship Cancell across state lines to people with cancer. Sopcak and Sheridan had never sold the product to anyone anyway, since they had always just *given it away* to people who needed it. But by prohibiting its "distribution," the injunction also effectively prohibited them from giving the formula away. What was the official injunction based on? It was based primarily on the fact that Jim had never had an LD-50 toxicity test run on the latest version of his formula.

Although Jim Sheridan never gave up trying to get Cancell officially evaluated and accepted, his successful, non-toxic formula for treating cancer was effectively kept from widespread availability to the public through a variety of "official" actions over a span of many years. As with other successful non-toxic alternative cancer treatments, his formula *should* have been immediately fairly evaluated by the official organizations and, if found effective, incorporated into mainstream medicine.

The *American Spirit Newspaper* published an interview with Ed Sopcak in their January/February issue of 1994. In the article, written by Nancy Burnett, Sopcak said,

> It's outrageous that we have in our files probably 10,000 people that we have helped and who are living today because of Cancell. And this was all done freely with no exchange of money involved. Now I am considered a criminal. That's how panicky these people are. You become a criminal to help your fellow man.

When asked *who* brought the lawsuit and injunction against him, Sopcak answered,

> Actually they didn't have a plaintiff. The FDA represented it but the FDA can not be a plaintiff. It really was the American Medical Association who uses the FDA as an enforcement arm. Furthermore, the National Cancer Institute lied and said they never ran the test.
> . . . When investigators for the FDA went out and interviewed people trying to find a harmed party they got all positive responses. They got the names illegally by going to the United Parcel Service and getting the names of the people I had sent it to. Then when they couldn't get a harmed party that way they solicited oncologists to try to get one to sign a complaint against me. But none of them would sign a complaint.
> So they went to trial without a plaintiff. And because they didn't have a plaintiff, there was never a hearing. I never saw the judge. They just did this all in paperwork and the judge illegally issued a permanent injunction. The law says I have a constitutional right to face my accuser. I didn't have that because there was no accuser. Furthermore, the law says the judge has to issue a temporary injunction to determine if the product does irreparable harm. He didn't do that. He issued a permanent injunction.

Referring to the 1990 tests that the National Cancer Institute performed in vitro on Cancell (graphs presented earlier), Sopcak stated,

> According to the law, if they find one positive result out of the testing done, one case where a tumor was reduced in size or eliminated, they have to continue testing. What they did in this case is they said there was no reason to do any further testing. And they dropped all tests. It was completely unlawful.

. . . We erroneously think that all we have to do is just modify the law. But they're not following the law anyhow. What difference does it make if you modify it?

Because of the FDA injunction to stop all distribution of Cancell, the exact version of Jim Sheridan's formula was not available for about seven years (between 1992 and 1999). But in April 1999, the Sheridan family was able to get the formula produced once again for marketing. This time it was named "Protocel" and was brought back on the market as a general health supplement to rid the body of non-productive anaerobic cells. It is now being legally sold in the United States by a company called Renewal and Wellness, LLC. However this company does *not* make any claims that the product cures cancer or any other disease.

As to the official toxicity test, another LD-50 test was requested and run on the formula before Protocel went into production. This time, the test was achieved without any difficulty. (Possibly, the test wasn't blocked this time because the FDA-approved laboratory that performed it did *not* recognize the "Protocel" name and did not know it was connected to the earlier Cancell formula. Or possibly the test was allowed because the Protocel product was not going to be sold as a cancer treatment.) At any rate, Protocel passed the test with flying colors! In fact, the LD-50 test results indicated that a quarter teaspoonful of Protocel taken four or five times a day is *less* toxic to the body than taking one aspirin a day. The non-toxic aspect of Protocel has also been verified by many people who have used it for years with no toxic side effects. There is even a report of one woman who did not understand the instructions and drank one-quarter bottle of the formula all at once (about a two-week supply), instead of one-quarter teaspoonful. She merely ended up with two hours of diarrhea, and then she was fine.

Although Jim Sheridan's formula was officially suppressed and successfully kept out of mainstream medicine, it did not die. Over the years, thousands of people have found one way or another to use the formula (either under the name of Entelev, Cancell, or Protocel) with amazing success.

CHAPTER 12

Protocel

How to Use Protocel Correctly

Because Protocel is not currently being sold as a cancer treatment, and any company distributing it cannot legally advise people about its use for cancer, I present some in-depth usage instructions in this chapter. These are instructions I put together, on my own, after talking to many different people who used Protocel for cancer. I also recommend visiting the private website http://www.elonnamckibben.com for more information. Additionally, there is an excellent Internet user support forum for people using Protocel, and you can access information and help from other current users there. Just go to http://www.protocelforum.com.

As already mentioned, Protocel is a liquid formula that is taken by mixing a small amount of it into water, iced tea, or juice. When using water, it is recommended to avoid chlorinated tap water if possible. (Distilled, filtered, or spring water are all okay, however.) Many people prefer to mix their Protocel into a small amount of juice (such as apple, cranberry, grape, or tomato) to cover the taste of the formula, and doing so can make it quite pleasant to take.

There are two slightly different formulations of the Protocel formula that are currently being sold. These formulations are called "Protocel Formula 50" and "Protocel Formula 23." (Or, in Australia, "Entelev Formula 50" and "Entelev Formula 23.")

Protocel Formula 50 is generally taken four times a day with each dose being a quarter teaspoonful (1/4 teaspoonful, 1/4 teaspoonful, 1/4 teaspoonful, 1/4 teaspoonful). These doses should be spaced out as equally as possible throughout each 24-hour period. For one person, taking it at 6 A.M., 12 noon, 6:00 P.M., and midnight might be convenient. For another, taking it at 8 A.M., 2 P.M., 8 P.M. and 2 A.M. might be easiest.

For optimum results, it is best *not* to let more than six hours lapse between any two doses. The goal with Protocel is to try to keep a steady therapeutic dose in the body at all times. Most people find that taking a dose in the middle of the night is not so difficult as it seems. Those who know they will be getting up during the night to use the bathroom may place their dose of Protocel in a cup or bottle of distilled water and leave this in the bathroom when they go to bed. Others may decide to set their alarm to be sure they get up and take their middle-of-the-night dose. Some make this dose easy to take by placing it in distilled water by their bedside so they don't have to get out of bed to take it.

Protocel Formula 23, on the other hand, is generally taken five times a day for cancer (1/4 teaspoonful, 1/4 teaspoonful, 1/4 teaspoonful, 1/4 teaspoonful, and 1/2 teaspoonful), and four times a day for auto-immune disorders and viral infections. These doses should also be spaced out as equally as possible throughout each 24-hour period. (Notice that the bedtime dose is generally a double dose, but if lysing starts going too fast, this can be reduced to 1/4 teaspoonful.) Again, never going more than six hours between any two doses is going to facilitate the fastest recovery. Thus, a sample schedule for Formula 23 for cancer might be 7 A.M., 11:30 A.M., 4:00 P.M., 8:30 P.M., and 2 A.M.

For *very* small children with brain cancer, dose size for both formulations may need to be smaller at first, then slowly worked up to 1/4 teaspoon for each dose. For example, for children under 60 pounds or so, some parents have found it best to use only 1/8 teaspoonful most doses. A recommended way to start very small children on Formula 50 is 1/8, 1/8, 1/8, and 1/4 teaspoonful each day. For Formula 23, 1/8, 1/8, 1/8, 1/8, 1/3 teaspoonful each day is a recommended way to start very small children. (Many parents wake the sleeping child up at some point during the night to administer the last dose. Often, the child does not completely wake up and easily goes back to sleep.)

Both Jim Sheridan and Ed Sopcak used to stress the importance of taking the formula doses with rigorous regularity around the clock every day. Sopcak would tell people that the formula metabolizes and dissipates from the body fairly quickly. He urged people to understand that, after about six hours, the amount of the formula in their bodies may become sub-therapeutic and that going longer than six hours could be counterproductive to healing. An explanation for this is the following: Protocel works by interfering with the ATP production of our bodies' cells. This does not bother our healthy cells, which have plenty of ATP energy to spare. But it *does* bother cancer cells a *lot* by interfering with their energy production enough to "starve them to death" over time. Beyond six hours after any dose, the level of Protocel remaining in your body may not be able to perform its job 100 percent. With the goal being to starve your cancer cells to death, going more than six hours between any two doses is like giving your cancer cells a little bowl of soup on the seventh or eighth hour. They are not going to starve to death so quickly if they keep getting a little bowl of soup every night. Thus, *don't give your cancer cells a bowl of soup!*

For adults and children, Protocel is best taken on an empty stomach whenever possible (about 30 minutes before a meal). But it will still work if there is food in the stomach, and sticking to an evenly spaced schedule is preferable to postponing or missing doses. One of the reasons we know that Protocel works even when food is in the stomach is because it has always been administered to pets by mixing the formula directly into their food, and this has consistently shown great results. (See upcoming section called "Protocel Works for Pets, Too!")

Although mixing Protocel into juice and drinking it immediately is fine, leaving Protocel in juice for hours is not recommended. If a person wishes to carry one or two premixed doses of Protocel in a small plastic bottle for a day trip, it is best to have the Protocel mixed into distilled water. These premixed doses can then be carried in one's pocket, purse, or glove compartment and kept for hours at a time. Or, a small plastic bottle of pure Protocel can be carried while traveling and mixed on the spot with juice to drink immediately. Protocel does not need to be refrigerated, but it should probably not be left in direct sunlight or high temperatures for long. It can easily be kept on a shelf or carried around on one's person under normal conditions.

When measuring out Protocel, be sure to shake the bottle vigorously each time, then quickly measure out your dose! The reason for this is that a small proportion of the ingredients precipitate out of the formula and form a sediment at the bottom of the bottle. If you do not shake the bottle vigorously right before each dose, then by the time you are into the latter half of the bottle, there will be a higher ratio of sediment to formula than there was in the first part of the bottle. Jim Sheridan and Ed Sopcak used to always tell people to shake the bottle vigorously, and virtually all the people who have used this formula successfully have done so.

Protocel Formula 50 and Protocel Formula 23 are virtually the same. They have the same ingredients and are made only slightly differently. Formula 50 is generally considered a little faster-acting in causing anaerobic cells to lyse, and this small difference provides people with a degree of control over how fast their lysing process goes. People with different health challenges have also found that one formulation or the other may actually work a little better for their specific condition. Thus, the choice between two formulations gives people more control over their own recovery process.

Since Protocel is *not* approved by the FDA as a cancer treatment and no official claims are made as to its use or effectiveness for cancer or any other serious illness, the following guide may be used for ascertaining which formulation to start with for various health conditions. This guide is based on customer usage (anecdotal information), and it is important for each individual to remember that they can try one particular formulation for a while, then switch to the other formulation if they need to according to how their progress is going. (If your particular health condition is *not* listed below, start with Protocel Formula 50.)

Anecdotal Guide for Which Formulation to Start With

Formula 50	*Formula 23*
Cervical cancer	Bladder cancer
Colon cancer	Brain cancer (primary)*
Esophageal cancer	Breast cancer
Leukemia	Kidney cancer (renal cell)
Liver cancer (primary)*	Multiple Myeloma
Lung cancer (even with mets to brain)	Neuroblastoma
Lupus	Prostate cancer
Melanoma	Wilmes tumor
Non-Hodgkin's lymphoma	Auto-immune disorders
Ovarian cancer	Crohn's disease
Pancreatic cancer	Endometriosis
Sarcomas	IBS or UC
Stomach cancer	Multiple Sclerosis*
Squamous cell cancer	Parkinson's
Throat cancer	Pets with any condition*
Uterine cancer	Psoriasis
	Viral infections*
	When kidneys are weak*
	Mononucleosis

* For people with primary brain cancer, Formula 23 has been the preferred version by most users to start with. The reason for this is that, as brain tumors lyse away, some amount of edema may occur. (Edema is a common possible occurrence whenever a space in the brain is created, and can occur as a result of surgery or radiation therapy as well.) Whenever dealing with cancer in the brain, one needs to be cautious of not promoting too much edema, and this is *particularly* true for anyone with a tumor in the brainstem area. Thus, using Formula 23 for most primary brain cancer situations has been known to make the lysing process and edema symptoms more manageable.

* For people with primary liver cancer, Formula 50 is recommended by some people, but must be tailored to the individual. If one has *advanced* primary liver cancer, one may need to use just 1/8 teaspoonful four times a day for the first few weeks, then slowly work up to 1/4 teaspoonful over the next few weeks.

* When a person *already* has weakened kidneys *before* starting Protocel, Formula 23 is generally the preferred version for *any* condition. This is because, when the kidneys are already in a weakened state, it is harder for the body to process out the lysed material in an efficient way. So, going a little slower may help keep the kidneys from being overwhelmed.

* Many people with multiple sclerosis have experienced wonderful improvements in their condition through the use of Protocel. Multiple sclerosis is so named because it is a condition where multiple areas of scar tissue (sclerosis) build up around neurons and this then interferes with proper functioning of the nervous system. The way Protocel helps people with MS is by breaking down the anaerobic scar tissue that has built up around their neurons. As this lysing process progresses, people find their normal functioning slowly returning. However, since Protocel cannot repair or rebuild the myelin sheath around damaged nerve cells, people using Protocel for MS may also want to supplement daily with: 1,000 mg borage oil, 3 tablespoons granular lecithin, and 2 tablespoons extra virgin cold pressed olive oil. These extra supplements are thought to help the body rebuild new myelin sheath. Cortisone medications and the "ABC&R" drugs often prescribed for MS are suspected to interfere with Protocel and should probably be avoided when using this formula.

* Many people with viral conditions have also experienced remarkable recoveries. The reason that Protocel can help the body overcome viral challenges is the following: When viral infections occur in us, the viruses must invade our normal healthy cells to replicate. While viruses circulate throughout our bloodstream, they have a special protein coating that protects them from attack by our immune system. But when they invade healthy cells to replicate, they have to shed their protective protein coating. These previously healthy cells then be-

come damaged, anaerobic cells after becoming viral-infected. Protocel causes these types of anaerobic cells to lyse and fall apart, just as it does with cancer cells. When the viral-infected anaerobic cells fall apart, the viruses are then released back into the body, but *without their protective protein coatings.* When this happens, the body's natural defenses can attack and destroy the unprotected viruses. Numerous people have experienced amazing improvements with their herpes, hepatitis, or other viral conditions. Some may even have experienced complete recoveries.

*   Pets often require fewer and smaller doses of Protocel for their recovery processes when given Protocel for cancer or other conditions. (See upcoming section called "Protocel Works for Pets, Too!" for more details.)

Because both formulations are so similar and both work for any condition involving anaerobic cells, the particular formulation one starts with is not as important as making sure to use Protocel correctly in general. Keeping to your daily schedule and not missing doses unless absolutely necessary is critical.

Also, only take Formula 23 or Formula 50 at any given time. In people's efforts to fine-tune their own lysing process and recovery, they may end up with part of a bottle of Formula 23 and part of a bottle of Formula 50. If this happens, do *not* mix the two formulations together. Formula 50 and Formula 23 should *always* be kept in separate bottles, and people should only use one or the other for any given period of time.

Finally, it is important to understand that certain supplements can interfere with Protocel's action on the cellular level and should therefore be avoided. Since Protocel works by depleting ATP energy production of cells, the types of supplements or herbs that tend to interfere are those that raise the ATP energy production of cells. These supplements can counteract the process of the Protocel formula to varying degrees.

The main supplemental items you should be sure to avoid are listed below.

Definitely Avoid While Using Protocel

Vitamin C
Vitamin E
CoQ_{10}
Selenium
Essiac tea
Ozone treatments

These items are certainly very beneficial when using a different approach to health improvement. But they have been known to seriously interfere with the action of Protocel. This is not because they are anti-oxidants, but because most of them raise the potential voltage of cells. So quite a few people prefer to stay away from supplemental CoQ_{10}, vitamin E, vitamin C, selenium, and cancer-fighting herbal mixtures altogether until they are cancer-free — just to be on the safe side.

If a person eats a healthy, well-balanced diet while using Protocel, the intake of the above nutrients in their natural food form will usually not be enough to interfere with the formula's effectiveness. Many cancer patients have proven this to be true time and again. However, it is recommended to keep the ingestion of those fruits that are *very* high in vitamin C to a minimum. In other words, while using Protocel, it is probably best to avoid a *high* amount of whole citrus fruits or fresh-squeezed citrus fruit juice. Both Jim Sheridan and Ed Sopcak used to discourage the use of supplements while using this formula and urged people to get balanced nutrients from their food instead.

The one exception in the above list, which does not raise ATP energy, but does interfere with Protocel, is ozone. Although ozone treatments administered to people *not* using Protocel can be very beneficial for many types of health recovery, they should be completely avoided when on Protocel. Ozone is the only known treatment or substance that chemically interacts with the Protocel formula directly in an undesirable way. Most supplements that help oxygenate the body, such as germanium, work fine with Protocel because they help to bring "O_2" to the cells. But because ozone is "O_3," it chemically interacts with the formula and this interaction produces toxic aldehydes as a byproduct. These toxic aldehydes are not good for the body. Worse yet, when ozone and Protocel are combined and they interact with each other, you no longer have ozone or Protocel left. Thus, you get neither the benefit from the Protocel *nor* the benefit from the ozone.

While it is important to avoid ozone treatments when taking Protocel, drinking water that has been "disinfected" with a small amount of ozone is fine. This is because, when ozone is used on municipal or bottled water for disinfectant purposes, the ozone has virtually always dissipated completely or converted back to O_2 by the time you drink it.

There are some other supplements that should *probably be avoided* as well (or at least limited to minimal amounts) because they are "suspected" to interfere with the way Protocel works. These supplements are suspected to work at cross-purposes with Protocel because there are indications that they raise the ATP energy level in cells. But keep in mind

that more research needs to be done with the following items before anything *certain* can be said about using them with Protocel.

Should Probably Avoid While Using Protocel

IP_6	Creatine	L-Cysteine
Alpha lipoic acid	Homeopathic remedies	Ginseng
714X	Poly-MVA	Any "Sulfhydril"
L-Carnitine	Taurine	antioxidant
L-Lipoic Acid	Glutathione	Rife treatments
Sea Silver	Acetyl-Cysteine	Cat's Claw
Acetyl L-Carnitine	Glutamine	

Because it is *so* important *not* to interfere with the way the formula
works, it is best to avoid any supplement or herb while using Protocel
unless you know from the literature sent with the product, or from anecdotal reports, that the supplement or herb you wish to take will not interfere with this formula. In other words, "When in doubt, do without."

On the other hand, there are certain excellent nutritional supplements that have been found to be *compatible* with the use of Protocel.
They are the following items

May Be Taken While Using Protocel

Any type of enzymes	Coral calcium (*without vitamin C*)
Shark liver oil	Pau D'Arco
Multiple B vitamin	Reishi mushrooms
DMSO	Willard's water (clear)
Ellagic acid	Vitamin D_3
Hydrazine sulfate	Potassium
Paw Paw*	Magnesium
Primrose oil	Calcium
Laetrile	Soy isoflavones
Borage seed oil	Indole-3-Carbinol (I3C)
Grape seed extract	DIM
Fish oils	Natural progesterone
Germanium-132	Ambrotose Complex
Low-Dose Naltrexone	Collostrum

*   In the case of Paw Paw, use cautiously—preferably not before the fourth
month on Protocel, and possibly never with brain cancer. (The combined effect

with Protocel can cause overly rapid lysing and one must be sure the body's detoxifying systems are not overwhelmed.) If used, Paw Paw should be taken *between* doses of Protocel with two to three hours between the Protocel and Paw Paw. Graviola is similar to Paw Paw, but the potency levels are not standardized, so Paw Paw from Nature's Sunshine is preferred.

These days, avoiding supplements that might interfere with Protocel can be difficult because we live in an age of nutritional supplementation, and many people who seek alternative approaches for cancer want to be able to supplement with as much as they can get their hands on. But this can *seriously backfire* for people using Protocel. Unfortunately, most supplements that show anti-cancer activity are much more publicized than Protocel is. This can cause people using Protocel to be inundated with suggestions from their doctor, family, or friends to supplement with this or that cancer-fighting agent. For instance, I heard of a man using Protocel for his cancer who also took high doses of vitamin E at the same time because his doctor said he should take E for his cancer. Yet, like many people, this man never told his doctor that he was using Protocel, and even if he had, the doctor would not have known that vitamin E can interfere with the formula. Unfortunately, this man did not have success with Protocel.

Protocel has a shelf life of many years. It does not spoil after the bottle has been opened, therefore it requires no refrigeration. The best way to store it is simply on a shelf or counter where it is not in direct sunlight. Middle-of-the day doses can be carried around in small containers, as mentioned earlier, and can be carried around for hours mixed in distilled water. Protocel can go through airport scanners without detriment to the formula, so it is easy to travel with.

Most prescription medications will *not* interfere with the action of Protocel, nor will Protocel interfere with their effectiveness. However, anecdotal observation has shown that the use of Protocel can often *improve* other health conditions a person may have, such as high blood pressure, arthritis, chronic fatigue, some forms of diabetes, Crohn's disease, multiple sclerosis, viral infections, endometriosis, hemorrhoids, and psoriasis. So it sometimes happens that while a person is using Protocel, he or she may see an improvement in these conditions and require less prescription medication over time. It is important, therefore, for people to be aware of this and carefully monitor the dosage of any prescription medications they may be taking—*especially* in cases where a person is taking blood pressure medication or insulin for diabetes.

People who require insulin should monitor their blood-sugar levels more than once a day while on Protocel until their levels have stabilized.

Using Protocel correctly is very easy. For best results, simply:

1. Space the doses out over each 24-hour period as evenly as possible and try to never go more than six hours between any two doses.

2. Shake the bottle vigorously immediately before each dose.

3. Make sure you are *not* taking any vitamin, mineral, herbal remedy, or other type of cancer treatment that might interfere with Protocel's action.

4. Be sure to drink plenty of good water each day, *besides* other liquids. (Preferably, as close to a gallon of water a day as possible.)

5. Try to promote at least one bowel movement *every* day to support your body's ability to process out lysed material. (Use extra roughage or a mild laxative if needed.)

Diet

In general, no specific dietary changes are required while using Protocel. As you can see from some of the recovery testimonials listed earlier, diets varied from person to person. Some people using Protocel choose to eat meat, while others choose to be vegetarian. Some people cut out all junk food, while others do not. (Most people drastically reduce their intake of sugar, however.) The best recommendation to anyone trying to improve their health using Protocel is to simply eat a sensible, healthy diet including: fresh organic vegetables and fruits, good sources of dietary protein (eggs, yogurt, cottage cheese, meat, fish, soy products, legumes), and plenty of water.

Because cancer is a chronic, metabolic disease that usually gets started when a person's body is out of balance or weakened in some way, it is wise to pick the most nutritious foods you can to support your body's healing. "Whole" foods will support your body better than refined foods. Organic foods will support your body better than inorganic foods full of pesticides or other pollutants. And "good" fats will support your body better than bad fats. Choosing a diet (and possibly some nutritional supplements) that will help to balance and support your particular body will optimize your chances for recovery.

The one dietary restriction that is *strongly recommended* (but not required for Protocel to work) is that anyone using this formula to rid their body of anaerobic cells would do best to reduce their intake of refined sugar and refined wheat flour. This is not because sugar and refined wheat interfere with Protocel's action, however. Rather, it is because all anaerobic cells thrive on sugar. (Remember, they use glucose, or glycogen, for energy.) So it just makes sense to take away the energy source that cancer cells thrive on while trying to reduce their energy production and cell voltage with Protocel. Refined wheat products tend to metabolize like glucose as they are digested in the body, whereas the more complex whole-grain wheat products do not. Thus, eating whole-grain breads while taking Protocel is fine. However, if total restriction of refined sugar and refined wheat causes too much stress for a person, then intake of these foods *in moderation* might be best, since stress can be a drain.

Lysing Symptoms

The Protocel formula produces no direct negative side effects. Any symptoms associated with taking Protocel are a result of the anaerobic cells of the body lysing and being processed out of one's system. Therefore, any symptoms that may occur during one's recovery process on Protocel are referred to as "lysing symptoms." In other words, a perfectly healthy person using Protocel will generally *not* experience any symptoms at all, because they won't be experiencing a lot of lysing. Protocel is non-toxic and *very* safe to use.

Lysing of anaerobic cells most likely begins within the first 24 to 48 hours of starting Protocel, but may not be noticed through outward signs or symptoms for a while. The onset of noticeable lysing symptoms will vary from person to person, with some people noticing lysing symptoms within a few days of starting Protocel, yet others not noticing any for weeks or months. Visible, outward indications of lysing are not always apparent, though, even when cancer cells are actively lysing inside. Some people have even fully recovered from their cancer with no outward signs of lysing at all.

Although visible signs of lysing should not be expected, when they do occur it can be comforting to the person with cancer to see them. Four common types of lysing symptoms that *may* occur are:

1. Initial tiredness in the first few weeks

2. Possible excretion of mucousy material in various ways

3. Possible initial tumor enlargement (along with reduced density)

4. Possible initial dramatic rise in cancer marker levels

The one type of lysing symptom that appears to be unique to Protocel is a mucousy excretion of egg white-like material that may be noticed draining out of the nose, being coughed up from the lungs, or coming out in the feces. This is because, as the cancer cells lyse, the body will try to process the "dead cancer cell parts," or protein material, out of itself through any orifice it can. A runny nose is quite common, and as long as the mucous is not a greenish color, it is usually an indication of lysing. (Greenish mucous from the nose may indicate a sinus infection.) For anyone using Protocel for cancer and having a clear, whitish, or slightly yellowish mucous draining from the nose, it is best *not* to use a cold medicine to dry this up. Just keep lots of tissues handy. Some people may also experience some crust around their eyes in the morning. These types of excretion are visual evidence that lysing is occurring and can be seen as a very *good sign* if it happens. It is simply the body's way of housecleaning the unwanted material as cancer cells break down.

Some other lysing symptoms that may be noticed are similar to common "detoxing" or flu-like symptoms. These may be short periods of mild nausea, elevated temperature, tiredness, upset stomach, or headache while the body is working on processing out lysed material. Usually these symptoms will not last long, or they may occur at certain times of each day like clockwork. Also fairly common are the following experiences due to lysing: "bubbly" or "foamy" urine or pimply bumps on the skin or temporary rash. Less common symptoms are excess earwax and vomiting. (Vomiting is not common, but if it does happen because of lysing, it will often contain unusual-looking material in it.) It seems our bodies have many ways to rid themselves of unwanted material.

For people using Protocel for brain cancer, there may be a short period of dizziness or foggy thinking around the fourth to sixth week after starting Protocel. This may result when the tumor or tumors are starting to lyse in the brain and the resulting effect from the tumor starting to break down is a mild edema. Most people will get through this period just fine if they know what to expect. If any of the lysing symptoms get to be *too* much, adults can reduce their Protocel dosage down to 1/8 teaspoonful four times a day until the lysing becomes more manageable, then work back up to the normal dose.

It is important for anyone using Protocel for cancer to be aware of the possible lysing symptoms. Otherwise, a person might misconstrue some of these symptoms as indications that their cancer is getting worse. In other words, cancer patients using Protocel need to learn how to distinguish between lysing symptoms and cancer progression. Usually, the best way to do this is to take note of diagnostic scans that can show whether the cancer is growing and spreading or not. Most people will find that within the first two to four months on Protocel, their cancer diagnostic tests will show a stabilization of their cancer, and their scans often show that previously aggressive tumors have stopped growing or spreading. This halting of the progression of the disease is a very good sign and means that the Protocel is working. At the same time, other types of lysing symptoms will often be noticed to confirm that the cancer is indeed breaking down. By the third month, or sometimes not until the fourth month, most people will start to see a decrease in tumor size.

However, interpreting scans can also be tricky. For instance, even if tumors do not decrease in size in the first two to three months, those same tumors may be decreasing *in density*. To note whether or not this is happening, you can request a "density reading" of your scans. Not all radiologists know how to do this, and in any case, will not perform it without your doctor requesting it. However, this is a much more meaningful type of scan for people using Protocel than the usual types that are done, where a radiologist simply measures the size of any tumors that show up and compare them to the sizes that showed up in the previous scan. In some cases, tumors will actually show up *bigger* on scans in the first few months on Protocel because, as tumors break down they may sort of liquefy and spread a little (like an ice cube melting and forming a puddle). But in these cases, the tumor will actually be less dense and in the process of breaking down, and simply needs more time on Protocel to complete the process.

So even though it is important to take note of scans, it is best to *not* expect scans to show a significant decrease in tumor *size* before the fourth month. Once tumors start to diminish, they will then usually continue to decrease steadily until they are gone. (For more information on how to interpret lysing symptoms, log onto http://www.elonnamckibben.com or access the Protocel User Support Forum by going to http://www.protocelforum.com.)

Cancer Marker Tests May Elevate

Another possible outcome of lysing that is extremely important to know about when using Protocel is that, as one's cancer is stabilizing and then starting to dissipate, one's cancer blood marker tests may begin to elevate. Doctors usually interpret higher cancer marker results as "more cancer." However, when using Protocel, this is not necessarily the correct interpretation. Most cancer marker tests are *general* indicators of how much cancer is in a person's body because they measure certain things that go along with, or are released by, particular types of cancer cells. For some types of cancer, the marker tests will be measuring a type of enzyme that is released by that particular type of cancer cell into the bloodstream. For other types of cancer, the marker tests will be measuring a type of protein released by the cancer cells, and so forth.

But when Protocel is doing its job and causing cancer cells to lyse and break down, the cancer cells *release* their enzyme or protein markers into the bloodstream even more quickly than they did before. This can cause marker test results to go dramatically higher for a period of time. If this happens, oncologists and cancer patients can get very worried. It is important at these times to determine from *other* means, such as results of scans or by how one is feeling overall, whether or not the cancer is actually progressing. If your scans show the tumors to be stable or getting smaller, then you can interpret the high markers as a sign that lysing is occurring, and that your cancer cells are actually falling apart and more actively releasing their markers into the bloodstream. These marker levels will eventually go down as the lysed material is processed out of the body.

For the cancer patient who wishes to use Protocel, it is *very* important to remember that Protocel operates in a *fundamentally* different way than doctors are used to. This means that lysing symptoms, such as temporarily elevated cancer markers, will not necessarily be understood correctly by oncologists and other doctors who are not familiar with Protocel.

How Long Does Protocel Take?

It is always impossible to give a time-scale for recovery that would apply to every cancer patient. Keep in mind that Protocel does not work as quickly as cytotoxic agents like chemotherapy. This is because it is not a fast-acting dangerous poison as most chemotherapy agents are. Instead, it is designed to work *with* the body toward health and long-term recovery, in a safe and effective way that the body can handle.

Some cancer situations respond with very fast recoveries, while others take longer. It is best to think of each person's recovery time as unique. There have been people who have become cancer-free using this formula in about six months time, while others have needed to use it for a year or more. There are always differing factors in each person's situation, including how much cancer they are starting with and how weakened their bodies are from previous conventional treatments, or from the cancer itself.

As a general rule, most people using Protocel for cancer will start to experience some lysing symptoms within a few weeks of starting the formula, and many will also experience a reduction of pain or an increase in well-being within the first month. But as mentioned in the previous section on lysing symptoms, the first two months or so may simply involve the Protocel formula stopping the progression of the cancer. This, in itself, is a wonderful thing. It generally takes *longer* than two months for most people to experience a noticeable reduction in the size of their tumors. But as already mentioned, tumors may be decreasing in *density* during the first two months, though this does not always show up on scans.

One woman named Elonna (case story #5), who recovered 14 years ago from a rare and "incurable" spinal cord cancer, aptly describes the patience that is sometimes required when using this formula. She suggests that people using Protocel for cancer think of themselves as being in a marathon race. As Elonna explains,

> You are in a marathon race (a race against time really). In this race, your cancer/disease is the lead runner and well ahead of the pack runners. You can think of the pack runners as your other body organs and even your immune system doing their best to stabilize your body functions and return them to normal. However, as the months go by, they are losing ground and the lead runner (your disease) is miles ahead.
>
> With your first dose of Protocel, the Protocel takes the position of the very last runner in this marathon. With each subsequent dose, and as the weeks go by, Protocel begins to move up in the race. At some point in time, it gets even with the midpack runners. Then it will move ahead of the pack and begin gaining on the lead runner. Eventually, the lead runner is in its sights and the process Protocel has instrumented in your body begins to overtake the leader (your disease). For some time, they run side by side. However, your immune system, with the help of Protocel, finally moves ahead. At this point in time, the cancer/disease does stop growing, and it is a matter of your body breaking down what is left in your body.[1]

It helps to keep in mind that the speed at which Protocel can totally rid someone of their cancer is still remarkably fast when compared to conventional treatments like chemotherapy and radiation. These conventional treatments may put someone into remission quickly, but because they so often do not completely get rid of the cancer, tumors will many times grow back and must be treated a second or even a third time over a several-year period. The initial reduction of tumors under these circumstances (called "remission") may be fast at first, but short-lived. Whereas, with Protocel, the reduction in tumor size may be slower at first in some cases, but *permanent* when one continues to use the formula correctly.

What About Doing Chemotherapy or Radiation at the Same Time as Protocel?

This is an important question. Low-dose or short-term radiation will not interfere with the action of Protocel, as long as it does *not* damage the vital organs or other parts of the body too much. In fact, it appears that in some ways radiation treatments work synergistically with Protocel. This is mainly because radiation also reduces cell voltage. But it is important to make an informed decision whenever considering the use of radiation treatments. Ask your doctor about all the side effects that are possible from the radiation treatments you are considering. If a tumor is so big or life-threatening that it needs to be dealt with through surgery or radiation to help ensure the survival of the patient or to give Protocel enough initial time to work, then it is probably a good idea. If this is not the case, then it might be best to either decline it or make sure that the radiation treatments are considered low-dose.

Chemotherapy, on the other hand, often works *against* Protocel. Years ago, Jim Sheridan himself wrote, "Chemotherapy can bring the percentage of success down, because chemotherapy changes the level on the oxidation-reduction ladder where Entelev/Cancell works."[2] Therefore, if at all possible, it is best to *not* combine most types of chemotherapy with Protocel. One exception to this rule may be when the chemotherapy agent is an "anti-metabolite." The anti-metabolite types of chemo agents push the energy level of cells down and therefore tend to work well with Protocel. However, anti-metabolite chemotherapies also damage normal, healthy cells, and can cause serious side effects and possible permanent damage to the body. The risks versus the benefits must be weighed. If chemotherapy is deemed necessary to give a person enough time for Protocel to work, then it is probably best to start on Protocel as soon as possible, even while doing chemo.

When to Stop Using Protocel

Most people using Protocel for cancer continue to take it for at least one year *after* their doctor has given them the "all-clear." (Some people prefer to use it for up to two years or more after the all-clear point, just to be on the safe side.) The reason for this is to make sure that all the cancer cells have completely lysed before stopping the treatment. Keep in mind that current diagnostic techniques may not always detect cancer unless there are about 10 million cancer cells or more all in one place. This means that if you have as many as 9 million cancer cells, *diagnostic techniques available today may not reliably detect them*. Therefore, if a person stops using Protocel as soon as their scans or other tests show no more signs of cancer, there may still be a small number of cancer cells in their body that are still alive and ready to begin proliferating again. So, continuing to use the formula rigorously for at least six months after the "all-clear" point is the best safeguard.

The one exception to this general rule is for people who have used Protocel to reduce and stabilize a large brain tumor that may be too big to be completely absorbed by the brain. Instead of completely disappearing, these brain tumors may shrink somewhat, then stop highlighting. In these cases, the person should most likely stay on Protocel indefinitely— as long as there is still a mass in the brain. As shown in case story #10, stopping Protocel simply because the mass is no longer highlighting can risk the tumor becoming active again after a while.

The length of time each person continues to take Protocel after their cancer is no longer detectable is up to each person. Since Protocel is not toxic to the body like chemotherapy or radiation, people can continue taking it indefinitely as a "cleansing agent," if they choose to. At least one woman has taken it for over 15 years with the only effect being that she feels great and never seems to come down with a cold or flu anymore.

Protocel Works for Pets, Too!

Many people have helped their beloved pets with Protocel, and it is exciting that some veterinarians have recently started using Protocel on their animal patients with cancer. These results have been very good, and it appears that many animals respond even faster than humans.

Although there is a lack of information about using Protocel for birds or reptiles, it is very easy to administer Protocel to a dog, cat, or horse since the formula can be mixed into any type of meat or other food the animal likes. Some animals will even lick it up straight from a plate. One colorful story comes from a family that treated their dog for cancer by putting a few drops of Protocel onto a piece of bread and throwing the bread up into the air. The dog would then happily leap up, grab it in his mouth, and gulp his cancer treatment down. Other pet owners may want to use canned pet food, baby food, or broth to get their animals to eat it.

A great success story involving a horse was told to me by one woman who treated her 20-year-old horse named "Lad" for melanoma with Protocel. Lad was a white Arabian-Bay mix (about 90 percent Arabian) and was suffering from a type of melanoma that light-skinned horses often get. Lad had melanoma spots on various parts of his body and one bulging tumor that had originated inside his right ear that was growing outward as well as inward. A biopsy was done on the tumor mass and the resulting diagnosis was "dermal sarcoid with acanthosis and hyperkeratosis." This type of melanoma is not necessarily fatal, but Lad's veterinarian said that if nothing was done, the mass would eventually cut off the horse's hearing in that ear. As the mass grew steadily larger and larger, Lad became more and more uncomfortable and could not tolerate anyone or anything touching that side of his face.

The woman who owned Lad had, herself, recovered from life-threatening cancer using Cancell and decided to try Protocel on her horse. Every morning and evening, she would core an apple, put 1 teaspoonful of Formula 23 into the inner part of the apple, and give the apple to her horse. (Thus, the horse received a total of 2 teaspoonfuls of Protocel each day). Lad loved the taste of the formula so much that if any accidentally spilled on the ground, he would eagerly lick it up. After about three to four months of doing this regularly, all of Lad's melanoma was gone, and he was a completely normal horse again with no spots and no bulging mass in his ear.

To confirm the stories I heard about using Protocel for pets, I called one veterinarian in Illinois who had been using Protocel on a few of his dogs and cats. An example of a success story he had was with an adult boxer dog that had been diagnosed in early January 2002 with adenocarcinoma of the stomach. The dog was extremely sick when diagnosed and was experiencing frequent vomiting. Within a month of starting Protocel (Formula 23), the dog was feeling a lot better and, in the second month, stopped vomiting altogether. The dog continued to feel better and better throughout the year, and by October 2002 all of his tests and bloodwork were completely normal. In about nine months, this extremely sick dog showed no more signs of cancer.

The most astounding recovery that this veterinarian observed, however, was when he used Protocel to try and help a small cat that was so sick from FIV (Feline Immunodeficiency Virus), that he was almost dead. This cat was not expected to live through the night, so the vet assumed it couldn't hurt to try one last thing. He began administering Protocel (Formula 23) to the cat. By the next morning, the vet was astounded to see the cat sitting up and drinking water. This alone was amazing. But by the third day on Protocel, the cat was energetic and eating normally. After only one more day in the hospital, the cat seemed to have made a full recovery and was sent home to its family. He has remained healthy ever since.

The most common dosing for pets has been the following:

- For cats and very small dogs: 1/8 teaspoonful of Protocel 23 every eight hours. (Three times, spaced as evenly as possible, over every 24-hour period.)

- For medium and large dogs: 1/4 teaspoonful of Protocel 23 every eight hours. (Three times, spaced as evenly as possible, over every 24-hour period.)

- For horses: 1 whole teaspoonful of Protocel 23 every 8–12 hours (Can be placed on the inner part of a cored apple or other treat.)

When dosing animals, however, the above instructions are only general. Pet owners may need to adjust the dose size or frequency to their animal's specific situation. If the above dosing only brings about stabilization, an extra dose can be administered and all doses can be spaced more frequently around the clock. Or Protocel Formula 50 can be tried instead of Formula 23.

How Effective Is Protocel for Cancer?

This is a difficult question to answer with specific numbers. Cancer is not a "simple" condition like a single virus infection. It tends to occur in bodies that are weakened or out-of-balance for one reason or another and can then debilitate the body in complex ways as it spreads. Therefore, as with any other approach to cancer recovery, conventional or alternative, there is no 100 percent guarantee. The most accurate description of Protocel's effectiveness with cancer might be to say that it has been observed to bring about very "real" and long-term recoveries for a majority of the people who use it correctly.

For those cancer patients who do not experience success, there may be a variety of reasons why this happens. One reason may be that some people start using Protocel when their cancer is already so far advanced that the formula does not have enough time to work effectively. Although there have been many recoveries of late-stage, metastasized cancer, there will always be some cases where the cancer has advanced so far that it has damaged the vital organs too much for a person to be able to recover using *any* method.

Another reason for some people not recovering, might be that they start using Protocel after they have already gone through so much chemotherapy and/or radiation that their bodies have been too damaged by these toxic treatments. Chemotherapy and/or radiation can sometimes damage vital organs or other parts of the body past the point of repair. And yet another reason might be that some people will use the formula *without* carefully looking into what supplements or herbs might interfere with it. For example, if a person uses Protocel while taking high doses of vitamin C, vitamin E, CoQ_{10}, selenium, or other nutritional or herbal supplements that can interfere with Protocel's process, then the formula may not be able to work to its fullest extent. (Be sure to review the lists of supplements and herbs to avoid.)

Last but not least, some people believe that cancer patients who have high levels of mercury or other heavy metal toxicity may exprience more difficulty recovering from their cancer using Protocel. This has not been proven yet, but it is theorized that high levels of heavy metals may chelate to, or bind to Protocel and render it less effective. Possibly people using Protocel should even avoid flu shots, since most flu vaccinations contain dangerous amounts of mercury.

Unfortunately, because the Protocel formula has been opposed by the ACS, FDA, and NCI in the past, no formal studies have been done on it to provide us with any sort of official statistics. But even so, many people are choosing to assess Protocel's success by investigating numerous real-life stories from people who have used it. As can be seen from the small sampling of true cases listed in this text, there have been many amazing recoveries that involved cancer patients who were not expected to live more than a few weeks or months. Many of these people faced the grim reality that there was nothing in conventional medicine that could save them and were told by their doctors that they should go home and get their affairs in order. In my search into alternative cancer treatments available today, I could *not* find any other approach that appeared to be more successful than Protocel for so many types of cancer, including late-stage cancer.

Resources:

Protocel is available for purchase in the United States as well as through a network of international distributors.

For purchases within the U.S., contact:

Renewal and Wellness, LLC
South Carolina, USA
(866) 776-8623 or (864) 962-8880
Mon.–Thurs. 8:30-6:00 / Fri. 8:30-4:00 EST

Orders can be placed by phone or over the Internet at: www.protocel.com

For purchases outside the U.S., contact:

International Internet Services
Central America
International Customer Service
Phone: +41-1355-3777

Orders can be placed by phone or over the Internet at: www.protocelglobal.com

Cost of Treatment: Protocel is extremely inexpensive—the average cost in the U.S. is approximately $55–$75 per month. (Dosage size and frequency may vary slightly for individual cases.) For inquiries as to international prices and distribution, go to www.protocelglobal.com.

Websites:

www.webnd.com
(Website for U.S. sales and information.)

www.protocelglobal.com
(Website for international sales and information.)

www.elonnamckibben.com
(For more details and important information about cancer recovery using Protocel.)

www.protocelforum.com
(Internationally Hosted User Support Site)

CHAPTER 13

Hospital Santa Monica and Oxygen Therapy

Hospital Santa Monica is a 60-bed facility located in Mexico, just over the San Diego–U.S. border. It is a modern hospital fully equipped with blood chemistry laboratories, pharmacy, physiotherapy programs, and large medical staff, and is one of the largest facilities worldwide to treat cancer holistically.

At Hospital Santa Monica, people with cancer can stay for weeks at a time as in-patients, can be treated with a variety of approaches, can be monitored by fully accredited doctors and technicians, can partake of healthful meals every day, and can interact with other cancer patients dealing with similar issues, all while staying at a beautiful location on the Baja coast. Hospital Santa Monica provides a broad holistic approach to cancer, but their special focus is on the use of oxygenation therapies.

The founder and director of Hospital Santa Monica is Dr. Kurt W. Donsbach, a naturopathic doctor and chiropractor. Dr. Donsbach is one of the leading pioneers in the use of oxygenation therapies. The three primary types of oxygenation therapy used at Hospital Santa Monica are:

1. Hydrogen peroxide

2. Ozone

3. Hyperbaric oxygen

The general purpose of these oxygen treatments (also called bio-oxidative therapies) is to increase the oxygen content in the bloodstream and around each cancer cell. As we know from previous chapters, cancer cells are primarily anaerobic. They do not thrive well in oxygen-rich environments and may sometimes even be completely destroyed by high levels of oxygen. According to the book *Oxygen Healing Therapies* by

Nathaniel Altman, bio-oxidative therapies have been studied extensively and used clinically for treating cancer in many countries, such as Russia, Germany, Cuba, Mexico, Italy, France, and Australia. Besides causing a hostile environment for cancer cells, bio-oxidative therapies have numerous cancer-fighting effects on the body, including (among other things):

- They stimulate the production of white blood cells.

- Ozone and hydrogen peroxide are virucidal, and thereby may be able to destroy micro-organisms related to cancer.

- Ozone and hydrogen peroxide treatments stimulate an increase in the production of interferon and tumor necrosis factor, both of which are used by the body to fight cancer.[1]

At Hospital Santa Monica, a specially diluted form of hydrogen peroxide is administered intravenously. (Drinking or injecting straight hydrogen peroxide from a drug store *is not* safe.) DMSO is also added to the treatment to potentiate the hydrogen peroxide. Ozone treatments are administered primarily by "insufflation." This is a procedure whereby ozone is introduced painlessly into the rectal area. In that area of the body, rich capillary beds efficiently absorb and utilize the oxygen.[2]

For Hyperbaric Oxygen Treatment, patients are placed in a pressurized type of chamber that has a higher concentration of pure oxygen than our normal environment. Once the patient is inside, the pressure in the chamber slowly increases to the equivalent of several hundred feet below sea level. This pressurized, highly oxygenated environment has the effect of forcing oxygen directly into the body through the tissues of the skin. Each treatment in the chamber typically lasts from 45 to 60 minutes and patients are often given multiple sessions per week.[3]

As well as the oxygen therapies, many other treatment approaches are used as well to treat cancer at Hospital Santa Monica. These include:

- Hyperthermia
- COX 2 Inhibition
- DMSO
- High Doses of Melatonin
- Thymus Gland Stimulation
- Anti-angiogenesis (through the use of Bovine Cartilage, Genestein, and Vitamin A)

- Microfrequency (Rife) Induction
- Micro-Dose Chemotherapy (IPT)
- BioMagnetic Therapy
- Nutritional Therapy
- Herbal Therapy (a variety including Black Salve)
- Immune-Stimulating Vaccines
- Far-Infrared Therapy
- UV Light Blood Irradiation

It is recommended that patients first stay at Hospital Santa Monica for an intensive two- or three-week period. This is done on an in-patient basis. After the initial intensive, each patient leaves the hospital with a specialized program to continue at home that is uniquely designed for his or her individual needs.

Dr. Donsbach and his staff at Hospital Santa Monica do not claim to "cure" cancer, but they have had success helping many people to attain either complete remission or stabilization of their cancer. Dr. Donsbach claims cancer recovery statistics to be difficult to ascertain, but has reported that, "Approximately 70 percent of our patients are alive three years after their first visit to our facility."[4] Although Donsbach admitted that not all these cancer patients were already in remission, one must remember that upon arrival, very few of them had been given more than just a few months to live by their conventional doctors.

Anyone interested in learning more about Hospital Santa Monica and the cancer treatment program offered there, can call for a free video and full information packet.

Resources:

Hospital Santa Monica
Administration Offices
870 Canarios Court
Chula Vista, CA 91910

(619) 482-8533
(800) 359-6547
www.hospitalsantamonica.com

For a *free* video and brochures about treatment at Hospital Santa Monica, call (800) 359-6547. Cost of treatment will vary depending on each patient's unique needs. However, in general, the initial two-week in-patient intensive costs approximately $12,000 and some cancer patients elect to stay a third week for an additional $4,000.

Books

Nathaniel Altman. *Oxygen Healing Therapies*. Healing Arts Press: Rochester, Vermont, 1998.

Websites

www.hospitalsantamonica.com

www.donsbach.com

www.oxygentherapies.com

CHAPTER 14

Dr. Budwig's Flaxseed Oil and Cottage Cheese Diet

A truly remarkable all-natural cancer recovery approach is German biochemist Johanna Budwig's "Flaxseed Oil and Cottage Cheese" diet. Dr. Budwig held a Ph.D. in natural science, went through medical training to become a physician, and was schooled in pharmaceutical science, physics, botany, and biology. Because of her important contributions to science and medicine, she was nominated by her peers to receive a Nobel Prize seven different times!

Dr. Budwig's most important contribution to the world involved her pioneering research into the roles of essential fatty acids. Her discoveries began in the 1950s, and over time, she illuminated a common causative factor behind many of our modern degenerative diseases, including cancer. In a nutshell, Dr. Budwig found that the widespread dietary habits of our modern world tend to promote a dangerous deficiency in the essential fatty acids so important to good health. She discovered that, as a result of modern food industry practices, we no longer eat enough good oils in their natural states, and instead, eat way too many chemically altered oils that are damaging to our health. This tends to create a situation where we become deficient in two of the most important categories of essential fatty acids: the omega-3 and omega-6 fatty acids.

Dr. Budwig found that in order to mass produce and distribute food products high in oils (e.g., salad dressings, cooking oils, margarine, etc.), modern food manufacturers put these products through chemical processes to deliberately alter the makeup of the oils. These alterations are done because most healthful oils easily go rancid once they are processed out of the natural foods they are found in, such as vegetables, fish, seeds, and nuts. Once these oils are exposed to heat and sunlight for periods of time, as they would necessarily be through shipping and storage, they can easily degrade into a spoiled state. Thus, manufacturers of common food products such as margarines and bottled oils used in cooking or salad dressings, must put the oils they market through chemical processes so they can be packaged, shipped, and left to sit on store shelves for long periods of time.

The process of chemically altering natural oils is good for the manufacturers' profits, but bad for the consumer's health because these processes turn good, healthful, natural oils into harmful oils, or "pseudo" fats, as Dr. Budwig called them. Some of the most health-damaging pseudo fats are the hydrogenated and partially hydrogenated fats and oils, but many of the processed poly-unsaturated fats can be harmful as well.

It might surprise many people that *all margarines* and *virtually all fried foods* include these extremely harmful fats. Many other common foods contain harmful fats as well. For instance, any solidified peanut butter, such as those commonly advertised on TV for children, that does *not* show a layer of oil at the top of the jar when sold is made up of altered, harmful oils.

History and Theory

It wasn't until the late 1920s that essential fatty acids were beginning to be understood and categorized by researchers. Although food industries were producing substances such as margarine since the 1930s, they did not understand all the effects these altered oils were having on people. When Dr. Budwig began studying them in the 1950s, she was able to discover much more about the metabolism of oils in the body than had previously been known to the scientific world. She began her research by first studying and categorizing thousands of blood samples from people who were seriously ill, then comparing those samples to the blood of people who were healthy. One of the things Dr. Budwig discovered was a strange greenish-yellow substance in the blood of people with debilitating chronic illnesses. This was *not* found in the blood of people who were healthy. And this greenish-yellow substance appeared in place of healthy, red oxygen-carrying hemoglobin!

Dr. Budwig saw this greenish-yellow substance over and over in the blood of people with cancer, particular. She also discovered a marked *lack* of phosphatides (an important fatty compound) and lipoproteins (fats bound to proteins) in the blood of cancer patients. After more research, Dr. Budwig discovered that these anomalies were linked to a severe deficiency of omega-3 and omega-6 essential fatty acids (EFAs).

There are a variety of omega-3 and omega-6 essential fatty acids which are found in many different natural foods that we eat. (They are called "essential" because they are critical to good health and are substances our bodies can't make and must be supplied through diet.) In general, certain ocean fish—particularly the oily, cold-water fish such as tuna, salmon, and mackerel—are the foods highest in the omega-3 essential fatty acids, and certain seeds and nuts are the foods highest in the omega-6 essential fatty acids. (I like to remember this general rule by saying to myself, "Omega-3 from the sea; omega-6 from the sticks.")

Some food sources have both types of EFAs, however. When Dr. Budwig discovered a deficiency of these essential fatty acids linked to degenerative diseases, she looked for a natural way to replenish them. She settled on flaxseed oil because it is an extremely rich source of both omega-6 and omega-3 fatty acids, and is *particularly* high in the very important omega-3's. Unrefined, cold-pressed flaxseed oil contains a whopping 15 to25 percent linoleic acid (omega-6), and an incredible 50 to 60 percent alpha-linolenic acid (omega-3). [*Note:* Flax seeds are called "linseeds" in many places, so the term "flaxseed oil" refers to the same thing as the term "linseed oil."]

Dr. Budwig discovered that omega-3 and omega-6 essential fatty acids are critical to our health, especially in their following three roles when it comes to cancer:

1. Their role in maintaining the health and integrity of cell walls

2. Their role in oxygenating cells

3. Their required role in the body's production of prostaglandins

She also found that people tend to be more deficient in the omega-3's than the omega-6's. This may be because people in the modern world tend to have more sources of omega-6 EFAs from other seed oils in their diets, such as safflower oil, sunflower oil, corn oil, sesame oil, and soybean oil.

Lipids and Cell Wall Integrity

Every cell in our body is covered with a protective membrane, or cell wall, that is made up of lipids. In his book, *How to Fight Cancer and Win*, William L. Fischer states:

Each cell in this miracle we call the body is protectively covered with a sheath of fats. The cell body (plasma) is interlaced with little lipid veins, often called the "nerves of the cell." These lipid veins are the connection between the nucleus and the outer membrane. They influence the care and feeding of the cell and the process of normal cell division by the use of tiny electrical impulses.[1]

Dr. Budwig came to believe that cancer was a result, not of "too much" cell growth, but of "faulty" cell growth, or cell division. She proposed that this faulty cell division was caused by not enough essential fatty acids in the cell membrane along with an accumulation of harmful manmade fats in the cell membrane. In her book, *Flax Oil as a True Aid Against Arthritis, Heart Infarction, Cancer and Other Diseases*, Dr. Budwig explains the important role of the cell, or "lipoid" membrane in the process of cell division:

> In growing cells, we find a dipolarity between the electrically positive nucleus and the electrically negative cell membrane with its highly unsaturated fatty acids. When the cell divides, it is the cell nucleus which begins this. The cell body and the daughter cell are then separated and tied off by the lipoid membrane. When a cell divides, its surface area is larger and must, of necessity, contain enough material in this surface with its fatty acids, to be able to divide the new cell completely from the original. Normal growth is always distinguished by a clearly defined course of action. In all our skin and membranes, in that of adults too, there are continual growth processes. The old cells have to be shed with new ones being formed underneath. When this process is interrupted, it means the body is beginning to die.[2]

Dr. Budwig reasoned that the common deficiency of essential fatty acids in cancer patients—evidenced by a marked lack of phospholipids in their blood—was why cancer cells often have multiple sets of chromosomes. The normal cell would attempt to divide but wouldn't have enough lipids necessary to complete the formation of the new cell membrane. Rather than one mother cell becoming two daughter cells, the mother cell would become one daughter cell—but the mother cell's chromosomes would have already divided and replicated themselves. Thus, according to Dr. Budwig, the daughter cell becomes an abomination with too many chromosomes due to lack of material for building new cell walls.

Lipids and Oxygenation

The oxygen utilization of every cell in our body depends on essential fatty acids. For instance, without natural, unaltered linoleic acid (omega-6), the body cannot produce hemoglobin. And without hemoglobin, the blood cannot carry oxygen to all the body's cells. Another way that EFAs oxygenate cells is by *attracting* oxygen to the cell via the cell membrane. When a cell has a normal and healthy cell membrane, this membrane is full of highly unsaturated essential fatty acids. The "unsaturated" aspect of the lipids means that they have lots of unbound electrons looking for something to bind to. One thing they love to bind to is oxygen. This then brings oxygen to the cell, which supports and stimulates the respiratory process of the cell itself.

Taking a closer look at the mechanics of cells, every cell wall (or cell membrane) is made up of lipids (or fats). The most common of these are the omega-3 essential fatty acids and cholesterol. The polyunsaturated EFAs found in virgin, cold-pressed, unrefined flaxseed oil are *electron-rich*. These natural polyunsaturated fats greedily bind to oxygen and proteins. When absorbed into cell walls, they attract oxygen to the cell. When bound to sulphur-based proteins, they are water-soluble and free-flowing and their electron-rich characteristic is reserved as a form of energy that the body can use when it needs to.

The problem with fats and oils that have been chemically refined and altered for marketing, is that, in order to extend the shelf life of these oils, the vital electron cloud of the essential fatty acids is destroyed. The resultant effect is that these essential fatty acids can no longer bind to proteins to make them more assimilable by the body, and they can no longer attract and bind to oxygen. William L. Fischer discusses this issue in *How to Fight Cancer and Win*:

> The chemical processing of fats destroys the vital electron cloud, demonstrated in the foregoing material to be of immense importance to the functioning of every cell in the body. Once the electrons have been removed, these fats can no longer bind with oxygen and actually become an obstacle to the process of breathing. The heart, for instance, rejects these fats, and they end up as inorganic fatty deposits on the heart muscle itself. As we pointed out earlier, a diseased heart and its aortas clearly show deposits of these worthless, electrically dead lipids.

Chemically processed fats are not water-soluble when bound to protein. They end up blocking circulation, and they damage heart action, inhibit cell renewal, and impede the free flow of blood and lymph fluids. The bioelectrical action in these areas slows down and may become completely paralyzed. The entire organism shows a measurable loss of electrical energy that is replenished only by adding active lipids to the diet.[3]

Unfortunately, the amount of manmade, partially hydrogenated oils known as "trans-fatty acids" is extremely high in modern Western diets. These trans-fats are so similar to cholesterol that our bodies cannot tell the difference. They are mistakenly used in place of good cholesterol to build cell membranes. This then causes these cell membranes to lack a vital electrical charge that would normally attract oxygen. Without sufficient oxygen, the cellular environment becomes more and more anaerobic. The damaging trans-fats also impede the cellular exchange of nutrition and waste products through the membrane, or cell wall. They may even contribute to adult-onset diabetes because insulin is a large molecule that cannot easily pass through cell walls made up of manmade "pseudo"-fats.[4]

As mentioned in previous chapters, Dr. Otto Warburg believed that insufficient oxygen was the *key* reason that normal cells turned into cancer cells. He also reportedly proved that by reducing the oxygen levels in tissues around 35 percent, he could consistently induce the development of cancer. Dr. Budwig stated that Dr. Warburg believed the insufficient uptake of oxygen by cancer cells was somehow linked to fat metabolism and that Warburg tried to prove this theory by working with oils. But according to Budwig, Dr. Warburg was not successful because he did not use the *right type* of oils in his studies.[5]

When Dr. Budwig discovered the role that omega-3 and omega-6 fatty acids played in oxygenating cells, she believed felt that she had found the missing link Dr. Warburg had been looking for. In other words, she had found the *reason* cells sometimes had to resort to anaerobic functioning!

Lipids and Prostaglandins

Another important function of the omega-3 and omega-6 essential fatty acids is that they are converted by the body into "prostaglandins." Prostaglandins are hormone-like substances that have far-reaching effects on many different systems of the body. There are more than a dozen different prostaglandins that our bodies manufacture, none of which can be biosynthesized without sufficient essential fatty acids from our diet. EFA-derived prostaglandins regulate kidney function, inflammation response, and immune functioning in our bodies. They also help to keep blood vessels elastic, regulate blood pressure, influence platelet stickiness, and are necessary for proper metabolization of cholesterol. (These last functions of prostaglandins are largely why sufficient EFAs in the diet are important to cardiovascular health.) Thus, the prostaglandins play many roles in a healthy, well-functioning immune system and help the body to resist the development of cancer. And natural, unaltered EFAs are critical to the production of prostaglandins.

What Does Cottage Cheese Have to Do With It?

By now, you are probably wondering what cottage cheese has to do with anything. Obviously, what Dr. Budwig discovered was how important essential fatty acids are. The way that cottage cheese comes into play is the following: In researching how to most efficiently get the depleted essential fatty acids back into our bodies, *Dr. Budwig found that the body's assimilation and use of essential fatty acids was greatly enhanced when the fatty acids were combined with sulphur-based proteins.* In fact, nature has provided this combination already for us since most of the natural sources of essential fatty acids, such as milk, nuts, and seeds, also contain sulphur-based proteins.

Sulphur-based proteins are also found in many other foods, such as onions, leeks, chives, garlic, and yogurt. In her attempt to reverse advanced degenerative diseases, Dr. Budwig believed she needed to quickly replenish her patients' bodies with sufficient EFAs, and flaxseed oil was the highest source around. Then, she searched for the richest dietary source of sulphur-based proteins to go with the flaxseed oil. She finally settled on a food called *Quark*. *Quark* is common in Germany and is similar to cottage cheese and yogurt. However, since *Quark* is difficult to obtain *outside* of Germany, cottage cheese is the next best food source and most commonly used option around the world. Next to *Quark*, cottage cheese is one of the richest sources of sulphur-based proteins to be found.

By combining flaxseed oil with the sulphur-based proteins in *Quark* or cottage cheese, the essential fatty acids bind to the sulphur-based proteins, and this makes them water-soluble and much more bio-available to the body. Dr. Budwig also discovered that there were certain vitamin and mineral "co-factors" that aided the body in its use of the essential fatty acids. The primary co-factors are vitamins B_3, B_6, and C, and the minerals magnesium and zinc. These nutrients are all required by the body, as well, to make prostaglandins.

Thus, though the essential fatty acids are the main dietary factor needed for recovery from degenerative conditions such as cancer, simply ingesting flaxseed oil alone will not work as well as combining the flaxseed oil with foods rich in sulphur-based proteins. In fact, there is some evidence that taking flaxseed oil daily *without* sufficient sulphur-based proteins in the diet may even be harmful. (This is why some recent scientific studies that test the use of flaxseed oil alone for cancer do *not* show results anywhere near what Dr. Budwig was able to achieve.)

In case after case, Dr. Budwig found that thoroughly mixed flaxseed oil with cottage cheese was an efficient and successful way of replenishing the body's levels of essential fatty acids. She proved that, through the use of her special dietary approach, the anomalous greenish-yellow elements in her patients' blood would disappear over about three months and would be replaced by healthy red blood cells. Normal levels of phosphatides and lipoproteins would reappear in the blood as well, and tumors would start to disappear. Dr. Budwig reportedly accumulated over 1,000 documented cases of cancer recoveries with her special dietary approach!

As a result of her in-depth research and clinical practice, Dr. Budwig claimed the following:

- Lipoproteins can be found in all biochemically active tissues and always contain highly unsaturated fatty acids and sulphur-rich proteins.

- Anesthetics and certain drugs, such as barbiturates, sleeping pills, and painkillers, can separate highly unsaturated fatty acids from sulphur-containing proteins.

- Hard carcinoma tumors can be dissolved with serums high in essential fatty acids and organically bound sulphur.

- Polymerized pseudo-fats of marine origin (such as fish and whale oils) that have been radically altered by being subjected to high temperatures for use in margarines, have been isolated from soft tumors.

Opposition and Suppression

History tells us that the many health benefits of flax have been appreciated for thousands of years. Flax was cultivated in Babylon as early as 5,000 B.C. Hippocrates wrote about the healing benefits of flax. And ancient scripts from India claim that a yogi must eat flax daily in order to achieve the highest state of contentment and joy possible.[6]

Unfortunately, in the modern world, big businesses have gotten in the way of some of our most ancient healing traditions. Dr. Budwig met with ferocious opposition from various powers in the food industry, particularly from the margarine producers. She was the first scientist to oppose the modern practice of altering of oils for commercial distribution purposes. Her conflicts started with Professor H. P. Kaufmann, who was the head of the German Institute where she was doing her research. Kaufman also happened to be a very famous lipid expert who had been nicknamed the "Pope of Fats and Oils." He held patents for some of the hydrogenation processes that produced the very polymers Dr. Budwig claimed were harmful to our bodies and which she had isolated from soft tumors. Thus, even though her research was sound, he had a strong financial interest in the use of these polymers, or pseudo-fats, particularly by the margarine industry.[7]

According to Johanna Budwig, Dr. Kaufmann tried to bribe her with money to keep her from publicizing her discoveries about oils. She refused his bribe, whereupon he supposedly denied her any further access to the research institute facilities he headed. When Dr. Budwig tried to move to another institute where she could continue her research, she found her access blocked by what she felt was an industry-wide conspiracy against her. Apparently, the "Pope of Fats" and margarine industry moguls had mobilized in some way to keep her from continuing her work in modern scientific laboratories. She also found herself blocked from publishing her research in scientific journals. Her only recourse then was to write books and share her information that way.

The one good that came from Dr. Budwig's banishment from further laboratory research was that she spent more time working with patients in a clinical setting. It is unfortunate, however, that she was not able to continue her formal research, which might have given us an even better understanding of fat metabolism and its connection with serious illnesses, such as cancer.

Dr. Budwig's Dietary Protocol

Anyone wishing to use Dr. Budwig's approach should be aware of the protocol she recommended. The *basic* rules of her approach are listed below, but I do not recommend that readers rely solely on what I have written here. If you are interested in using flaxseed oil and cottage cheese to recover from an illness, please refer to the books and Internet sites listed at the end of this chapter for more detailed information.

Primary ingredient: Thoroughly mix low-fat cottage cheese (preferably 1 percent organic) with unrefined, virgin, cold-pressed flaxseed oil. The ratio of these two items may vary depending on the severity of disease, but the most commonly agreed upon ratio is 1 tablespoon flaxseed oil to 1/4 cup cottage cheese. For patients with serious illnesses, Dr. Budwig suggested anywhere from 3 to 6 tablespoons of flaxseed oil per 1/2 cup of cottage cheese. Using a blender or other sort of electrical mixer is important to optimally bind the essential fatty acids with the sulphur-based proteins. Various fresh or frozen fruits, honey, and/or stevia can be added to the mix to make it tasty. Lowfat or skim milk or unsweetened fruit juice can also be added. Keep the blended mix refrigerated and eat it throughout the day.

If preferred, lowfat plain yogurt may be substituted for cottage cheese. However, since yogurt is not quite as high in sulphur-based proteins as cottage cheese is, one should triple the amount of yogurt used. In other words, use at least 1 tablespoon flaxseed oil to 3/4 cup yogurt.

For people who are allergic to dairy products, other sources of sulphur-based proteins may be used instead of cottage cheese or yogurt, though it may be difficult to achieve the optimum effect with other substitutions. One non-dairy substitution is tofu, but it is unclear as to the amount required. Another substitution for dairy would be a special supplement in capsule form that contains dried sulfurated proteins. "Nature's Distributors," based in Arizona, sells this type of supplement. Their phone number is (800) 624-7114, and their non-dairy substitute for cottage cheese sulphurated proteins is called "Companion Nutrients." Nature's Distributors claims that one capsule of Companion Nutrients can activate the essential fatty acids in one tablespoon of flax oil.

Along with eating one of the above mixtures every day, Dr. Budwig included some dietary restrictions in her healing approach to help promote recovery. These restrictions were the following:

Foods to Completely Avoid

- Refined sugar (Unsweetened grape juice and honey okay)
- All animal fats
- All salad oils, including commercial mayonnaise
- All meats containing chemicals, hormones, or preservatives
- Butter
- Anything "hydrogenated" (such as margarine or fried foods)

Fresh vegetable juices, such as carrot, celery, apple, and red beet, are fine. Dr. Budwig also thought it essential to drink a warm tea, such as peppermint, rose hips, or grape tea, three times a day. (Black tea before noon is okay.) For those who would sorely miss butter and mayonnaise, there is a special flaxseed oil "spread" that can be prepared and used ,as well as a special flaxseed oil "mayonnaise." (To get more details on how to prepare these, go to www.positivehealth.com/permit/Articles/Nutrition/turner60.htm, or refer to Chapter 7 of Fischer's book, *How to Fight Cancer and Win*. For an in-depth description of Dr. Budwig's entire protocol for cancer, read both Chapters 6 and 7 of Fischer's book.)

Remember to use only unrefined, cold-pressed flaxseed oil that is sold in a dark (light-blocking) bottle and kept refrigerated at all times. Barleans is an excellent brand and produces very high-quality oil. For best results, use the bottled liquid oil rather than capsules and keep the bottle refrigerated. It takes about 14 capsules of flaxseed oil to equal just 1 tablespoon of the bottled oil, and many times the bottles of capsules are allowed to sit on store shelves or warehouses in the heat. Flax seeds freshly ground at home in a coffee grinder and *used immediately* can be added to the daily mixture. But do not grind your flax seeds at a health food store, then drive home and expect them to still be good. Dr. Budwig claimed that the oils in freshly ground flax seeds can go bad in just 10 to 15 minutes! There are more details to this diet that can be obtained from the resources listed in the back of this chapter. These should be studied and followed carefully if you have life-threatening cancer and choose to use this approach.

Although some people have a remarkably fast disappearance of tumors using this approach—sometimes in just a few months—others may take longer. Dr. Budwig recommended that people using this dietary treatment for serious illnesses stay on it for three to five years to achieve true healing. According to Dr. Budwig, people who break the rules of the diet (for example by eating preserved meats, candy, etc.) may grow rapidly worse to the point where they cannot be saved. However, some people have just used flaxseed oil thoroughly mixed into cottage cheese on a daily basis, without adhering to the other aspects of Budwig's dietary protocol, and they have done quite well.

Here are two simple recipes that can be tried. The first creates a soft-yogurt consistency and can be poured into a bowl to eat with a spoon. The second creates a milkshake consistency and can be poured into a glass to drink.

Mix in a blender for at least 30 seconds these five ingredients:

> 1 cup lowfat, organic cottage cheese
>
> 4 tablespoons unrefined, cold-pressed flaxseed oil
>
> 2 fresh peaches (sliced), or other fresh fruit
>
> 1 tablespoon honey
>
> Juice from 1/2 lemon

Mix in a blender for about a minute these nine ingredients:

> 1 cup unsweetened grape or pineapple juice
>
> 1 banana, cut up
>
> 1 1/2 cups frozen, dark cherries
>
> 1/2 cup lowfat cottage cheese
>
> 1 cup plain, nonfat yogurt
>
> 1/4 cup freshly ground flaxseeds
>
> 2 tablespoons raw wheat germ
>
> 2 to 3 tablespoons flaxseed oil
>
> 1 to 2 tablespoons honey

You can create your own unique recipes for combining flaxseed oil and cottage cheese. Just be sure to also supplement with co-factors that help the activation of the essential fatty acids. A daily multiple B vitamin (or wheat germ) and a daily multiple mineral supplement of some sort are a good idea. There are some excellent cancer recovery stories to be found in Fischer's book, *How to Fight Cancer and Win*, and there are many others that can also be found on the Internet. The following case stories were recorded from interviews with people I contacted directly.

Case Stories

Case Story #1 — Metastasized Prostate Cancer

Cliff Beckwith is an American man who has done a great deal to spread the word about the use of flaxseed oil and cottage cheese for cancer. (I use his full name here because he publicly posts his story on his website: www.beckwithfamily.com.)

In January 1991, Cliff was diagnosed with prostate cancer. Initial bone scans and other tests indicated that the cancer had not spread, so surgery was recommended. During the operation, however, Cliff's surgeon discovered that his cancer had in fact metastasized to his lymph glands. Because of this, Cliff was diagnosed as stage IV, and the operation was *not* completed. His doctor said that, since the cancer was in his lymph system, it would not do any good to cut it out locally at the prostate gland.

At that point, it was decided to use the drugs Lupron and Eulexin to cancel the male hormones. Cliff was told that male hormones do not *cause* cancer, but if cancer is present, then they act like kerosene thrown on fire. Cliff went on the drugs, but in the meantime, he also found out about Dr. Budwig's flaxseed oil and cottage cheese approach. He read that most people are about 80 percent deficient in omega-3, and that Dr. Budwig had worked with cancer patients who sometimes had only a few hours to live and restored them to health.

So Cliff gave it a try. For two-and-one-half years he put about half a cup of cottage cheese and some fruit, such as crushed pineapple or frozen strawberries, mixed with just 2 tablespoons of flaxseed oil and a little honey, in the refrigerator. He ate that throughout the day. When he was first diagnosed, Cliff's PSA count was 75. After just six months of eating the flaxseed oil and cottage cheese on a daily basis, Cliff had another PSA test done. He got a call from his doctor's office the following Monday and the office girl exclaimed, "Mr. Beckwith! Your count is completely normal!" Cliff's PSA was down to 0.1.

For the first four years, Cliff continued to get PSA readings at six-month intervals, and every time, his count was between 0.0 and 0.16. He had continued on the hormone blockade throughout these years, so the flaxseed oil and cottage cheese mixture was *not* the only thing he was doing. Cliff knew that the hormone-blocking drugs could also effectively lower PSA counts for a while. But when he asked his doctor if he had expected the counts to go down that much, the doctor said, "No way!"

After 1995, Cliff was no longer on the Eulexin and Lupron and was just using flaxseed oil and cottage cheese. In the years since stopping the hormone-blocking drugs, his PSA level has varied a bit more. As of this writing, in August 2003, Cliff is still doing great and has no clinical signs of metastasis to other organs. He is 82 years old, and his PSA count has remained in a normal range for a man of his age. Best of all, Cliff has already lived about 12 years longer than his doctor thought he would.

Over the years, Cliff has helped many people with his Internet site and also with an audiotape about flaxseed oil and cottage cheese that he created to give out to people who needed information. He has known of over 100 people who have successfully used this method of treatment to help them recover from all types of cancer. He has even known some stories of flaxseed oil and cottage cheese working to help dogs recover from cancer.

Unfortunately, Cliff has *also* known people who were getting well using the FSO/CC combination (their cancer markers were going down, symptoms were going away, etc.), but were convinced by their doctors to do more chemotherapy or radiation. Many of these people who had been beating their cancer by replenishing their essential omega fatty acids then died after doing conventional treatment. Apparently, many of these people's doctors could see that their patient was recovering from cancer but couldn't accept that they were doing it without the help of conventional medicine.

Case Story #2 — Metastasized Pancreatic Cancer

William is a 72-year-old man whose friends and family have always called "Huck." About 10 years ago, at the end of 1993, Huck suddenly became very ill. He was overcome with extreme pain and nausea, and was rushed to a nearby hospital emergency room. Doctors there were unable to find the problem, so they sent him home. However, the symptoms kept returning, with Huck suffering from about a half-dozen painful attacks by the end of January. He was finally admitted to the hospital in late January 1994 to undergo more tests. The doctors suspected a problem with his pancreas but hospital tests still showed nothing. A CT scan also showed nothing unusual.

Because of his severe pain, Huck requested that his gallbladder be removed in case that was the problem. This surgery was done on February 7 and went smoothly. For a few days, Huck seemed to feel better, but then the pain returned in the same place it had been before. He saw some other specialists, but they couldn't find anything, either. Toward the end of April, Huck had lost 50 pounds and suffered his worst attack of pain ever.

Finally, in May 1994, another CT scan was done, and this time it showed some serious changes in his pancreas. The doctors could now see that Huck's pancreas had tripled in size since his first scan in January. He was referred to a pancreatic surgeon, who tried an endoscopic procedure to learn more details of what was going on. Unfortunately, that did not reveal anything either. So the next day, Huck went into surgery. After opening him up, the surgeon found malignant pancreatic cancer that had metastasized (stage IV). Huck's primary tumor in the pancreas was about the size of two slightly flattened lemons. It was also obvious now that the tumor had reached out and grown around the blood vessel running between the pancreas and liver, as well as around another primary blood vessel. The surgeon knew there was no way he could surgically remove all of the cancer and didn't even try to cut it out. The only thing the surgeon did before sewing Huck back up was to take a few fine needle biopsy samples. (The needle biopsies came back from the lab indicating that the type of pancreatic cancer was "adenocarcinoma.") After surgery, Huck was told he would probably not live more than three months. Huck and his wife, Nan, were told that neither chemotherapy nor radiation would help, so no treatment was recommended.

Huck and Nan left the hospital with a terrible diagnosis, but they didn't give up. They looked into alternative approaches. First, Huck started drinking six 12-ounce glasses of fresh vegetable juices each day and improved his diet. By the end of June, he also started getting Laetrile treatments at an alternative clinic. Every day (except Sundays) for three weeks, he received intravenous Laetrile along with DMSO and massive amounts of vitamin C. After that, Huck switched to oral Laetrile tablets. Huck added other supplements to his daily regimen, too, as well as Essiac tea. Then, around mid-August, Huck and Nan found out about flaxseed oil and cottage cheese, so he started taking 1 tablespoon of flaxseed oil with 1 tablespoon of cottage cheese after every meal. His total intake of oil was 3 tablespoons a day.

Huck never did any conventional treatment for his cancer but gradually began to feel better and better. In December 1994, he was feeling very well and had put back on 25 pounds. Another CT scan was performed, and unbelievably, just seven months after being diagnosed with metastasized pancreatic cancer, his doctor could not find anything abnormal on the scan at all! The doctor was stunned. He called in the radiologist to look at the scan with him, but the radiologist could not find any cancer or anything else out of the ordinary, either.

On December 28, 1994, a blood test was taken to measure levels of a pancreatic cancer marker. This test is called the CA-19-9. For this test, the normal range is between 0 and 37. Huck's test came back at 17. Over the years, Huck continued to get regular CT scans. Every time, the results showed him to be clear of cancer. In April 1997, he had another CA-19-9 test done. His count this time was 14.

Over a few years, Huck gradually stopped using the flaxseed oil and cottage cheese as well as the Laetrile tablets. He went back to eating a normal, healthy diet, and he continues to take some supplements. He has had no recurrence of cancer since, and his doctor has had a hard time believing it. At first, Huck would receive a phone call from his doctor's office about every three months, just to see how he was doing. After a while, his doctor's office only called him every six months, then once a year. Finally, the doctor's office stopped calling him.

Huck's story is truly an amazing one. People who are diagnosed with stage IV pancreatic cancer are given virtually no chance for long-term recovery by standard medical practices. Probably, everything Huck did worked together to help him get well. Laetrile treatment can be a very powerful approach but does not appear to have high success rates for metastasized cancer when the intravenous part of the treatment is only done for three weeks. Usually, patients must keep coming back for intravenous Laetrile treatments in order to fully recovery. Although it is hard to be sure, Huck and Nan believe the flaxseed oil and cottage cheese combination had the biggest impact.

Case Story #3 — Breast Cancer

Huck's wife, Nan, now has her own cancer story. In October 2002, Nan's breast started hurting and she noticed a big lump that had not been there before. She had undergone a mammogram just a couple of months before, and, strangely, it had showed her to be fine. But with the lump clearly observable now, she was given an ultrasound. The ultrasound showed that Nan most definitely had a tumor, and a needle biopsy came up with the diagnosis of "lobular infiltrating carcinoma."

Nan's doctor immediately recommended a mastectomy followed by chemotherapy. Nan had seen too many other people die after going through chemo for cancer, and she had also seen her own husband recover without it. So, she refused all surgery and chemotherapy. She started eating flaxseed oil and cottage cheese every day instead. Her conventional doctor refused to monitor her progress if she didn't do the standard treatments, so she had to look around for another doctor who would. Luckily, she found one with whom she could work.

Nan did not do any Laetrile treatments as her husband had done because the doctor who administered them to Huck had since moved. She started with 6 tablespoons of flaxseed oil mixed with cottage cheese every day. She also cleaned up her diet, avoided all junk food, and took lots of vitamin and mineral supplements. After a few months, Nan reduced her intake of flaxseed oil to 3 tablespoons a day.

When Nan had been diagnosed with breast cancer in October 2002, her tumor was almost as big as a golf ball. Another ultrasound in January 2003 showed that the tumor was stable in size (showed no increase). A full-body CT scan was done, and there was no indication that the cancer had spread to any other areas. In July 2003, the breast tumor was down to the size of a marble. The pain in Nan's breast has been gone since mid-November, and she feels great otherwise. Nan continues to diligently eat her flaxseed oil and cottage cheese on a daily basis.

Case Story #4—Prostate Cancer

Because of Cliff Beckwith's influence, many other American men with prostate cancer have found out about using flaxseed oil and cottage cheese and have their own great success stories. Seventy-eight-year-old Chester is one of them. Seven years ago, Chester was diagnosed with prostate cancer. At diagnosis, his PSA count was 24. Chester's doctors administered radiation five days a week for a total of 39 treatments. Chester also started taking flaxseed oil and cottage cheese on a daily basis.

For the first five months or so, Chester took 6 tablespoons of flaxseed oil a day. After that, he went down to 2 tablespoons a day and has stayed on that ever since. Chester just puts the oil in a bowl, stirs in about half a cup of cottage cheese, and eats it. From 24, his PSA count went down to 12, which is the level it stayed at for over three years. Then, his count went down even more, and for the last few years has remained at five.

Chester feels great and still works in his own barbershop, where he tells anyone who is interested about the healing wonder of flaxseed oil and cottage cheese.

Case Story #5—Brain Cancer

Tom Rolland was only 37 years old when, on February 10, 2002, he was rushed to the hospital with a splitting headache and projectile vomiting. He thought he just had a very bad migraine, but was to find out instead that he had a malignant brain tumor. Two days later, he was rushed into surgery, and the resultant biopsy on his tumor came back with a diagnosis of "glioblastoma multiforme," stage IV.

Although Tom's surgeon said he had removed all of the cancer he could see, Tom was told he would probably only live about six months if he did *not* undergo post-operative radiation treatments, and only about a year if he *did* do the radiation. This prognosis was due to the reality that glioblastomas virtually always grow back quickly, even if all the "visible" tumor has been removed. And radiation is only a palliative treatment in these cases, not a curative one. Tom gave the radiation a try, but stopped it after only five days of treatments because it made him feel so awful.

Being Christians, Tom and his wife, Kelly, decided it was time to seek guidance, and they went to their church. They had Tom anointed with oil and hands laid on in prayer by the elders of the church (according to James 5:14). They also began to look into holistic methods of fighting cancer. After all, there was nothing conventional medicine could do that would offer him a chance of long-term cure.

Through other members of the church, Tom and Kelly then found out about Dr. Budwig's flaxseed oil and cottage cheese treatment and they started Tom on this in March 2002. For the first three months, Tom mixed 1/4 cup of lowfat (2 percent) cottage cheese with 1 tablespoon of flaxseed oil twice a day. Thus, every day he took a total of just 2 tablespoons of flaxseed oil with cottage cheese. He also took three 750 milligrams of shark cartilage capsules three times every day. On top of that, Kelly frequently rubbed frankincense oil on Tom's head because they had heard that this oil has anti-cancer properties.

Three months after his diagnosis and surgery, Tom's MRI looked very good. His brain was clean and the hole where they had removed the tumor was empty except for a tiny line around a portion of the inside. Tom's doctor thought this line could be either (1) scar tissue, (2) a benign bit of tumor, or (3) re-growth of the glioblastoma. After the three-month mark, Tom and Kelly added Graviola tincture to his daily regimen. (Tom took the Graviola for about nine months.) They also had Tom take daily supplements of borage seed oil, CoQ_{10}, and a barley/mineral supplement called "AIM Garden Trio." And he cut back on his intake of meat and sugar.

At the six-month mark, Tom had another MRI, and this time his brain was completely clean! There was no cancer visible anywhere. Tom's doctor said it was a miracle, and that in 14 years of practice, he had never seen anything like it. All of Tom's MRI's since then have been clean, and he just had his 18-month MRI. *Still no sign of cancer.*

Tom has been given his life back, and he and Kelly have posted his story on the Internet to help others. Their website address is: www.flax-oflife.com. They don't know what caused his brain tumor at such a young age, but they suspect that it may have been caused by artificial sweeteners. Before he was diagnosed, Tom had been regularly drinking at least 2 liters of diet soda every day. Now, of course, he no longer ingests artificial sweeteners, and he, Kelly, and their two children are *very* happy he found out about flaxseed oil and cottage cheese. Tom and Kelly feel very strongly that their prayers were answered and say, "We believe that the Lord provided all of the information to get Tom well and we have to give Him the Glory."

Cliff Beckwith reports that most of the people he has seen recover from cancer by using flaxseed oil and cottage cheese did *not* know about Dr. Budwig's other rigid dietary requirements. Thus, it appears that it is possible to get well without following her full strict protocol. But according to Cliff, some of those who did *not* keep up the flaxseed oil and cottage cheese after their cancer went away found themselves facing a recurrence of cancer in a few years. It is possible that if one does *not* follow Dr. Budwig's full dietary protocol for three to five years to fully heal the body, then one may have to stay on the daily flaxseed oil and cottage cheese indefinitely to avoid having their cancer come back.

Some experts believe that although flaxseed oil is effective in treating degenerative diseases, it might be too rich in omega-3 fatty acids to be used on a daily basis for more than five years. In other words, at some point, a person should go back to consuming a two-to-one ratio of omega-6's to omega-3's. Udo Erasmus, author of *Fats That Heal, Fats That Kill*, states that a person using flaxseed oil as their "sole" source of essential fatty acids will develop an omega-6 deficiency over time. He claims to have remedied this problem by creating his own mixed oil blend with added sunflower and sesame oils. This product is called "Udo's Choice Blend." It also contains the omega-9 essential fatty acids, and may be something to consider using once normal health has been regained.

However, it is rare that a person will be using the flaxseed oil as his or her sole source of EFAs. This is because most people do get some significant amounts of the omega-6 fatty acids from other dietary sources. For anyone wishing to check the levels of omega-3 and omega-6 fatty acids in their bodies, there is a laboratory in Asheville, North Carolina, that can tell you what your levels are from a simple blood test. (For contact information, see end of chapter.)

It is still somewhat unclear as to why Dr. Budwig chose flaxseed oil as the best way to replenish EFA deficiency when much of her research seemed to indicate that the omega-6 EFAs were the *more* important deficiency involved in cancer. It is speculated that, though the omega-6's are extremely important, we tend to be more deficient in omega-3's. This may be because there are numerous other vegetable oil sources of omega-6's in our diets. Thus, we tend to be much more deficient in omega-3 than omega-6. Regaining a balance between these two EFAs is very important in the process of regaining health. Dr. Budwig's clinical results from working with very ill people certainly proved that the flaxseed oil combination of essential fatty acids is extremely effective.

Treatment

Unfortunately, Dr. Budwig died in 2003 at the age of 94. She had suffered a fall from which she was unable to recover. Specific doctors or clinics that specialize in the use of Johanna Budwig's approach to healing are virtually impossible to find, so the flaxseed oil and cottage cheese diet is almost always a self-administered cancer therapy at this point. The one exception I found is Las Mariposas Clinic in Spain. It uses an omega-3 approach, along with other supportive non-toxic techniques, and I have heard they have a very high cure rate for cancer.

For those people who are not able to attend the Las Mariposas Clinic, there are some helpful Internet support groups dealing with the use of flaxseed oil and cottage cheese. These might be worth searching for and joining. To obtain more information about this approach, one can also search the Internet using the common abbreviations "FSO/CC," or "FO/CC." For people who are so ill that they are unable to hold down food, a daily enema of flaxseed oil and skim milk may be used until the person is strong enough to eat the cottage cheese and oil mixture.

Resources:

Las Mariposas Clinic   Phone: (34) 952-057171 or (34) 619 966281
Malaga, Spain   www.mariposasclinic.com

To Measure Your Omega-3 and Omega-6 Levels Contact:

Great Smokies Diagnostic Lab   800/522-4762, Ext. 343 or 828/253-0621
Clinical Support Department

Books

William L. Fischer. *How to Fight Cancer and Win.* Baltimore: Agora Health Books, 2000. (ISBN 1-891434-01-2)

Udo Erasmus. *Fats That Heal, Fats That Kill.* British Columbia, Canada: Alive Books, 1993. (ISBN 0-920470-38-6)

Dr. Johanna Budwig. *Flax Oil As a True Aid Against Arthritis, Heart Infarction, Cancer, and Other Diseases.* Vancouver, Canada: Apple Publishing, 1994. (ISBN 0-9695272-1-7)

Websites

www.whale.to/cancer/budwig.html

www.aspartame.ca/page_c1.htm

www.positivehealth.com/permit/Articles/Nutrition/turner60.htm

www.beckwithfamily.com

www.mnwelldir.org/docs/cancer1/budwig.htm

www.houseofsteed.com/sons/budwig.htm

www.road-to-health.com/news/36/budwig.htm

www.fatsthatheal.com

CHAPTER 15

The Rife Machine

I n this chapter, we will look at another of the early non-toxic cancer treatments. This treatment approach may have been one of the *most* effective methods of treating cancer ever developed, but for reasons that will be presented here, it is a difficult approach to recommend these days.

In the 1920s and 1930s, an American named Royal R. Rife developed an audio frequency-emitting device that, when directed at a person with cancer, was able to send frequencies into the person's body that would destroy micro-organisms he found to be causally associated with cancer. Over a number of months of treatments, cancer patients of all types got well. This approach involves a theory of cancer that we have not yet discussed in detail. The theory behind it has to do with the concept that certain types of micro-organisms are involved in the development of cancer. It may sound hard to believe, but the fact is that research by numerous highly respected scientists has supported this theory repeatedly.

To the misfortune of the entire world, Rife's approach was never fully accepted into mainstream medicine and never got into widespread use. However, there are still some forms of Rife Machines in existence today and some people claim to have achieved complete cancer recovery through their use. The current difficulty for cancer patients is determining *which* of the machines available today are similar enough to the original Rife Machine to be effective. It appears that *none* of the machines today is exactly the same as the one Royal Rife developed and used. Although some modern Rife Machines may be close to the original and be effective for some people, others may be quite far from authentic with little effectiveness.

Therefore, if you are considering using a Rife Machine for cancer, it is important to understand the history and issues to look into. Hopefully, someday, the original Rife method will be resurrected in all of its authentic aspects and will once again be available to the world.

History and Theory

Royal Raymond Rife was born in the late 1800s and was undoubtedly one of the great scientific geniuses of the 20th century. At a young age, he became interested in becoming a medical doctor and attended Johns Hopkins University to pursue this dream. During his studies, he realized he was really more interested in the field of bacteriology, and decided to specialize in that instead. Rife began photographing specimens for Heidelberg University, and because of his great contribution to that institution, he was awarded an "honorary" doctorate of parasitology in 1914.[1] Realizing the restrictions of microscope technology, Dr. Rife became very involved in the field of microscope development, and studied for a while with some of the world's top German microscope specialists.

Jobs in bacteriology were scarce, however, so when Dr. Rife returned to the United States he took a position as a chauffeur for a wealthy businessman in San Diego, California. This businessman was Henry Timkin, a leader in the ball-bearing industry. Timkin discussed with Rife some of the production problems he was having, and Dr. Rife was able to develop and machine a new type of motor for Timkin's business. The motor and other innovative improvements to Timkin's ball-bearing business ended up saving Timkins millions of dollars and, in appreciation, Timkin set up a life-time stipend for Dr. Rife.[2] The stipend's monthly payments allowed Rife to focus his efforts on his work in bacteriology. A number of other wealthy people also believed in Rife's abilities and helped finance a privately owned and fully equipped laboratory.

Finally free to do his work in microbiology without restriction, Rife began to experiment with a bold new idea he had been toying with — that of electrically stimulating various micro-organisms as a means of killing them. Rife then made a discovery that should have been heralded later in all the history books. He discovered that, by using audio frequencies, he could actually kill micro-organisms. Finding that different frequencies were required to kill different organisms, he named each specific frequency the "M.O.R.," or "Mortal Oscillatory Rate," for each particular organism.

Rife soon faced a big problem, however. He wanted to include viruses in his study and realized that, in order to see such small organisms, he would have to somehow get around a limiting problem. This was the problem that standard microscopes could only magnify up to

2,500 times diameter. It was a mechanical problem that resulted from how microscopes were made, and was due to the limiting factor that no micro-organism could be seen if it was smaller than half a wavelength of light in size.[3]

By 1920, Rife had solved this problem by single-handedly developing a new type of microscope. Rife's innovative microscope could magnify up to 9,000 diameters with clarity! This was far more powerful than any other microscope yet developed in his time. He then began seeing and categorizing forms of micro-organisms that had never been clearly observed by anyone before.

But Rife soon encountered another problem. There were even *more* micro-organisms that he and other researchers could not see because the organisms themselves were smaller than the molecules in the dyes or acids used to stain specimens for observation. To get around this problem, Rife devised and patented a totally new way to observe specimens under a microscope *without staining* by focusing on the spectrographic light properties which coordinated with the chemical makeup of the micro-organisms he was trying to study.[4] To do this, he employed numerous quartz lenses immersed in glycerin. What Rife did is difficult to explain in simple terms, but basically he figured out a way to "stain" his specimens with light instead of dye. Rife's new microscope was eight times more powerful than the best microscopes used by physicists of his day.

Throughout the 1920s, Dr. Rife kept searching in his laboratory for the cause of cancer. He believed it would be a virus-like organism. In 1932, he found two forms of just such an organism. One form, which he called "BX," was the organism that caused carcinomas, and the other form, called "BY," was the organism that caused sarcomas. He also found that this virus-like organism was pleomorphic. In other words, the cause of cancer was an organism that could take more than one form. In one form, it was benign and *not* cancer-causing—in another form it *was* cancer-causing.

As briefly mentioned in Chapter 2, "pleomorphism" was an idea argued by the 19th-century French scientist, Antoine Bechamp. In those early days of microbiology, Antoine Bechamp and Louis Pasteur were the leaders in a huge battle of ideas regarding the forms microbes could take. Pasteur believed that microbes were distinct organisms with distinct, or unchanging, characteristics. In other words, every microbe is either a particular form of bacteria, or a particular form of virus, yeast, or fungi throughout its life cycle, and there is *no* crossover between forms. Pasteur's theory of microbes is referred to as "monomorphism."

Bechamp, on the other hand, argued that micro-organisms may not necessarily be limited to one distinct form. In his view, micro-organisms were capable of being pleomorphic, or capable of having more than one form in a given life cycle. This meant that the *shape* of a microbe could drastically change (i.e., a rod-shaped bacteria could turn into a spheroid-shaped bacteria) and the *size* of a microbe could drastically change during the life-cycle of a single organism. Bechamp argued that micro-organisms could undergo these changes in response to the state of health of the host organism in which the microbe lived.[5] Bechamp believed that a bacteria could actually "devolve" into a much smaller form which he called "microzymia."[6] His theory of pleomorphism included the possibility that bacteria could turn into virus-sized organisms in some situations as a response to their environment.

A key turning point in history occurred when Pasteur's ideas won out, which caused monomorphism to become the basis of today's modern views in microbiology. But many reputable scientists of the 20th century have proven Bechamp's ideas of pleomorphism to be correct and have continued to debate the issue.

One important aspect of Rife's work to understand is that, in the early 1930s, viruses were just beginning to be defined. Scientists knew quite a bit about bacteria already and had devised special filters that could filter out certain bacteria from the media or environment they were in. The size of an average bacteria is about 1 micron (or 1/25,000 of an inch in length). But the largest virus is only about 1/4 to 1/3 this size.[7] This means that most viruses are too small to be seen by any normal light microscope. (Although they *can* be seen now under an electron microscope, the electron microscope kills the specimen, so they can not be seen in their *alive* state.)

Because viruses could not be seen in the early 1900s, scientists had to rely on the process of *filtering out* viruses from cultures and then detecting them by other means. The filtering process was done using filters with pores too small for bacteria to pass through. Scientists decided that anything that passed through these special filters *must* be something different from bacteria, and they referred to the organisms that passed through as "filtrable viruses." (Eventually, the word "filterable" was dropped and they were just called "viruses.") In the early days, this filtering process was the *only* way to designate the difference between bacteria and viruses. Although more ways of defining viruses have since become accepted, there is still debate as to whether certain organisms are actually viruses or bacteria, and some organisms previously categorized as viruses have since been proven to be "filtrable" bacteria instead.

Given the many shortcomings in microbiology in the 1930s, Dr. Rife's discoveries were phenomenal. He was not only able to *find* a micro-organism involved in the development of cancer for the first time in history, but he was also able to *prove* the organisms to be pleomorphic, with the smaller life-cycle forms having the characteristics of a virus! Eventually, Dr. Rife identified four distinct forms that this cancer-causing organism could take within its life cycle:[8]

1. The BX virus (cause of carcinoma)

2. The BY virus (cause of sarcoma and larger than BX)

3. Monococcoid form (can be seen through standard microscopes in the blood monocytes of more than 90 percent of cancer patients)

4. Crytomyces pleomorphia fungi

Amazingly, Dr. Rife was able to culture the BX cancer virus from a fungoid organism. He then used this virus to *directly* produce cancer in hundreds of laboratory animals. He also proved that any of the above four forms of one organism could change back into the BX cancer virus within 36 hours. In fact, he was able to complete the cycle of virus to cancer and back to virus 104 times. He could observe and document all of this with his powerful microscope, something other scientists could not do. There is no doubt that Rife found a micro-organism involved in the development of cancer. His discovery was verified and documented by other prominent microbiologists who visited his laboratory.

Even now, with the electron microscope, the back and forth culturing of a micro-organism from bacterial form to viral form *cannot* be observed because the electron microscope virtually destroys any virus that is put under it. What Dr. Rife discovered was—and still is—ground-breaking news. However, although he proved a micro-organism connection to cancer, he also discovered that this did not mean cancer is an "infectious" disease. The key is that the organism is pleomorphic and only takes a cancer-causing form when a person's inner environment, or state of health, is poor or unbalanced.

Royal Rife was not some unheard-of "kook" who did his work in some seedy cellar. Over the years, he was given 14 government awards for scientific discoveries, was visited and acclaimed by world experts in medicine and microbiology, and had his accomplishments written up in many newspapers and magazines. A prominent professor, Arthur I. Kendall, Ph.D., and a prominent physician, Milbank Johnson, M.D., soon began collaborating with Dr. Rife. Drs. Kendall and Rife both observed normal tuberculosis bacteria convert to a filtrable type of bacteria the size of a virus, something not previously observed. Dr. Kendall, Dr. Johnson, and many other medical specialists were *extremely* impressed with Dr. Rife's accomplishments and wholeheartedly supported his work.

But Dr. Rife did not stop at simply *finding* the pleomorphic micro-organism responsible for cancer—he also found a way to destroy it. To do this, Rife experimented with a wide variety of audio and light frequencies to find just the right frequency, or M.O.R., that would kill what he called the "cancer virus." He only used "sine waves," which are pure tones or frequencies. (Most sound is made up of a jumble of frequencies, as is most light. However, a sine wave is a single frequency.) X-ray tubes were the prominent medical technology of the day, so Rife worked with that mode of delivery. Once he found the cancer virsus's M.O.R., he could then deliver that devastating frequency to the organism. Rife could literally *see* cancer viruses moving around, alive, under his microscope, then briefly zap them with the correct frequency from his "ray tube," and immediately observe that all the viruses on the same slide, which had been moving around only seconds before, were now dead!

Since audio waves do not broadcast efficiently, more research and experimentation was required for Rife to be able to successfully deliver the mortal oscillatory rate of frequency to cancer organisms *deep* inside tissues of living animals. Rife solved this problem of delivery by using a "carrier wave." In other words, the audio frequency which turned out to be the specific M.O.R. for the cancer virus would not penetrate deep tissue, so Rife ingeniously modulated (or "piggy-backed") the desired audio frequency to another frequency that *could* penetrate deep tissue. (If he hadn't done this, he would have only been able to treat cancers on or near the surface of the body.) The two frequencies travel together but remain separate and distinct. Rife's records later showed that he used frequencies ranging from the audio range to 17MHz, and that he also experimented with many different carrier frequencies.

Rife's theory that the BX virus caused cancer was proved to be sound when he injected 411 laboratory mice with the BX virus and produced 411 corresponding tumors.[9] Then, he was able to use his ray tube to completely eliminate the cancers in many of these animals. Rife's method was *not* directed at the cancer cell itself. Rather, he found the BX or BY virus to be *inside* each malignant cancer cell, and that killing this micro-organism would cause the malignant cell to also die off.

In 1987, after doing a great deal of research, author Barry Lynes wrote the definitive book on Royal Rife and his cancer cure. This excellent book, *The Cancer Cure That Worked: Fifty Years of Suppression,* is packed with fascinating information and is available today and well worth reading. According to Barry Lynes, "By the end of 1932, Rife could destroy the typhus bacteria, the polio virus, the herpes virus, the cancer virus and other viruses in a culture and in experimental animals."[10]

In 1934, Dr. Milbank Johnson set up a committee of leading medical experts to oversee human trials in a southern California clinic where Rife could start treating terminally ill patients who had no other hope for cure. The initial results were astounding. In just 70 days of treatment, this committee of physicians pronounced 14 out of 16 patients with terminal cancer "cured." Thus, this first human trial showed a success of 87.5 percent. Moreover, after 60 more days of treatment, the remaining two patients from the original trial were also pronounced cured. This meant that within 130 days, or just a little over four months, all 16 terminally ill cancer patients were pronounced cured by the committee of medical experts![11] After this amazing success, other doctors obtained ray tubes and operated them in their own clinics with a success rate of about 90 percent.

The cancer treatment itself was totally non-toxic. It caused no tissue damage whatsoever, and a person receiving Rife's frequency treatment could not feel or hear anything. They merely saw a tube light up for three to five minutes, and the treatment was done. The only slightly toxic aspect of the treatment resulted from the die-off of the cancer micro-organisms. In fact, Rife discovered with his human cancer patients that the treatment was *most* effective when given at the rate of only three to five of minutes exposure to frequency *every other day.* This was because he found that if he treated his patients every day, the toxins released by the dead micro-organisms accumulated too fast in the patients' bodies and caused toxic overload.[12] When he limited treatment to every other day, however, patients responded with incredible recoveries.

During the 1930s, Rife collaborated with many cancer researchers and doctors. Several reputable physicians began using Rife's frequency instrument on their patients with great success. They began seeing cancers of all sorts disappear. They also observed other conditions unexpectedly resolving after treatments with the ray tube. These other conditions included syphilis and gonorrhea.[13]

But the original ray tube Dr. Rife built was too cumbersome and expensive to market to doctors and clinics worldwide. It filled almost a whole room. So he signed an agreement with business colleagues to form a company called Beam Ray Corporation that would begin building Dr. Rife's frequency instruments for the purpose of selling them to medical practitioners. But unfortunately, not all of the businessmen involved were conscientious enough to make sure the machines were built correctly, according to Rife's specifications. His first business partner, Philip Hoyland, built the machines to emit *harmonics* of frequencies in order to save money, rather than building them to just emit specific, clean frequencies. Beam Ray Corporation's machines understandably performed poorly and Dr. Rife was not happy with what the corporation was doing.

Then, events took place that ended up bringing about the final downfall of the Rife frequency technology. These events began when Morris Fishbein, the head of the AMA, tried to buy into Beam Ray Corporation. Basically, Fishbein was attempting to take control for his own financial gain, but he only wanted to give Royal Rife a small royalty on the machines. (This was the same man who had tried to gain ownership of the Hoxsey therapy for his own profit.) After all Dr. Rife's work, the business deal Fishbein offered was scandalous. Dr. Rife refused Fishbein's business deal, and as a result, Fishbein went all out to destroy Beam Ray Corporation. The AMA filed expensive lawsuits and Beam Ray went bankrupt as a result of legal battles. To complicate matters, Philip Hoyland reportedly turned against Rife and also tried to take over total control of Beam Ray Corporation. Court transcripts from a 1938 trial show that Hoyland even tried to claim that he was the originator of some of the technology, instead of Rife.

Later, in the 1950s and early 1960s, Dr. Rife worked with another man, John Crane, with whom he formed a company called "Life Labs." They modified the technology again to produce a slightly different version of his instrument. This one was also portable but used round disks that came in contact with the body. But once again, although Dr. Rife was director of research, Crane disregarded some of his suggestions. Then, Crane started making changes he did not tell anyone about. For instance, he lowered Rife's frequencies *by a factor of 10* so that the machines would fall below the 10,000 hertz level. It is believed that Crane did this to avoid FCC regulations that were in place at the time. This drastic lowering of frequencies meant that the 1950s Rife machines could no longer achieve the impressive results of Rife's earlier 1930s technology.

Thus, Life Labs Rife Machines were not working as well as they could have. At the same time, Morris Fishbein was continuing to do everything he could to stifle Dr. Rife's technology. Doctors were put under pressure from the AMA to *not* use Rife's machines anymore. As with

Harry Hoxsey's herbal remedy, Morris Fishbein used his power as head of the AMA to stop any progress on treating cancer that he could not profit from. Then, with just the right timing to put the final blow on Dr. Rife's technology, penicillin and other marketable antibiotics began to take the limelight in medicine. Since Rife had refused to sell Beam Ray Corporation to Fishbein, Fishbein made sure that the AMA pushed the concept of fighting diseases with antibiotics rather than with Rife's technology. Fighting microbes with frequencies soon fell out of medical favor.

But Dr. Rife did not give up. He continued to improve his machine, and in the 1950s, he tried again to get the medical community interested in his methods. Dr. Rife had developed a smaller and less expensive form of equipment to try to entice doctors to buy them. Unfortunately, doctors were still being influenced to use antibiotics, and the medical community never showed significant interest in Dr. Rife's technology again. In 1971, Rife died without ever seeing a widespread use of his incredibly successful method of treating cancer.

In his book, *The Cancer Cure That Worked*, Barry Lynes sums up Morris Fishbein's influence as follows:

> . . . within the few, short years from 1934 to 1939, the cure for cancer was clinically demonstrated and expanded into curing other diseases on a daily basis by other doctors, and then terminated when Morris Fishbein of the AMA was not allowed to "buy in." It was a practice he had developed into a cold art, but never again would such a single mercenary deed doom millions of Americans to premature, ugly deaths.[14]

Partly as a result of Barry Lynes's book, an "underground" interest in the Rife Machine sprang up once more in the late 1980s and 1990s. Many different engineers started building Rife Machines according to blueprints and records from Rife's original papers. I have heard both pros and cons about current-day Rife Machines, some seeming to work well and others seeming to not work at all.

One problem is that many of the modern frequency machines claiming to be Rife Machines do *not* use a carrier wave at all. Yet, the carrier wave was an important aspect of Rife's technology and the only way to get the M.O.R. to deep tissue cancers. Another problem is that some current-day machines use technology that does not transfer the frequencies properly. Even though the specific frequencies that Rife discovered to be M.O.R.s for many different organisms and diseases are actually presented on the Internet, the method of delivery is critical for these frequencies to be effective. And this appears to be the reason many modern Rife devices are not as effective as they could be.

It is worth mentioning once more that, although Rife found a micro-organism to be a causal factor to cancer, this did *not* mean he was proving cancer to be an infectious disease. In fact, it is likely that the cancer-causing micro-organism Dr. Rife identified is within each and every one of us. Rife agreed with and confirmed Bechamp's earlier theory that it is a body's *inner* environment which ultimately influenced which form the pleomorphic cancer organism would take. If a person's inner environment was healthy, then it would remain in its harmless form. If, on the other hand, a person's inner environment was *not* healthy, it could devolve into one of the forms that might cause cancer. (See the next section on 714X for a similar conclusion made by the French hematologist, Gaston Naessens.)

Thus, to some extent, both Rife and Antoine Bechamp looked at various pleomorphic forms of bacteria as the "symptom" of disease, not the "cause" of disease. Royal Rife, himself, said:

> In reality, it is not the bacteria themselves that produce the disease, but the chemical constituents of these micro-organisms enacting upon the unbalanced cell metabolism of the human body that in actuality produce the disease. We also believe if the metabolism of the human body is perfectly balanced or poised, it is susceptible to no disease.[15]

Thus, it is best to *not* conclude from this chapter that cancer is a disease that can be "caught" by being near someone who has cancer. Instead, we need to realize that our common ideas about how micro-organisms are linked to diseases have been molded by one narrow viewpoint—that of monomorphism. We must be open to the reality that ideas in science get molded by various ideas of the times. Barry Lynes makes the very astute observation that Pasteur's view that all micro-organisms are monomorphic probably won out for two main reasons: (1) It was a simpler theory and much easier to understand, and (2) it applied more directly to *infectious* diseases which were the biggest problem of that era. (I would also add that monomorphism won out as the reigning viewpoint in part because no one had a microscope capable of "seeing" micro-organisms change from one form to another.)

It is time for medical science to rethink its reigning theories, especially since a huge problem of *our era* happens to be chronic degenerative disease in its many forms—and some degenerative diseases may be better explained by Bechamp's theory of pleomorphism.

Last but not least, scientists still need to have the right type of microscope in order to view pleomorphism, and even today that type of microscope is not prevalent. Rife's "universal microscope" was virtually lost to medical science, and I have heard that there is only one original Rife microscope left in existence today. According to Barry Lynes, the powerful Memorial Sloan-Kettering Cancer Center in New York is currently a leading institutional opponent of the concept of pleomorphism—even though, in 1975, Sloan-Kettering's *own* studies reportedly showed pleomorphic bacteria-virus in *all* of their cancer blood tests. According to Barry Lynes, Sloan-Kettering *buried* these laboratory results.[16]

Although the average person probably believes that modern medical practices are always based on "true science," there is a great deal of evidence indicating otherwise. A certain amount of medical practice is based on professional biases and profit margins of big business.

Antibiotics were highly profitable for pharmaceutical companies to market. They also happened to work quite well for infectious diseases, so it was easy for doctors and the public to wholeheartedly support them. But the downsides to antibiotics are showing up more and more with virulent drug-resistant bacteria becoming more prevalent and side effects to antibiotics taking their toll. Medical frequency technology, such as Rife created, is much cleaner with no side effects, and does not create drug-resistant bacteria. Moreover it works on viruses, which antibiotics and modern medicine *still* have not been able to fully conquer.

It is very interesting to note that, in the May 2003 issue of *Reader's Digest*, there is an article about some new and promising treatments for breast cancer. On pages 64–67, the article talks about one of these "new" treatments, called "RFA" (radiofrequency ablation). RFA is a recently developed technique whereby a probe is inserted into or next to a tumor and a certain radio frequency is then emitted for about 23 minutes. With an ultrasound, the technician performing this procedure can then see the dark tumor mass become the same grainy gray as the rest of the breast tissue. Surgeons can then simply go in and remove the tumor, which has become dead tissue.

This *Reader's Digest* article states that RFA has also been used on liver cancer since the early1990s, and is currently being tried on breast, kidney, and lung cancer. One study at Houston's MD Anderson Cancer Center is referred to where 20 women with breast tumors were treated with RFA. This study was small but achieved great success. Out of the 20 subjects, 19 were shown to have had the cancer completely killed! The current success of RFA shows that Rife's frequency technology was based on sound principles, but I wonder if Rife's discoveries will ever be given credit. No mention of Rife is made in the *Reader's Digest* article and the modern RFA procedure is referred to as "experimental." Too bad the article does not mention that an even more powerful form of frequency treatment for cancer was administered totally noninvasively as far back as the 1930s.

Maybe one day, we will yet again have Rife's original technology available to us. Until then, I strongly recommend that if you are considering using a Rife Machine type of device for cancer, you should thoroughly research the *specific* device you are considering using, and *make sure that it has been used successfully by other people for your type of cancer.*

Resources:

Book

Barry Lynes. *The Cancer Cure That Worked!* Ontario, Canada: Marcus Books, 1987. (ISBN 0-919951-30-9)

Video

"The Royal Rife Story: Historical Documentary," 60 minutes. To order, call (800) 550-5119. [This is an excellent production packed with fascinating information.]

Websites

www.biolectric.ws/eng/pplo.html

www.scoon.co.uk/Electrotherapy/Rife/BeamRay/

www.scoon.co.uk/Electrotherapy/Rife/BeamRay/Analysis/index.htm

www.Rife-Crane-Rockwell.com

CHAPTER 16

714X

nother unique and fascinating approach that also addresses the relationship of micro-organisms to cancer is 714X. It was developed by Gaston Naessens, a French biologist. In France, Naessens developed two anti-cancer products that created quite a stir. One was called "Ana-Blast" and the other was called "GN-24." In 1964, Naessens emigrated to Quebec and introduced his innovative treatments to Canada. In the 1970s, Naessens replaced Ana-Blast and GN-24 by what he called 714X, which has now been used by thousands of people to help them recover from cancer and other degenerative conditions. Considered by many to be a genius, Naessens has become known in the world of alternative cancer treatments as "French Canada's Wizard."

Naessens's personal background illustrates his creative intellect. He was born in 1924 and, as young as five years old, built a small functional, automobile-like vehicle. Next, he built a homemade motorcycle. At age 12, Naessens built an air plane that flew![1] When Naessens was old enough to attend college, he studied physics, chemistry, and biology, and later went on to study hematology (the study of blood).

Early on, Naessens had a "premonition" of sorts that there were tiny particles moving around in blood. But with normal light microscopes of the 1940s, nothing like that could be clearly discerned. So, like Royal Rife, Naessens decided a more powerful microscope (in terms of resolving power) was needed and he enlisted the aid of some German optical specialists to manufacture aluminum mirrors for him. The optical specialists were not aware of what Naessens was going to do with the mirrors, but they were to go in the new microscope that Naessens was developing.

Naessens's new microscope, which he called the "Somatoscope," was much more powerful than any other light microscope in use at the time. It used an innovative combination of laser and ultraviolet light technology and produced a magnification of 30,000 times with a resolution of

150 angstroms! Any light microscope with a darkfield condenser can observe live material, so that aspect of the Somatoscope was not unique. However, the conventional field of hematology has generally shown little interest in observing live material and the observation of living specimens has been a foreign concept to their staining methods. The Somatoscope did *not* require staining a sample before viewing it as other microscopes did, and this made a big difference in observing living organisms in blood.

The ability to observe behavior and life cycles of living microscopic organisms in blood made the Somatoscope in some ways superior to the electron microscope, which was developed later. As mentioned in the previous chapter, the electron microscope can achieve much higher magnification (enlargements into the millions of times), but can only observe dead or static specimens. Thus, it is of little value in observing actual behavior changes or life cycle changes that might occur in microscopic organisms.

Using his special microscope, Naessens was able to study the tiny blood particles he had previously noticed. He could now observe them with detail and clarity in their living state. Eventually, he identified a number of different micro-organisms that he concluded were all stages of development for one sub-cellular organism commonly found in blood. Naessens called this organism a "somatid." He believed that somatids were distinct from bacteria and viruses and, because he could observe these organisms in their alive state, he was able to discern two separate life cycles for them. One life cycle tended to occur in the blood of *healthy* people and the other life cycle tended to occur in the blood of *unhealthy* people. (This corresponds closely to what Royal Rife discovered.)

In healthy individuals, the somatids appeared to display what Naessens called a "microcycle" consisting of three different forms the somatids would take. In *unhealthy* individuals, however, the somatids appeared to display a much longer "macrocycle," consisting of 16 different forms that the somatids would take. This macrocycle was a more complex life cycle that Naessens observed in the blood of people with degenerative diseases. Naessens theorized that somatids play an important role in the body and that it is normal for them to be found in everyone's blood in their *microcycle* life stages. But he theorized, when somatids are exposed to trauma, such as pollution, radiation, and so forth, they can then enter into a wild and uncontrolled growth cycle (the macrocycle), which can lead to cancer.[2]

Just as interesting as Naessens's find that somatids have different life cycles in healthy versus unhealthy people was his discovery that somatids are *everywhere* in nature and seem to be an integral part of everything. In the human body, he found that somatids play a role in the cell division process of normal cells. According to one source,

> What Naessens discovered was that somatids were everywhere, in the sap of plants, in the blood of animals, and even in lifeless organic matter like ashes. When he cultured the somatid life cycle, he discovered that somatids are resistant to acids and bases as well as heat and that they cannot be cut with a diamond. Cell division cannot take place without the somatid. Somatid, according to Naessens's theory, releases the growth hormone trephone, which enables cells to divide and multiply. Naessens believes that the electrically charged somatid is the original spark of life, the point in which energy condenses into matter.[3]

In other words, Naessens believed somatids to be "basic living particles indispensable to life,"[4] and by culturing the somatids and using his special microscope he could verify their "micro" and "macro" cycles. (Apparently, other scientists who observe these same particles with normal microscopes generally refer to them as "fibrin formations.") In terms of how they are involved in the division of normal healthy cells, Naessens's theory proposes that when somatids are in their healthy three-stage microcycle, they produce just the right amount of a growth hormone-like substance. This substance keeps healthy body cells reproducing at their correct rate. Naessens called this hormone-like substance "trefons." However, when a person's body is seriously stressed or weakened, then the somatid shifts into its longer "unhealthy" 16-stage macrocycle that includes forms resembling bacteria, viruses and yeasts. In this extended cycle, the somatids produce excessive amounts of trefons and cause normal, healthy body cells to undergo abnormally fast cell growth, which can then develop into cancer.

Naessens theorized that a healthy body can hold somatids to their three-phase cycle by having ample "blood inhibitors" to keep the somatids functioning normally. These blood inhibitors in a healthy person consist of certain enzymes, hormones, and minerals. Naessens believed that inadequate nutrition and stress could *reduce* the amounts of these inhibitors in the blood and thus allow somatids to shift into their longer 16-phase cycle.

Naessens's theory of reduced blood inhibitors being a contributing factor to cancer is consistent with many of the nutritional deficiency theories of cancer development. And his observation that, at different life cycle stages, the somatids could resemble either bacteria, yeasts, or fungi, is also consistent with many findings over the last century that have indicated a connection between cancer and various bacteria, yeasts, or fungi.

Thus, there was no doubt in Naessens's mind that the somatid microbes were involved in the development of cancer, but it was not in the way that we normally think of microbial involvement. As Dr. Rife's research suggested, Naessens's research also suggested a type of "pleomorphism" whereby common microbes (somatids) in every person's body could, under certain conditions, *change into a different form of microbe that can cause cancer*. Some of these forms could be so different from the original microbe that, to any observer, it would appear that a common bacteria was actually "pleomorphing" into a virus or fungus.

An important aspect of Naessens's discovery was that when the somatids switched to their longer life cycles as a result of trauma and/or not enough blood inhibitors to control them, they then started secreting *excess* amounts of their hormone-like substance, which would cause cells to replicate too fast. The resultant effect would be a conglomerate of cells multiplying at an accelerated rate in close proximity to each other and beginning to form a tumor.

Once Naessens had formulated his theory on how cancer gets started, what was the solution he came up with? To understand this, we have to understand another interesting fact Naessens observed. He realized that fast-replicating cancer cells required much more *nitrogen* to survive than normal cells do and that they would often "steal" the nitrogen away from healthy cells in order to subsist. Naessens also observed that, in a healthy body, the immune system usually attacks and destroys any out-of-control conglomerate of cancer cells before the conglomerate gets too big. But if this group of renegade cells is able to reach a "critical mass," then the conglomerate of cells (or tumor) starts to act like its own *entity* and begins to emit a substance Naessens called "Co-carcinogenic K Factor" (CKF). Theoretically, CKF paralyzes the immune system by masking the cancer cells from recognition by the body's defenses. CKF thus frees the young tumor from attack by the body and the cancer cells are able to steal as much nitrogen as they need from surrounding healthy cells.

Naessens felt that if he could *stop* cancer cells from producing this Co-carcinogenic K Factor, then a person's immune system would be able to recognize and attack the cancer cells. He did this by developing an aqueous solution he called 714X. 714X is an innovative mixture of camphor, nitrogen and mineral salts specifically created to supply the cancer cells of the body with the extra nitrogen they need so the tumor does not have to excrete CKF in an attempt to obtain more nitrogen. When it does not secrete CKF, it is not hidden from the immune system and the body's own defenses can then attack the cancer. Thus, the main way that 714X works against cancer is not by directly killing cancer cells, but by debilitating the cancer's ability to mask itself. The immune system then kills the cancer cells.

Naessens found that camphor has a special affinity for cancer cells, so he used natural camphor as the base to carry the nitrogen to the cancer. Naessens also included ammonium salts in 714X because he believed that they could help to liquefy the lymph fluid and increase lymphatic flow. This could help the lymph system deal with toxins better and could activate certain "kinins" that inhibit abnormal cell growth.[5] Also found in the product are 18 different minerals in trace element form.

Gaston Naessens designed 714X to improve the natural defenses of the body and to stimulate the immune system. It does *not* kill abnormal or cancerous cells, but rather helps the body defend against them and heal from degenerative diseases and immune-deficiency disorders. 714X is administered by injection directly into the lymph system. As a general agent for healing, it performs two distinct functions:

1. It removes toxins from circulation by liquefying the lymphatic fluid.

2. It helps the body to repair itself.

714X is not a cytotoxic product, such as chemotherapy, and can be used safely for any length of time with no negative side effects. Injections are self-administered just under the skin with a very small 3/8-inch needle and "perinodally" around a lymph node in the groin area. It is sold by Cerbe Distribution, Inc., located in Quebec, Canada. The product comes with very clear instructions on how to use it, and Cerbe also offers a phone service that answers inquiries.

The use of 714X involves a perinodular injection once a day for 21 days straight. After two days of rest, the injections are repeated again for 21 days, and this cycle is repeated over and over until one is disease-free. The perinodular injections are the *main* treatment and cover the main large lymphatic circulation. In some circumstances, where the disease is localized in the upper body and/or in the upper right areas, 714X may be given by inhalation as well to cover the small lymphatic circulation. This inhalation, or nebulizer method, is considered an "add-on" treatment to be used along with the injection, not instead of it. The nebulizer add-on is recommended when there is cancer in the right breast, the lungs, the esophagus, or anywhere in the head.

How long the treatment takes for each individual will vary. This is partly because each person metabolizes the product at his or her own pace, and also because the body tends to "clean" itself before repairing itself. Thus, the more a person has used toxic treatments such as chemotherapy or radiation prior to starting 714X, the more cleaning out needs to be done by the body before repair can begin. It is probably safe to say that the prognosis is best when 714X is started immediately after diagnosis. 714X can also be used safely while doing conventional cancer treatments, and in those cases, it can reduce the side effects of the toxic treatments. Cerbe Distribution recommends that 714X be used for a minimum of six to eight consecutive cycles when a confirmed cancer diagnosis has been received. Once a person is cancer-free, then a maintenance program of one or two cycles twice a year is recommended.

There is no doubt that 714X has brought about truly astounding recoveries for many people with late-stage cancer. Most of these people had reached the point where their disease was *not* responding to conventional treatments and their doctors had no other options to offer them. Many of these remarkable case stories have been documented by physicians or other reliable sources, and many others can be found throughout the Internet. Some examples that I found are the following:

Jacques Viens was 39 years old when he had seven-eighths of his stomach removed, according to writer Stephanie Hiller. The cancer had already spread to the lymph. Since there seemed to be no hope of recovery, his doctor offered him 714X. Four months after taking 714X he was healthy enough to go hunting and soon resumed his job. Marcel Caron had intestinal cancer but refused to have his intestine removed. His wife's breast cancer had been successfully treated with 714X and so he tried it as well. Sixty-five days after he started treatment, no cancer was found in Caron's body. Eight years later he is still healthy. Anne Vignal, wife of the former French Counsel General in Quebec, sought out medical opinions and was told she could not conceive children. She was also told that her infertility was due to a lethal form of leukemia and she had only three to five years to live. She took 714X. She is now cancer-free and the mother of a healthy son.[6]

The story of a 17-year-old boy named Luke Stevens is yet another remarkable story. In August 1995, Luke (the son of a South African chiropractor) developed a giant cell tumor on his knee. This grew so rapidly that it destroyed most of Luke's upper tibia. According to one source, "Surgeons removed the tumor and rebuilt the boy's tibia. Four months later, Mr. Stevens's body rejected his bone graft and the tumor returned with a vengeance, breaking through the skin and growing into a hideous, fist-sized mass. Stevens's father grew disillusioned with oncologists, ignoring their advice to amputate his son's leg and begin massive chemotherapy."[7]

Luke's father found out about 714X and his son began that treatment instead of undergoing amputation and chemotherapy. Luke's condition rapidly improved and, according to the same source as above, "the tumor disappeared. Subsequent X-rays documented 100 percent bone regeneration, considered medically impossible. Today, at 21, Mr. Stevens attends university and rows on his school's team. He gives all the credit to Dr. Naessens's therapy."[8] About two-and-one-half years after he was diagnosed with cancer, Luke's diagnostic tests showed him to be cancer-free and he has been cancer-free ever since.

Here are 714X testimonies from two different physicians:

> Dr. Florianne Pier, a Belgian physician, reported that over a four-month period she had treated seven cancer patients with 714X. "The product prolonged the lives, and eased the deaths, of two terminally afflicted patients," she said, "and has allowed the other five who came to me with seriously advanced cancerous states, to see every one of their symptoms disappear and to take up their lives as if they had never incurred the disease."[9]

> Dr. Raymond Brown of New York City, a former Sloan-Kettering cancer researcher, told a pretrial press conference how he had treated one of his own patients with 714X for a pancreatic cancer that had proven resistant to all other forms of treatment. Naessens's therapy had prolonged the patient's life well over expectancy and kept him free of side effects, he said. Dr. Brown declared that while 714X was not a panacea, it deserved a place in the arsenal of weapons available to official medicine.[10]

In Canada, 714X is still not a fully approved cancer treatment. It is only allowed for use against cancer "on an emergency basis" through the Canadian government's Special Access Program. This means that any Canadian physician wishing to *officially* use 714X for a cancer patient must request special authorization to do so on compassionate grounds. Since January 1990, when 714X was introduced as an emergency drug in Canada, to June 2003, 18,366 authorizations were given to 1,684 doctors to use 714X on behalf of 4,030 patients.

714X can also be obtained by individuals outside of Canada *without* a physician's authorization. Although 714X is not approved as a cancer treatment in the United States, people in the United States can order this non-toxic compound by simply phoning Cerbe Distribution in Quebec and having it mailed to them. The promise of cancer recovery through this form of treatment is somewhat difficult to ascertain for any particular person, and may have a lot to do with how soon one starts to use it after diagnosis. Unfortunately, since the law in Canada only allows 714X to be prescribed by doctors as an emergency drug, it is often given to patients who are so far along in their disease that they are beyond recovery through any means. However, even in these cases, 714X has often been known to improve the patient's quality of life (less pain, more appetite, more energy, etc.). In these cases, there is no risk associated with using 714X because there are no adverse side effects.

Many of the full recoveries involving 714X have been achieved without any other treatment used. But there have also been people who achieved remarkable recoveries when they combined 714X with other alternative, non-toxic treatments. For example, there is one well-known story of a teenage boy, named Billy Best, who was cured of his Hodgkin's lymphoma in just two and one-half months by the combined use of 714X, Essiac tea, nutritional supplements, and a healthy diet. His story is presented at www.grand-strand.com/suebest/.

As we have seen with many other effective alternative non-toxic cancer treatments, the general rule is that there will be attempts at suppression. Gaston Naessens, unfortunately, had to deal with this as well. In the mid-1950s, Naessens started to have trouble with the medical authorities in France. When his unorthodox methods began having incredible success in the 1960s, his laboratory was closed by these authorities, his equipment was confiscated, and he was fined for practicing medicine without a license. This prompted Naessens to move to Canada in 1964 where he was able to continue his work for a number of years in a privately funded laboratory outside Montreal. However, in 1989, Naessens was brought to trial by the Quebec medical authorities. It was a long and difficult trial where testimony was heard from both patients and physicians who had used 714X for cancer, AIDS, and other degenerative conditions. Dozens of demonstrators rallied outside the courthouse throughout the proceedings and carried banners in support of Naessens.

Some impressive cancer recovery stories were brought to light throughout the court battle. For example, one man named Roland Caty testified that he had been diagnosed with adenosarcoma of the prostate. His conventional doctor recommended he have all of his sexual organs removed. When Roland refused, his doctor told him he'd be dead in three months. Instead, Roland began to inject himself with 714X and achieved a complete recovery. At the trial, Roland Caty told the press, "And here I am testifying to you, eleven years after I got well."[11]

Marcel Caron, another ex-cancer patient, testified with his story. Marcel had been diagnosed with cancerous intestinal polyps eight years earlier. As with Roland Caty, surgery was recommended to Marcel by his conventional doctors. However, Marcel refused because his brother had died after surgery years before for the very same condition. According to Marcel's court testimony, he used 714X instead, and after just 21 days of treatment he was cancer-free.[12]

Fortunately, this trial resulted in acquittal for Naessens in December of that same year (1989). In fact, the jury turned in "not-guilty" verdicts on all counts. In January 1990, the Canadian Federal Government then hurriedly introduced 714X for use as an Emergency Drug.

So, how has Canada's powerful neighbor, the United States, reacted to 714X? In 1974, Dr. Raymond Brown from New York's Memorial Sloan-Kettering Cancer Center visited Gaston Naessens and investigated 714X. He was *very* favorably impressed and wrote an extremely enthusiastic memorandum about Naessens's work. Below is an excerpted paragraph from what Dr. Brown wrote:

> What I have seen is a microscope that reveals with spectacular clarity the motion and multiplicity of pleomorphic organisms in the blood which are intimately associated with disease states. The implications . . . are staggering . . . It is imperative that what its inventor, a dedicated biological scientist, is doing be totally reviewed. I am convinced that he is an authentic genius and that his achievements cut across and illumine some of the most pertinent areas of medical science.[13]

At first, Memorial Sloan-Kettering was reportedly very interested in Dr. Brown's report, at first. But then they supposedly lost interest in pursuing 714X. Some speculations are that Sloan-Kettering dropped their interest in 714X like a hot potato when they found out that the American Cancer Society had "blacklisted" Naessens. Apparently, the American Cancer Society was Sloan-Kettering's biggest monetary contributor in the 1970s.

Then, in 2001, the U.S. National Cancer Institute suddenly put 714X on a "fast-track" for review. This was supposedly in response to patients in Massachusetts and media reporters making allegations that an investigation of 714X had been covered up the Dana-Farber Cancer Institute in Boston. In August 2001, Cerbe, Inc. submitted 16 in-depth cases of patients who had used 714X successfully for long-term recovery. Gaston Naessens and his wife, Jacinte Naessens, attended a press conference in Boston, and were accompanied by successfully treated 714X patients.

One of these patients, 14-year-old Katie Hartley, spoke at the press conference. In April 1995, when Katie was seven years old, she was diagnosed with a malignant tumor (undifferentiated sarcoma) that was growing inside her head. It was first noticed when one of Katie's eyes started to protrude from its socket. The sarcoma was the size of a tangerine, and Katie's doctors from the Dana Farber Cancer Institute prescribed chemotherapy. Katie went through nine of the 13 weeks of chemo that had been prescribed. She had to stop it early because of debilitating side effects of the treatment.

Next, Katie went through six weeks of radiation, after which she was too weak to continue any further conventional treatment. Her tumor began to grow again and her doctors sent her home and told her family that she only had a couple of weeks to live. Katie's mother frantically searched for other options, and in January 1996, started her on 714X. They gave her injections in the morning and nebulizer treatments at night. A year and a half later, tests showed that Katie's cancer was completely gone.[14]

The NCI's Office of Cancer Complementary and Alternative Medicine (OCCAM) initially was responsible for the review of 714X. After that, it was supposed to go to the Cancer Advisory Panel for Complementary Alternative Medicine (CAPCAM). At this point in time, it is unclear as to what the results of the NCI investigation have been.

714X is extremely inexpensive compared to conventional cancer approaches and costs about 300 U.S. dollars per 21-day cycle. The number of cycles required for recovery will vary from case to case, but is usually six to eight cycles, or until conventional tests show remission. No significant dietary changes are required, though it is recommended to reduce one's intake of red meat and dairy products. In terms of other supplements that may or may not be used in conjunction with this treatment, it is merely suggested that people using 714X stay away from supplementation of the following: vitamin E, vitamin B_{12}, and all antiangiogenic herbs or drugs (e.g., bindweed, shark or bovine cartilage, or thalidomide). The amount of vitamin E or B_{12} ingested from a normal diet, however, is fine.

Gaston Naessens is considered by many to be a great contributor to the field of microbiology, and his work impacts the treatment of not only cancer, but other terrible diseases including HIV/AIDS as well. (These other applications of 714X are beyond the scope of this book.) Christopher Bird, co-author of the best-selling book *The Secret Life of Plants*, wrote a detailed book about Gaston Naessens and his struggles with organized medicine. His book is called *The Persecution and Trial of Gaston Naessens: The True Story of the Efforts to Suppress an Alternative Treatment for cancer, AIDS, and Other Immunologically Based Diseases*.

For those people who have used 714X for cancer, the recoveries have sometimes been astounding. Thus, this non-toxic cancer treatment approach is definitely worth considering.

Resources:

CERBE Distribution, Inc. (819) 564-7883
5270 Mills Street, Rock Forest www.cerbe.com
Quebec, J1N 3B6
Canada

Book

Christopher Bird. *The Persecution and Trial of Gaston Naessens*. Tiburon, California: H. J. Kramer, 1991. (ISBN 0-915811-30-8)

Video

For around $10, you can purchase an information and instruction video about 714X by calling the above phone number.

Self-Treatment at Home: 714X is relatively inexpensive and costs only about $300 per month (and an extra $150 for those who also need to use the nebulizer). The number of months of treatment will vary for each individual.

Websites

www.cerbe.com/en/web_review.html

www.healing.bc.ca/therapy_714x.shtml

www.sph.uth.tmc.edu/utcam/therapies/714x.htm

www.luminet.net/~wenonah/new/naessens.htm

www.sonic.net/sentinel/gvcon4.html

www.grand-strand.com/suebest/boywho.htm

www.bccancer.bc.ca/pg_g_05.asp?PageID=1708&ParentID=2

www.cancerinform.freewebsites.com/naessens.html

www.prevention.com/cda/feature/0,1204,3847,00.html

CHAPTER 17

Cesium High pH Therapy

C esium high pH therapy is yet another powerful and highly impressive approach for outsmarting your cancer. For cancers outside the brain, this alternative, non-toxic treatment must certainly be considered one of the best. It has brought about incredible recoveries for people with primary cancers as well as for late-stage, metastasized cancers. (This approach may also work well for people with cancer in the brain, but ample evidence that cesium effectively crosses the blood/brain barrier is not yet available.)

The good news is that cesium high pH therapy is *particularly* effective at reducing large tumors quickly and also at quickly reducing the severe pain that often accompanies advanced cancer. Thus, for people whose disease is so far advanced that they may not have time for another alternative approach to work, or are in such severe pain that they are on heavy narcotics, which may be shutting down their bodily functions, cesium high pH therapy may be their best treatment option.

Like Protocel, this approach specifically targets anaerobic cells. But, whereas Protocel interferes with the cell respiration process of cancer cells until they no longer have enough energy to hold themselves together, cesium high pH therapy directly raises the alkalinity within cancer cells until they can no longer function. The premise for this approach is based on the fact that anaerobic cancer cells are also much more acidic than normal, healthy cells and must maintain their acidic intracellular environment in order to survive.

Cesium high pH therapy has been known about and used to treat cancer since the 1980s. But it has recently been made easier and more effective as a treatment with the development of "liquid ionic minerals." And as you will see, it is because of this liquid ionic form of cesium that this approach is now taking off and bringing about truly astounding recoveries for cancer patients.

History and Theory

The pioneer of cesium high pH therapy was physicist Aubrey Keith Brewer, Ph.D. Dr. Brewer lived from 1893 to 1986 and was a highly esteemed American physicist who focused his research on the study of cell membranes. For a period of time, he held the position of chief of the National Bureau of Standards Mass Spectrometer and Isotope section.

Dr. Brewer proved with spectrographic analysis that cancer cells have an *affinity* for cesium—meaning they readily absorb cesium through their cell walls. (The fact that cancer cells have an affinity for cesium is also evidenced by the current-day use of a radioactive isotope of cesium as a common marker in conventional oncology for tracing how well chemotherapy agents get into tumors.)

Dr. Brewer developed his theory of how cancer could be treated with cesium (the non-radioactive form) based on his understanding of the physics of cell membranes and the fact that cesium is the most alkaline mineral. He wrote a number of scientific articles on his theory, and in the late 1970s, initiated animal research studies at three U.S. universities—first using rubidium (the second most alkalizing mineral), then using cesium salts. All three university studies proved that high pH therapy was, indeed, effective against malignant tumors in mice. In fact, these tests showed marked shrinkage of mice tumors within just two weeks. Then, in 1981, Dr. Brewer initiated a series of human clinical trials using cancer patients who had been given up on by modern conventional doctors. They all showed great success.

In 1984, Dr. Brewer published his findings in *Pharmacology Biochemistry and Behavior*.[1] In the article, Dr. Brewer explained his approach in great scientific detail, and also proposed his understanding of how normal cells can become cancer cells. Starting with the widely accepted knowledge that normal healthy cells have membranes which allow the free exchange of both oxygen and glucose and maintain stable intracellular environments at around 7.35 pH, Dr. Brewer proposed that there is a sequence of four main steps that could occur as the healthy cell turns into a cancer cell. These steps are summarized below:

How a Healthy Cell
Becomes a Cancer Cell

1. When carcinogenic materials, such as environmental toxins, attach themselves to the outer surface of the cell membrane, the membrane may become damaged. This involves two factors:

(a) the presence of carcinogenic-type molecules primarily of the polycyclic type, and (b) an energized state of the membrane, which may result from prolonged irritation.(H. E. Sartori, M.D., a physician who supervised some of the human clinical trials on cesium, added that X-rays, parasites, or other factors may also damage the cell membrane.) At some point, the membrane may become so damaged and altered that it can no longer pass certain materials easily. In particular, the damaged cell membrane may no longer be able to readily pass magnesium, calcium, or sodium into the cell. Since oxygen transport depends on two of these elements, calcium and magnesium, the cell then becomes oxygen deficient. However, a damaged cell membrane *can* still pass potassium, cesium, and rubidium. Since glucose transport depends on potassium, glucose continues to be fully supplied to the damaged cell while oxygen is no longer being fully supplied. Without sufficient oxygen to maintain aerobic functioning for energy, the cell reverts to the *fermentation of glucose* for energy in order to survive. Thus it turns into an anaerobic cell.

2. Fermentation of glucose produces "lactic acid" as a byproduct, and this lowers the *intracellular* pH of the cell. The cell pH drops internally from the normal 7.35 to around 7, and then to the extremely acidic pH level of about 6.5. In very advanced stages of cancer, the cell pH may drop even further to 5.7. Thus, the damaged cell has not only become an anaerobic cell, but it has also turned into a cell with a highly acidic internal environment.

3. In the acid medium of the anaerobic cell, the genetic blueprint of the cell (DNA and RNA) is easily altered, resulting in impairment to the cell's control mechanism. With the control mechanism for growth now damaged, the cell rapidly duplicates and grows out of control as a cancer cell.

4. Various cell enzymes are also completely changed in the acid medium of the anaerobic cell. Lysosomal enzymes are changed into toxic compounds, which kill the cells in the main body of the tumor mass. (A tumor therefore consists of a thin layer of rapidly growing cells surrounding a dead mass.) The acid toxins leak out from the tumor mass and poison the host. This is also the source of much of the pain associated with cancer. These acid toxins can then act as carcinogens on other healthy cells, in part by lowering

the extracellular pH of normal healthy tissues to the point where that environment becomes oxygen deficient as well.

The above sequence of steps is how Dr. Brewer theorized that a normal cell becomes a cancer cell. His concept of how cesium can then be used therapeutically to *treat* cancer is based on the fact that cesium is the most alkaline (or alkalizing) of all elements. In fact, when taken up by cancer cells, cesium is able to *radically* raise the intracellular pH of the cancer cells to the very alkaline range of between 8.0 and 9.0. In this range, according to Dr. Brewer, the life of the cancer cell is short—a matter of days at most. The cancer cell soon dies and is absorbed by the body fluids and eliminated from the system.

It is important to realize that, when a cancer patient alkalizes his or her body through diet changes and the use of supplements other than cesium (or rubidium), the effect on the cancer cell is not as profound. It is widely accepted that cancer cells thrive best in highly acidic *extracellular* fluids and do not thrive as well when their extracellular fluids are optimally alkaline. This is why, no matter what treatment a cancer patient is using, it is almost always a good idea for the person to attempt to alkalize their body in general. (See Chapter 18 for more details.)

However, in most alkalizing programs, it is the *extracellular* environment of one's cancer cells that is being influenced the most. But with the use of cesium or rubidium, a person is able to impact the *internal* pH of their cancer cells so powerfully that their cancer cells quickly begin to die off. Also, cesium is able to limit the transport of glucose across the cancer cell's membrane. This causes an immediate decrease in fermentation and a resultant decrease in lactic acid formation. Since a large part of the pain associated with cancer is due to lactic acid build-up, cancer patients using cesium often find their pain subsiding within about 12 to 24 hours.[2]

Dr. Brewer also determined that there were some other key nutrients that, when administered in conjunction with cesium, enhanced the cellular uptake of the cesium. These are vitamin A, vitamin C, zinc, and selenium. He suspected that the administration of Laetrile would also greatly enhance the uptake of cesium by the cancer cells. Dr. Brewer wrote:

> The therapy I am proposing is one of changing the pH of the cancer cell from acid to alkaline. This is entirely possible since as already stated, the cancer cells have lost their pH control mechanism . . . .There are areas of the earth where the incidences of cancer are very low. An analysis

of the foods in these areas shows them to be very high in cesium and rubidium. It is these elements, which are absent in modern commercial foods, that prevent cancer growth. I am convinced that it is food that causes cancer, but it is the food we don't eat and not the food we do eat.[3]

Clinical Trials

As mentioned earlier, Dr. Brewer initiated a number of human trials in 1981. In his summary of one of the trials involving 30 cancer patients, Dr. Brewer stated, "In each case the tumor masses disappeared. Also all pains and effects associated with cancer disappeared within 12 to 36 hours; the more chemotherapy and morphine the patient had taken, the longer the withdrawal period."[4]

Another clinical trial on 50 patients studied over a three-year period had similarly impressive results. This trial was overseen by Dr. Sartori and written up in his book *Cancer—Orwellian or Utopian*. All of the 50 subjects were terminal cancer patients with metastastic disease. Forty-seven of the 50 had received maximal amounts of conventional treatment. Three of the subjects were comatose, and 14 were already suffering from previous treatment-related or cancer-related complications. After cesium treatment was started, pain in *all* 50 subjects disappeared within one to three days! Thirteen of the subjects died within the first two weeks, which was most likely due to the treatment simply coming too late for them. But, over the next three years, 50 percent of the original 50 survived.[5] This was an incredible survival rate given that all the patients were very late stage, had exhausted all conventional forms of treatment, and were all originally expected to die within weeks. Moreover, post-mortem examinations done on those subjects who died showed substantial shrinkage of those patients' tumor masses.[6]

Well-known German cancer researcher and physician, Dr. Hans Neiper, also conducted studies on cesium high pH therapy in Germany. Like the U.S. studies, Dr. Neiper's trials were extremely successful.

In Kathleen Deoul's revealing book, *Cancer Cover-Up*, Deoul presents the story of her husband, Neal Deoul, and his battle with the cancer industry's efforts to suppress effective natural and non-toxic cancer therapies. In 1996, Neal Deoul had provided financing which enabled a Maryland company, T-Up, Inc., to become a primary distributor of cesium and concentrated aloe vera, each sold as natural dietary supplements. (The form of aloe vera sold was found to have the ability to greatly stimulate the immune system and had proven to be very beneficial for both cancer and AIDS patients.) The cesium and aloe vera were obviously working for people because T-UP, Inc., had hundreds of testimonies on file from consumers who claimed life-changing beneficial results. T-UP also had never received a single consumer complaint.

But "big business" was not interested in whether cesium or aloe vera were beneficial to T-UP's ailing customers. And, even though Neal Deoul was *not* receiving profits from the sale of T-UP's products, he was targeted as a financier of the company and taken to court for bogus reasons. Ironically, in January 1999 while Neal Deoul was battling his case in court, he himself was diagnosed with prostate cancer. Believing in T-UP's products, Deoul immediately started administering cesium high pH therapy to himself along with the aloe vera concentrate. By October of that same year, his PSA was down to normal levels and there were no more indications of cancer. Neal's complete story is presented in Kathleen Deoul's revealing book, *Cancer Cover-Up*.

Dr. Brewer wrote numerous scientific articles and papers, one of which was titled "Cancer Its Nature and a Proposed Treatment." In *Cancer Cover-Up*, Deoul describes one of the cases reported in this paper as the following:

> The patient [an individual suffering from lymphoma who arrived in a comatose state] had a massive tumor in his abdomen, as well as an enlarged liver and spleen. After three months of the High pH therapy, the tumor had been virtually eliminated, and the liver and spleen were returned to near normal size. Three years after the treatment the patient was still alive.[7]

Deoul states, "Clearly, the tests had shown that the High pH therapy kills cancer. But 'Big Medicine' ignored and continues to ignore these dramatic results."[8]

Treatment

Until recently, the cesium used to treat cancer was a powdered form of cesium chloride. Usually given to patients in capsules, it was effective but somewhat risky to use. This was because the powdered form could build up to toxic levels in the body. It could only be safely administered under a doctor's care, and some doctors believed cesium should not be used for longer than one month.

Although some cancer patients continue to successfully use the powdered form of cesium, the use of liquid ionic cesium is becoming more and more popular. When cesium is administered in liquid ionic form, it is thought to be more easily assimilated by the body and a smaller amount of cesium can be used to achieve the same results as larger amounts of the powdered version.

An ionic mineral is an element that has a positive or negative electrical charge, meaning it has either too many or too few electrons. In this unstable state, the element bonds readily with water. Because the liquid ionic cesium delivers cesium in a form that is bonded to water molecules, it enters the bloodstream faster than the powdered form, which the body would have to dissolve in the stomach first. The liquid ionic form of cesium is also thought to penetrate cancer cell walls more easily, causing it to be more completely absorbed by the cancer cells. As to toxicity, a dose amount of 6 grams of liquid ionic cesium per day is only about 5 percent of the minimum toxic level. Thus, when liquid ionic cesium is used correctly, there appears to be no danger of toxicity.

The most important aspect about using cesium safely is making sure that enough potassium is supplemented along with it. This is because taking high doses of cesium causes the body to leach out potassium and a severe potassium deficiency will result if high doses of potassium supplementation are not also taken. The danger of potassium deficiency cannot be overstated, since severe potassium deficiency can easily result in death. The prime cause of death from this sort of deficiency is heart attack. Thus, although a common ratio of potassium to cesium supplementation for high pH therapy is usually around three to one, patients with weak hearts may need to use a ratio of more like five or six to one of potassium to cesium.

Any distributor selling liquid ionic cesium will also sell liquid ionic potassium, and this is the form of potassium supplementation preferred when using liquid ionic cesium. People using cesium (either in capsule or liquid form) should always have their blood potassium level checked on a regular basis to be sure they are getting enough potassium and not developing a potassium deficiency. For optimal effectiveness, cancer patients usually also make positive changes in their diets and take other supplements as well to enhance their overall health and immune system.

Even though the therapy is non-toxic, cesium in the amounts required to kill cancer cells can cause stomach upset or nausea if taken on an empty stomach. The reason that cesium may cause nausea is because, as nature's most alkaline mineral, it reacts with anything that is highly acidic, including stomach acids. This type of discomfort is generally avoided by only taking cesium right after a meal.

Patients taking cesium may also experience some diarrhea and/or temporary numbness of the lips and tip of the nose for about 20 minutes after the intake of cesium. These numbness or tingling sensations, however, are not indicative of long-term damage, but are simply a result of cesium being a mild nerve stimulant. People with high blood pressure or other heart conditions should be sure they are under the supervision of a physician while using cesium.

Case Stories

Case Story #1 — Lung Cancer Metastasized to Bones and Liver

In April 2003, at the age of 82, Olga was diagnosed with advanced lung cancer. She had such a large tumor in her lung that it could be easily felt from the outside around her ribs. She underwent chemotherapy and radiation. But these treatments were ineffective, and by June 2003, Olga's doctors proclaimed that her cancer had spread to every bone in her body and to her liver. The family was told she would be dead by September

Because of her age and advanced state of illness, Olga was too weak to undergo any more conventional treatments. With no further treatment, her cancer began to progress quickly. Soon, Olga was having so much difficulty breathing, she had to be hooked up to oxygen 24 hours a day, seven days a week. She was also on heavy pain medication. Since the diagnosis, however, Olga's daughter, Trish, had been trying to find something else that could be done for her mother. Luckily, in late August 2003, when Olga's doctors thought she had only a few more weeks to live, Trish found out about cesium high pH therapy using liquid ionic minerals. She contacted someone who had experience and knowledge about how to use this approach safely and started her mother on it immediately.

Because Olga did not want to take too many different supplements, her treatment protocol was extremely simple. She just took 1 tablespoon of liquid ionic cesium and 1 tablespoon of liquid ionic potassium every morning right after breakfast and every evening right after dinner. She simply stirred the liquid minerals into juice and drank them down. She also took a coral calcium supplement. Olga used no other treatments, but she did drink chocolate whey protein mixed into whole milk on a daily basis to make sure she was getting adequate protein and to help her gain weight. She also ate red beets every day to help support her liver.

When Trish started helping her mother to take the cesium and potassium, she had to quickly lift the oxygen mask off her mother's mouth and nose to give it to her, then quickly put the oxygen mask back on. It was so difficult for Olga to breathe that she could barely get by without the oxygen long enough to take the minerals. After just a few days of taking cesium and potassium, however, she was not so desperate for the oxygen and could breathe without it for a few extra minutes whenever she took her minerals. Amazingly, only 10 days after starting the liquid ionic cesium and liquid ionic potassium, Olga was able to go off the oxygen altogether and hasn't needed it since. Trish says, "It was like a miracle!"

Olga continued to feel better as she kept taking the cesium and potassium. Soon, she was out of bed walking around. Within a few months, Olga was back to being active and living her life almost normally. In mid-December 2003, another MRI was done. This time, only three-and-one-half months after starting on cesium high pH therapy, the MRI showed a very different picture. The cancer in Olga's lungs was gone, her liver looked good, and almost all of the spots on her bones had disappeared. It looked like her advanced, metastasized cancer was almost all gone, and the only problem she was experiencing was some severe bone pain that was either due to some bone fractures caused by the cancer or the fact that she might still have a small amount of cancer in her spine that had not yet had enough time to go away.

Unfortunately, in February 2004, Olga contracted a bad case of the flu that quickly developed into pneumonia. She was rushed to a hospital and put on intravenous antibiotic treatment along with respiratory therapy. She showed signs of improvement, but after being sent home with oral antibiotics, she began to decline again. Her body just could not withstand the infection and she passed away. Olga's daughter, Trish, related the following, however: "They scanned Mom's lungs at the hospital, and her brain was free of cancer and so were her lungs. Her nurse told me point blank, 'As far as the cancer goes, you were there!'"

Case Story #2 — Multiple Myeloma Metastasized to Bones

Jim was 57 years old when he went to a doctor because he was experiencing terrible pain in his neck. Tests revealed that he had a tumor on the C3 vertebra that had nearly destroyed the vertebra itself. More scans showed that he also had tumors on his pelvis, thigh bone, and a few other bones in his body. A bone marrow sample was then taken through the hip into the pelvis. This was biopsied, and the official diagnosis came back "multiple myeloma — IGG, stage III."

Multiple myeloma is a malignant cancer of the bone marrow, and this was considered the primary location of Jim's cancer, with metastases to other bone locations. The "IGG" is a particular type of multiple myeloma that is determined through a blood test, and his IGG count was high at 5,720. Jim's oncologist recommended radiation, chemotherapy, thalidomide, and a stem cell transplant. The doctor also told Jim, "We can't save your life; we can only prolong it. You have from a few months to a few years to live."

Jim was not happy with his prognosis. He had already looked into coral calcium for another condition he'd had, so he knew about the importance of alkalizing the body. However, he also knew that taking the coral calcium had never been enough to keep his pH in the optimal range unless he took about nine capsules a day. He found out about cesium high pH therapy and learned that, as opposed to some of the old powdered forms of minerals, liquid ionic minerals do not build up to a toxic level in the body. Jim worked with someone who knew a lot about liquid ionic minerals, and he started the therapy using liquid ionic cesium as his main cancer-fighting agent. The only conventional treatment he did was one week of radiation right after his diagnosis. According to Jim, when he turned down all conventional treatment and started on the liquid minerals, it was "much to the dismay of his oncologist."

Jim took the liquid ionic cesium and liquid ionic potassium three times a day. In general, Jim's protocol consisted of a variety of minerals in liquid ionic form that included cesium, potassium, germanium, sodium, silver, zinc, boron, and iron. He also supplemented with coral calcium, vitamin D, and a few other vitamins and enzymes. Before Jim was diagnosed, he drank only a glass or two of water each week. He drank a lot of soda and coffee, and rarely ate fresh fruits or vegetables. When he started cesium high pH therapy, he cut out all soda and coffee and drank lots of good water instead. He avoided sugar and refined carbohydrates, and reduced his intake of red meat while eating more fish and chicken. He also greatly increased his intake of fresh fruit and vegetables and started juicing mostly green vegetables as well.

Unbelievably, just 24 hours after starting on the cesium, Jim's terrible neck pain was completely gone. About four days into his program, he felt that he was already detoxifying dead cancer cells out his body. Some of his detoxing symptoms included a tired, weak feeling, loose stools, night sweats, and increased urination. But the symptoms were mild and not even as bad as flu symptoms.

Jim had started cesium high pH therapy in January 2003. In March 2003, he went back to his oncologist to be tested again. A blood test this time showed his IGG count to be down to 1,520, which is actually in the normal range for a healthy person. His oncologist told Jim he was "blown away" by the test results. Jim told his doctor all the things he had done. The doctor said, "Well, I don't know why it's working, but keep doing it."

About a year after his cancer diagnosis of "incurable" multiple myeloma, Jim is back to living a normal life and his scans no longer reveal any cancer. He plans to continue taking the liquid minerals and to maintain a healthy diet to keep the cancer from coming back.

Over the year that Jim was recovering through the use of cesium high pH therapy, he only experienced minor aches and pains, which he attributes to his bones rebuilding. He also felt a slight tingling in his neck and hips at times in the places where his tumors were, and he sometimes experienced a slight numbness in his lips and nose for about 20 minutes after taking the cesium. But all of these symptoms were easy to go through and simply a part of his healing process.

Jim says that, because he was going against conventional establishment, he had to have faith that he was doing the right thing by following the alternative approach that he chose. He credits his ability to stay with the approach to his belief that God was guiding him and putting him in touch with the right method that could help him to fully heal!

Case Story #3 — Non-Hodgkin's Lymphoma of the Stomach

LaVaughn had been a welder for an oil company for many years and breathing a variety of toxic substances on the job may have had something to do with the cancer he was diagnosed with in April 2002, at age 47. Before consulting a doctor, LaVaughn had started having excruciating pain in his stomach and was sometimes throwing up blood. LaVaughn and his wife, Cindy, thought he probably had a bleeding ulcer.

When his condition worsened, LaVaughn went to a doctor. Nothing abnormal showed up on the CT scan or the MRI, so an endoscope procedure was performed. With the endoscope, LaVaughn's doctor could visually see a huge tumor in his stomach. Right in the middle of the tumor mass was a constantly bleeding ulcer about the size of a silver dollar. A sample of tissue from the ulcer was biopsied, and the diagnosis came back "non-Hodgkin's lymphoma of the stomach." It was considered to be of a medium to aggressive variety.

LaVaughn's doctors did not want to try to surgically remove the tumor because it involved too many large blood vessels and there was too high a risk that LaVaughn would bleed to death. He started on nutritional therapy immediately and began juicing and taking some herbs to strengthen and support his body. He felt better right away, as the pain left and his energy returned. However, the tumor continued to grow until it blocked the lower stomach. LaVaughn was no longer able to eat and had to be put on intravenous feeding. He began chemo in June, thinking that might cause the tumor to shrink enough so he could begin eating again. He knew that if he could eat again, he would then become more aggressive with the nutritional therapy.

Unfortunately, the chemo was not effective and on October 1, 2002, another endoscope procedure showed that the tumor was bigger than ever. It had been five weeks since the last chemo treatment, and LaVaughn was too weak to undergo any more chemo at this point. He was in terrible pain and had not be able to keep any food or drink down for 16 weeks. His oncologist suggested to LaVaughn that the only option was to surgically remove his entire stomach.

LaVaughn did not want to undergo stomach removal surgery. Cindy had been searching for alternative options throughout his battle and finally found out about liquid ionic cesium and potassium. On September 29, 2002, she started LaVaughn on cesium high pH therapy. He was extremely weak and lethargic at this point, and his duodenum was now completely blocked. Since nothing was going through his stomach, Cindy decided to spray the liquid minerals on his skin and let them absorb into his body that way. She sprayed the liquid cesium on his chest and back and sprayed some of the other liquid minerals on his arms and legs. She did this four times a day for two days. By the end of these two days, LaVaughn's stomach had started gurgling and his vomiting had stopped. On the third day, Cindy was able to start carefully giving the minerals to LaVaughn orally in juice, along with spraying them on him. It seemed like, each day after that, his stomach was able to handle more and more food and drink, and he gradually gained his strength back.

LaVaughn's treatment focused around using liquid ionic cesium and liquid ionic potassium, as well as other liquid ionic minerals. After a while, Cindy also started him on Dr. Kelley's enzymes, Essiac tea, and a variety of other supplements. But he never stopped taking the liquid minerals.

Incredibly, about six weeks after beginning cesium high pH therapy, LaVaughn felt well again. Two weeks after that, at the eight-week point, another endoscope procedure was done. It was the day before Thanksgiving 2002. This time, the endoscope showed that the tumor was completely gone and the central ulcer part had shrunk down to the size of a pencil eraser. A biopsy accompanied the scoping, and the resulting pathology report stated that the cancer was now benign and no helicobacter pylori bacteria were present.

LaVaughn has not had any more endoscope procedures done, but he has continued to take the liquid ionic minerals and has continued to feel great. In fact, he now says he feels 15 years younger than he did before his diagnosis. In October 2003, he had a general physical and his doctor could not find anything wrong with him or any signs of cancer. Even the hernias that had developed because of the chemo were gone.

LaVaughn's treatment approach involved a three-to-one ratio of potassium to cesium at first. But he eventually switched to an even higher ratio of potassium to cesium to be sure he did not suffer any potassium deficiency. Although not everyone does this, LaVaughn also decided to follow the practice of taking the cesium for five days, then skipping it for two days every week. During the two days of not taking the cesium, however, LaVaughn would still take all his other minerals, including the potassium.

LaVaughn and Cindy believe that when a person is on cesium high pH therapy and starts to experience numbness or tingling in the mouth and nose, or a general disoriented, dizzy, or shaky feeling, it's an indication of low potassium. They believe that using the cesium "five days on, two days off" helps to avoid potassium deficiency and also gives the body time to detoxify or flush out the dead cancer cells.

As of February 2004, LaVaughn is still feeling great, and as far as anyone can tell, is completely cancer-free. His wife, Cindy, is now a distributor of liquid minerals, and her contact information is listed at the end of this chapter.

Case Story #4—Non-Hodgkin's Lymphoma, Grade III

"Cheddy" is the nickname for a woman who was also diagnosed with a form of non-Hodgkin's lymphoma. Her diagnosis came in February 2002, when she was 70 years old. Cheddy had gone to her doctor because of a lump on her arm that had appeared and was about the size of a nickel. Her doctor removed the lump and had it biopsied. The resulting diagnosis was "non-Hodgkin's lymphoma, grade II." Cheddy was immediately referred to an oncologist who did more scans and tested her bone marrow to see if her cancer had metastasized. Luckily, these tests indicated that the cancer in her lymph system had not metastasized to other parts of her body. She was advised to have a small amount of radiation done on her arm for one month, which she did. After this, her doctor pronounced her clear of cancer.

Just three days later, however, the cancer reared its ugly head again as three new lumps appeared on her neck. Needle biopsies proved these to be a recurrence of her lymphoma, and it was obvious that the radiation had not fully gotten rid of her cancer. Cheddy's oncologist wanted her to do chemotherapy. But Cheddy did not want to do chemo and told her doctor that she wanted to look into a nutritional approach instead. Her doctor replied, "I don't know anything about nutrition, and I don't *want* to know anything about it."

Cheddy pursued nutritional support on her own for about a year. She made major changes in her diet and took lots of supplements including liver capsules, CoQ_{10}, and garlic. Throughout this year, her approach seemed to be successful at keeping the cancer stable, but she still had tumors on her neck and one inside her throat.

In mid-March 2003, Cheddy found out about liquid ionic cesium and potassium and started taking those. She also took other minerals in liquid ionic form, including germanium, trace minerals and selenium, plus an immune support supplement. After about six months of doing this, Cheddy's lumps started going down, so she patiently kept doing her program. Her persistence paid off as she saw the tumors go away, and she says she experienced very little in the way of side effects. She had no nausea, no numbness or tingling in the mouth or nose, was simply a little more tired initially, and had bowel movements that were a little looser.

By September 2003, all the lumps on her neck and in her throat were completely gone and she had no indication of cancer whatsoever. In February 2004, she continues to feel great and show no further signs of cancer.

Case Story #5—Prostate Cancer

At age 56, Gerry was feeling so tired and depressed all the time, that he was contemplating early retirement. But he knew that if he gave up his job, he would need to get health insurance coverage from some other source. He decided to see if he could get medical coverage from a VA hospital. The application for coverage required a medical exam, so he underwent the exam. Gerry was checked for polyps and given an ultrasound to check his prostate gland. Unfortunately, the ultrasound showed a tumor on his prostate, and Gerry was diagnosed with prostate cancer. This was in mid-November 2002. About a month later, a needle-biopsy was performed on the tumor and Gerry's cancer was officially verified and classified as 7 on the Gleason scale. However, even though Gerry definitely had prostate cancer, his PSA count was only .9.

Gerry's oncologist suggested that they perform surgery to remove his entire prostate gland and to also remove any surrounding lymph nodes if, during the surgery, it appeared necessary. But just about everyone in Gerry's family had died of cancer after going through conventional treatment, so, he was extremely reluctant to go through it himself. Instead, he declined surgery and searched for alternative options. Gerry found out about liquid ionic cesium and potassium and started taking those in January 2003. When he told his oncologist about cesium high pH therapy, the doctor was appalled and actually mailed Gerry a letter urging him not to do it, writing, "You are making a big mistake."

But Gerry was steadfast in his decision to decline conventional treatment. Along with the liquid ionic cesium and potassium that he began to take, he also took other liquid ionic minerals, including calcium, magnesium, germanium, sulphur, and vanadium. Plus, he used a "rebounder," which is a mini-trampoline that can be used for mild exercise indoors, and started walking a lot outdoors. Gerry radically improved his diet and cut his bread and sugar intake to almost zero. He also bought a magnetic mattress pad for his bed.

About four months later, Gerry went back for another ultrasound, and this time no tumor showed up at all. He continued to eat well, exercise, and take liquid ionic minerals. After about six months, he was able to cut back on the amounts of the liquid minerals, continuing them at lower dosages. Gerry would have liked to continue to get ultrasounds and PSA tests to monitor his progress, but his doctors refused to do these tests on him anymore. They seemed to believe Gerry still had cancer and that more ultrasounds or PSA tests will not change their minds about this.

Gerry now realizes that the extreme tiredness and depression that had made him want to retire from his job early had been partly due to the cancer. About a month or two into his cesium high pH therapy, he began to feel a lot of energy and felt the depression go away. Now, at the beginning of 2004, he has so much energy that he jogs between 6 and 9 miles every day and is scheduled to run in this year's New York Marathon. He thinks his positive attitude and diet changes were very important to his healing, but he credits the bulk of his recovery to cesium high pH therapy and liquid ionic minerals.

Case Story #6—Ovarian Cancer

Sixty-one-year-old Merille (pronounced Marilee) had not been feeling well for some time when she went to her doctor in January 2002. A CT scan showed fluid in her lungs, and since one of the causes of this could be cancer, she was referred to a specialist at the Mayo Clinic. More tests at the Mayo Clinic revealed tumors on both of Merille's ovaries as well as in her lymph system. A blood test for the ovarian cancer marker "CA-125" showed her to have a count of almost 800. (The normal, healthy range for the CA-125 is a count of around 34 or below.)

Merille was rushed into surgery to have her uterus and ovaries removed. After the surgery, biopsies were done on the tumors and the diagnosis came back "ovarian cancer, stage IIIC." At this point, Merille's oncologist recommended chemotherapy but told her there was no cure for her type of cancer. The implication was that the best conventional medicine could do would be to manage her cancer for as long as they could, but that she would always have it. Merille did not know of any other option but to go with her doctor's recommendation, so she followed her surgery with six rounds of chemotherapy.

When the chemotherapy was completed, Merille's CA-125 had gone down to a count of 9 and she was pronounced in remission. But as is common after chemotherapy, her count immediately started going back up. By March 2003, her CA-125 was up to 84 and her cancer was obviously back. Merille now had new tumors in her abdomen and also in her neck area around her collar bone. Her Mayo Clinic oncologist pronounced that "the chemo had failed." At this point, the doctors performed more surgery on Merille, but they could not remove all her cancer. They recommended more rounds of chemotherapy, but at the same time told Merille that there was a significant risk that further chemo would damage her heart. Merille was forced to make a difficult decision and she decided to decline more chemo and look for alternatives instead.

Merille's daughter found out about cesium high pH therapy using liquid ionic minerals. Merille was able to contact an experienced consultant and start on liquid ionic cesium and liquid ionic potassium immediately. She also began to take other supportive liquid minerals and supplements. Within three months, all her tumors disappeared and her cancer marker test had gone from 84 down to 23. Now her CA-125 was back in the normal range. Merille's doctor at the Mayo Clinic was amazed and wondered what she was doing. When she told him, he just said, "Keep doing what you're doing!"

Merille reduced her dosage of liquid minerals at this point, but her next CA-125 test three months later showed her marker results to be up another 10 points. So she went back on the full dose of cesium and other minerals and her marker results began to go back down again. By January 2004, her CA-125 marker was all the way down to 12, and she had no clinical signs of cancer at all. The latest CA-125 test, taken in April 2004, was 6.4—the lowest it has ever been.

Merille did nothing other than the cesium high pH therapy while she was recovering from her metastasized ovarian cancer. To ensure that she stays free of cancer, she is continuing to take the liquid minerals and supportive supplements. Merille says she took the cesium five days out of each week, followed by two days off. (During those two days, she continued the liquid ionic potassium and other supplements, though.) She took potassium four times a day and cesium twice a day with the ratio of potassium to cesium being five to one. This way, it was easy to avoid potassium deficiency.

Merille also says that she felt very good during her treatment, with only mild detoxing symptoms and sporadic diarrhea. And she only experienced a little tingling and numbness around the nose and mouth at times. All in all, it was a truly easy and miraculous recovery! (Merille is now distributing liquid minerals, and her contact information is listed at the back of this chapter.)

The real-life experiences of people who have used cesium high pH therapy show that, when administered correctly, it is safe and non-toxic. But like other alternative, non-toxic approaches, it is not approved by the FDA as a cancer treatment. Thus, it cannot be legally prescribed by most physicians. Also, distributors of cesium are not legally allowed to advise people of its use as a cancer treatment. However, they *can* advise people as to how to use cesium and other minerals for raising one's pH levels.

For those people who choose to use cesium to raise their alkalinity, seeking the guidance of a qualified practitioner or consultant to find out how to use it safely and effectively is advised. Taking precautions to not become potassium deficient is the only serious, concern and because of that, it is *always* advised to get regular blood tests to check your potassium levels. If you have any type of heart condition, you should be under a doctor's supervision while using cesium.

As long as one is getting adequate guidance, this is an easy and extremely effective approach to self-administer at home. It appears to work well for all types of cancer outside the brain, and its effectiveness for brain cancer may also be substantiated in the future. Overall, it is certainly one of the most impressive, quick and easy approaches for "out-smarting" cancer available today.

Resources:

To Contact Consultants/Distributors of Liquid Ionic Minerals:

(888) 336-4972   Ask for Cindy, or email Cindy at lcyordy@swbell.net
(866) 776-8623   Renewal & Wellness, LLC

Cost of cesium high pH therapy: This varies, depending on how many other liquid minerals or supportive supplements are used along with the cesium and potassium. The cost ranges from approximately $200 per month for just cesium and potassium, to up to about $650 per month when a variety of other minerals and supplements are added.

Books

Kathleen Deoul. *Cancer Cover-Up.* Baltimore: Cassandra Books, 2001.

H. E. Sartori, M.D. *Cancer Orwellian or Utopian?* Life Science Universal Inc., 1985.

For Historical Documentation and Papers by Dr. Brewer:

A. Keith Brewer Library   (608) 647-6444
325 N. Central Avenue
Richland Center, WI 53581

Websites

www.mwt.net/~drbrewer/highpH.htm

www.mwt.net/~drbrewer/brew_art.htm

www.cancer-coverup.com

www.essense-of-life.com

www.advancedhealthplan.com/2cesiumchlorideforcancer2.html

www.mwt.net/~brewer/intro.htm

www.thewolfeclinic.com/cesium.html

SECTION III

Key Cancer
Recovery Issues

CHAPTER 18

To Alkalize or Not to Alkalize

I f you have cancer and you are not using cesium high pH therapy, should you still try to alkalize your body? This is an important question, and the answer in just about all cases is a resounding *yes!* Most alternative cancer practitioners agree on this issue because cancer cells thrive best in acidic bodies. It is also known that, in general, cancer patients are much more acidic than non-cancer patients—even to the point of being 1,000 times more acidic!

Do cancer patients start out with more acidic bodies in the first place? Often they do—especially when cancer develops in adults. (When it develops in children, however, this many not be the case.) It is theorized that overly acidic body tissues are prone to developing cancer. And once a person *has* cancer, the body may become even *more* skewed toward the acidic end of the scale due to the cancer cells themselves producing lactic acid. As discussed in Chapter 17, lactic acid is a byproduct of cancer cell metabolism that causes the cellular environment to become more acidic than it was before the cancer started.

Of course, the reason that overly acidic bodies are good environments for cancer is because acidic tissues carry less oxygen than optimally alkaline tissues. (Again, the anaerobic nature of cancer cells is key.) The extracellular and intracellular fluids of tissues are what we must look at for a better understanding of this issue.

Cells and Homeostasis

Most of us could go our whole lives without wondering how our extracellular and intracellular fluids are doing. Normally, we shouldn't *have* to worry about them because these fluids are usually well-maintained by the body through a process called "homeostasis." But if we want to understand cancer, we have to get down to the cellular level and understand what our cells need and want from their immediate environment. To do this, it helps to look at how multicellular organisms developed in the first place, and I'd like to present the scientific evolutionary viewpoint on this. (If this does not agree with your own belief system about how life developed on earth, remember that this is just a theory. It does, however, give us one way of understanding cells that seems to make sense.)

From a scientific evolutionary viewpoint, life on Earth first evolved in the primordial waters of our planet, which became our oceans. This ocean environment was perfect for fragile, single-celled organisms to develop in because it was so constant in temperature, pressure, and nutrient availability. Living in the ocean was like being in a womb for these early single cells. Chaotic characteristics of the dry land environment, such as weather fluctuations, landslides, earthquakes, floods, and so forth, were not felt in the ocean womb. Thus, in this ideal environment, single-celled organisms thrived, and the entire surface area of each cell could happily interact with the outside watery environment to allow food in from the ocean as well as to expel waste back out into the ocean.

Being in such a good situation, these early single-celled forms of life evolved and progressed eventually into more complex life forms. They became "multicellular" organisms. But amassing more than one cell together risked cutting some cells off from their watery environment which each cell needed so much to survive. In essence, multicellular organisms solved this problem by creating an *inner* fluid environment for all the cells to interact with—an "inner ocean," so too speak, that they could carry around with them. In fact, this "inner ocean" probably mimicked the original pH, osmotic pressure, ionizing capabilities, mineral composition, and other features of the outside ocean of primordial days.

Since those days, after billions of years, some of the characteristics of Earth's oceans have changed quite a bit. Evaporation, erosion of land into the water, and climate changes causing large portions of water to be frozen into polar ice caps, have all contributed to the oceans of today being saltier than they used to be when single-celled organisms were evolving. But the original "inner ocean" that multicellular organisms developed is still a part of our physiology today, and still allows each individual cell to gain its nourishment from and excrete its wastes into the fluid around it. It is called the "extracellular fluid" of our bodies. Our cells depend on it to survive. This fluid is maintained by the body at constant conditions through a process called "homeostasis." Homeostasis is carried out in *other* ways in the body, as well. Six overall examples of homeostasis processes are[1].

1. Keeping the body temperature constantly around 98.6 F°
2. Keeping blood acidity/alkalinity levels constant
3. Keeping certain chemical concentrations in body fluids constant
4. Keeping the glucose level of the blood constant
5. Keeping the levels of oxygen and carbon dioxide constant
6. Keeping the volume of blood and body fluids constant

All the above processes of homeostasis could be said to be the body's way of mimicking the constant conditions of earth's primordial waters wherein life first developed.

The Body's Acid/Alkaline Balancing Act

Of course, *all* of the above constant conditions are important to the functioning of a healthy body. But many believe that the acid/alkaline balance of the intracellular and extracellular fluids is of *particular* importance to whether or not normal cells turn into cancerous cells, as well as to whether cancer cells, once established, rage out of control.

The body has a variety of ways that it maintains proper pH levels, but the primary way that it does this is through the use of minerals from the diet. Contrary to what some people might believe, however, it is *not* the acidity or alkalinity of the foods we eat that keeps us in balance. In other words, whether a food is acidic or alkaline *before* it goes into our bodies is not an indication of whether it will make us more acidic or alkaline once that food is digested. For example, citrus fruits such as limes and lemons are very acidic *outside* the body, but they promote alkalinity when they are broken down and digested *inside* the body. This is because certain minerals, such as calcium, magnesium, potassium and iron, among others, are very alkalizing to the body's inner environment and many fruits and vegetables (including limes and lemons) tend to be high in these alkalizing minerals. Thus, the digestion of fruits and vegetables tends to have an overall alkalizing effect on the body, even though some of them may be quite acidic before we ingest them.

Basically, what a food breaks down into when digested is the key factor when it comes to influencing body pH. Therefore, it is best to forget about whether a food is acidic or alkaline itself, and instead, look at which foods are "acid forming" or "alkaline forming" in the body. Unfortunately, typical dietary habits in the modern industrialized world generally include high quantities of refined and processed foods. These foods tend to be robbed of their natural minerals, vitamins, and enzymes. Very refined foods, such as white sugar and white flour, are so severely stripped of their mineral content, they are virtually all acid-forming in the body.

In contrast to refined sugars, raw fruits (which are also very sweet due to their fructose content) are accompanied by such an abundance of alkalizing minerals that the total fruit is alkaline-forming in the body. Also, when people no longer had to work hard to hunt down their meat and could buy it instead from a grocery store or fast-food restaurant, the consumption of meat became easier and more frequent. Animal foods such as meat, fish, poultry, and eggs are acid-forming in the body, primarily because of the extremely acidic byproducts that are produced during digestion. These byproducts, such as sulphuric acid, phosphoric acid, and uric acid, tend to overwhelm the alkalizing effects of the minerals contained in these foods.

A brief look at some common acid-forming and alkaline-forming foods and beverages can give us a quick understanding of one way that people's acid/alkaline balance can get skewed over many years of modern eating habits. The modern tendency toward acidity as a result of diet is then *compounded* by the fact that chronic stress contributes to acidity in the body as well, as do almost all prescription medicines.

In certain details, lists of acid-forming versus alkaline-forming foods may vary slightly from source to source, but the following foods and beverages are most commonly listed as they are below.

Acid-Forming Food

all meats	most nuts and seeds
fish	peanut butter
poultry	lentils
eggs	most legumes
margarine	soft drinks
most commercial cheese	coffee
pasteurized milk	commercial teas
most processed grains	most alcoholic beverages
pastas	ice cream
crackers	chocolate and cocoa
noodles	tobacco
refined sugar	NutraSweet, Equal, Sweet'N Low
pastries and candies	most prescription drugs

Alkaline-Forming Food

most raw vegetables	olive oil
most ripe, raw fruits	goat cheese
sprouts	raw milk
sprouted whole grains	honey
wheatgrass	molasses
sauerkraut	maple syrup
apple cider vinegar	stevia
algaes and sea vegetables	spices
miso	herbs and herbal teas
soy sauce	green tea

Almost Neutral (slightly alkaline-forming)

soured dairy products (yogurt)
butter
almonds
buckwheat, millet

Optimally, people's diets in general should be made up of approximately three-quarters alkaline-forming foods, and approximately one-quarter acid-forming foods to maintain a healthy pH balance. Yet, looking at the above lists, it is clear that most Americans ingest way too many acid-forming foods and beverages, and not nearly enough alkaline-forming foods and beverages. Just think about how many people eat sugary cereal or refined wheat toast with coffee and maybe eggs for breakfast, a meat sandwich with refined wheat bread and a soda for lunch (maybe along with a little salad). Then, for dinner, there is often a main course of meat, fish, or pasta, possibly followed by a sugary dessert. Not to mention the common extra cup of coffee or soda in the afternoon with a candy bar as a pick-me-up.

In general, understanding which foods tend to be acid forming and which tend to be alkaline forming is important. But these types of lists can only give us a *partial* understanding of how the acid/alkaline balance in the body can become skewed. For instance, if a deficiency of certain key nutrients builds up over time, then some important alkalizing features in the body may not be able to do their job no matter how many alkalizing foods you ingest. A good example of this is illuminated by the research of Dr. Johanna Budwig and her flaxseed oil and cottage cheese approach (see Chapter 14). Her findings show us that people who become severely deficient in omega-3 and omega-6 essential fatty acids can develop low oxygen cellular environments because their cell membranes cannot attract as much oxygen to their cells when they don't have enough of these vital, electron-rich substances to build their cell membranes with. Thus, it is somewhat ironic that fish, for instance, is acid forming in general, but a prolonged deficiency of the essential fatty acids that are found in some fish and other foods can promote acidity in the body as well.

And diet is not the *only* source of acidity in our bodies. There is chronic stress, which is rampant in modern living. Stress triggers the sympathetic nervous system, which increases cellular metabolism, which in turn increases acidity.[2] Also, chronic dehydration is a more and more common problem for modern people who are rushing around between working, taking the kids to school, talking on the cell phone, and so forth, while keeping themselves going with caffeinated drinks that are diuretics and deplete the body of its water even more. Chronic dehydration can promote acidity in the body, too. Certain toxins in our bodies promote acidity, chronic infections can promote acidity, and even allergic reactions to foods can promote acidity.

Oxygen, Alkalinity, and the Heart

So why is it that overly acid environments in the body are also low oxygen environments? The answer to this question is somewhat detailed on a biochemistry level, but basically it is because all acidic conditions consist of excess hydrogen ions. In the absence of sufficient minerals to neutralize this acidity, the body must combine these excess hydrogen ions with any oxygen that is available, thereby creating water as a harmless by-product. Thus, if a person is continually creating an acidic inner environment because of their diet, toxins, or other lifestyle factors, and they *don't* have enough alkalizing minerals in reserve from their diet, then their body is constantly having to neutralize their overly acidic state by depleting the body's internal oxygen.

However, if there are enough alkalizing minerals available for the body to use first, such as calcium, magnesium, or potassium, then it is not necessary for the oxygen of the body to be used up in order to maintain the correct alkaline balance. According to Robert Barefoot and Carl J. Reich, M.D., authors of *The Calcium Factor: The Scientific Secret of Health and Youth*, calcium is the most important alkalizing mineral we can get from our diets. They claim that "calcium to acid, is like water to a fire."[3]

A body pH level of 7 is considered neutral on a scale of 0 to 14. The more you go down the scale from 7 (toward 0), the more *acidic* you are. The more you go up the scale from 7 (toward 14), the more *alkaline* you are. Our bodies "like" to be slightly alkaline to function optimally. All of our cells and enzymes function best in slightly alkaline environments. The pH level of our blood, however, is the *most* important for our bodies to maintain at a constant level of about 7.4. This is partly because it is so critical that the blood be able to maintain sufficient oxygen in it in order to circulate oxygen to all of our cells. Also, if the blood becomes too acidic, the heart might relax to the point where it could cease to beat. If the blood becomes too alkaline, on the other hand, the heart might contract to the point where it could cease to beat.[4] Thus, the blood pH *has* to be given priority over pH anywhere else in the body.

There are numerous ways that our bodies maintain a virtually constant blood pH of about 7.4. (It literally must be maintained at the very narrow pH range of 7.35 to 7.45.) If necessary, the pH of the rest of the body will be "sacrificed" so that the pH of the blood can be maintained at its critical level. Our bodies do this by using up reserves of alkalizing minerals from other parts of the body. These alkalizing minerals may come from body tissue such as the bones, teeth, cartilage, muscles, kidneys, and liver, among other places. Thus, a person's tissues and extracellular fluids can become way too acidic for good health throughout many areas of the body, even though the blood remains at a constant alkaline/acid balance.

The constant optimum pH level of the blood, along with the constant optimum oxygen level of the blood, is probably why cancer of the heart is virtually unknown. This is helped by the fact that blood flowing into the heart comes directly from the lungs and has the highest pH and oxygen levels of any blood within the body.

But *all* of our bodies' cells are highly sensitive to proper pH levels of the fluid environment around them, and they will not function well if this environment becomes overly acid. Robert Barefoot and Dr. Carl Reich explain the above concepts in the following passage from their book *The Calcium Factor*:

> In chemistry, alkali solutions (pH over 7.0) tend to absorb oxygen, while acids (pH under 7.0) tend to expel oxygen. For example, a mild alkali can absorb over 100 times as much oxygen as a mild acid. Therefore, when the body becomes acidic by dropping below pH 7.0 (*note*: all body fluids, except for stomach and urine, are supposed to be mildly

alkaline at pH 7.4.), oxygen is driven out of the body thereby, according to Nobel Prize winner Otto Warburg, inducing cancer. Stomach fluids must remain acidic to digest food and urine must remain acidic to remove wastes from the body. Blood is the exception. Blood must always remain at an alkaline pH 7.4 so that it can retain its oxygen. When adequate mineral consumption is in the diet, the blood is supplied the crucial minerals required to maintain an alkaline pH of 7.4. However when insufficient mineral consumption is in the diet, the body is forced to rob Peter (other body fluids) to pay Paul (the blood). In doing so, it removes crucial minerals, such as calcium, from the saliva, spinal fluids, kidneys, liver, etc., in order to maintain the blood at pH 7.4. This causes the demineralized fluids and organs to become acidic and therefore anaerobic, thus inducing not only cancer, but a host of other degenerative diseases, such as heart disease, diabetes, arthritis, lupus, etc.[5]

Although our bodies' cells, in general, require a slightly alkaline environment to function optimally, there are certain systems of the body that have differing acid/alkaline ranges. Here is an overview of *all* the body's pH ranges[6]:

Common pH Ranges

Blood	7.35–7.45
Saliva	6.50–7.50
Urine	4.50–8.40
Liver bile	7.10–8.50
Stomach fluids	1.00–3.50

Thus, the stomach is the only part of the body that is supposed to be extremely acidic because it needs to be this acid in order to digest foods.

Over-Acidity and Cancer

Many people believe that normal cells become cancer cells in the first place (at least in part) because their intracellular and extracellular environments are too acidic. Although it is unlikely this is the only reason healthy cells become cancer cells, it may be a prime reason. The Nobel Prize winner, Dr. Otto Warburg, believed that cancer cells are normal cells which have been forced to adapt to a low oxygen environment in order to survive. Could it be that, by switching to anaerobic functioning, these normal cells are simply "remembering" how they once functioned in the primordial oceans when they were single-celled organisms? This might be true because, according to current scientific theory, *all the cells that existed at that time were living in an anaerobic environment.*

We don't generally think about this, but oxygen did not become prevalent in the earth's atmosphere until after plants evolved, so all single-celled life before plants *had* to function anaerobically. It may be that every cell in our bodies retains the ability (a "memory," if you will) to function anaerobically if it needs to in order to survive. Another example of normal, aerobic cells of the body turning to anaerobic functioning under adverse conditions is seen with muscle cells. When we exercise so strenuously that the supply of oxygen to our muscles is not sufficient for normal functioning, then our muscle cells switch to anaerobic functioning. This involves utilizing glucose for energy, instead of oxygen, and it results in the production of lactic acid — just as in cancer cells. It is largely this production of lactic acid in the muscles that causes muscle soreness after strenuous exercise.

Thus, the low-oxygen content of overly acidic bodies is an important cancer-contributing factor. But there are other aspects of too much acidity that need to be understood as well. One of these aspects is explained by author Keiichi Morishita.

Keiichi Morishita wrote in his book, *Hidden Truth of Cancer*, that when the condition of the blood starts to become too acidic, then our bodies deposit the excess acidic substances in various other places in the body. Wherever this deposit occurs, those tissues may become so acidic that cells in that area may start to die due to lack of oxygen. In turn, the dead cells themselves turn into acids, and contribute to the overly acidic conditions. However, some cells will eventually survive by becoming abnormal, anaerobic cells, and will use the process of glucose fermentation (glycolysis) for much of their energy needs. According to some researchers, the lactic acid produced by this fermentation can also break down, or damage, the DNA and RNA in cells. The DNA and RNA contain the control mechanisms that modulate the growth of cells, so once they are broken down or damaged, those cells may multiply out-of-control because they no longer have functioning control mechanisms. Thus, overly acid conditions not only contribute to cancer development by being low-oxygen environments, but may also result in damage to DNA and RNA, thereby promoting uncontrolled cell growth.

Another problem that over-acidity may cause is related to the fact that enzymes of the body do not function well in acidic environments. Thus, some of the body's best defenses against cancer are neutralized. And yet another problem may be related to micro-organisms. There are some researchers who believe that, when the pH balance of the body is skewed, certain harmless micro-organisms can then change form, become pathogenic, and thrive. We saw in the chapters on Royal Rife and Gaston Naessens that some micro-organisms can change into cancer-causing forms when conditions are unhealthy in the body.

It is also interesting to note that how fast-growing or how slow-growing a tumor is directly correlated with the degree to which it uses anaerobic functioning. Some cancer cells rely more on anaerobic functioning than others. Decades ago, two researchers at the National Cancer Institute performed some experiments where they actually measured the fermentation rate of different cancers known to grow at different speeds. What they found was that the more aggressive (fast-growing) a cancer was, the higher its glucose fermentation rate was, and that the slower-growing a cancer was, the lower its fermentation rate was.[7]

How to Test Your pH Balance

In the early 1970s, Dr. Reich discovered that the pH level of saliva is an outstanding indicator of ionic calcium levels in the body. And he was able to validate clinically that a simple three-second test of the saliva, done under the right conditions with litmus paper strips, could indicate whether a person was functionally deficient in calcium or not. He found that the pH of saliva for healthy people is generally 7.0–7.5. On the other hand, when a person was deficient in ionic calcium, he found their saliva pH would be about 4.6–6.4 (much more acidic).[8] Reich was able to prove that a few weeks to a few months of supplementation, along with dietary changes, would produce a gradual increase in saliva alkalinity and a corresponding increase in wellness.

The pH strip testing is very easy to do, and strips usually come with a color-coded chart. According to Barefoot and Reich, a healthy person with sufficient alkalinity and ionic calcium levels will generally show a result of dark blue on the pH strip. Most children test dark blue. But over 50 percent of adults are green-yellow, indicating a pH of 6.5 or lower and calcium deficiency. Amazingly, according to Barefoot and Reich, "terminal cancer patients are usually a bright yellow, a pH of 4.5. This is more than 1,000 times the acidity level of a normal healthy individual at pH 7.5, causing the body to self-digest."[9]

Strips for testing saliva pH levels are very inexpensive and generally available in many health food stores as well as from a number of sites on the Internet. It is suggested that pH strips with a range of 4.5–7.5 are best. Since eating certain foods or drinking certain beverages can temporarily influence the pH in the mouth, it is best to test your saliva pH first thing in the morning or two hours after eating. Wait at least 15 seconds for the color on the strip to form. It is also important to notice whether the color-coded chart you are using indicates optimum color ranges for saliva or for urine, since they are different. The optimum pH for urine is much more acidic than for saliva. For saliva testing only, the optimum pH is between 7.0 and 7.5. There is another way to test pH that is sometimes suggested, as well, and that involves separately testing your saliva and urine (with separate pH strips), and then taking the average of the two. When done this way, the average would be an optimum pH level of around 6.8.

How to Alkalize Once You Have Cancer

Although poor diet can contribute to overly acidic bodies, which in turn can contribute to damaged cells and cancer, *once a body is very out-of-balance, it can be difficult to regain an optimum acid/alkaline balance through diet alone.* This is especially true for cancer patients because the cancer cells themselves contribute even more to the acidity of their bodies by creating lactic acid through their respiration process. So, it would be a mistake to use acid-forming and alkaline-forming food charts and diet changes as the *only* way to try to correct the imbalance once you have cancer.

Simply put, once a person is dealing with cancer and an overly acidic body pH, it is often necessary to use more powerful means than diet alone to correct the pH imbalance. The most powerful means, other than cesium high pH therapy, involves supplementation of the alkalizing minerals: calcium, magnesium, and potassium. Of all the minerals common to our day-to-day diets, utilizable calcium is *the most important* mineral for alkalizing the body and may also be one of the key nutritional deficiencies for many people in the modern world. (As we shall see, this is not due to a lack of calcium in our diets, but results more from insufficient vitamin D and magnesium, both of which are required to make calcium utilizable.)

An understanding of the health benefits of calcium was first developed by named Dr. Carl Reich. Dr. Reich was a medical maverick who, in the early 1950s, suspected that most of the diseases of his patients could be related to overly acidic bodies and calcium deficiency. In fact, Reich worked together with the Nobel Prize winner, Otto Warburg, for many years to formulate an understanding of the role of ionic calcium and cancer.

Dr. Reich started his medical practice in 1950 in Calgary, Canada. When he suspected calcium deficiency in his patients, he began to experiment with prescribing several times the RDA of calcium, magnesium, vitamin D, and other nutrients to his patients. Reich was immediately rewarded with a high percentage of his patients (who were suffering from a variety of chronic degenerative diseases) getting better. By the 1980s, Dr. Reich had cured thousands of suffering patients. He did not specialize in cancer, so most of his patients received treatment for conditions such as asthma, arthritis, colitis, dermatitis, rheumatism, migraine, fatigue, and depression. But his findings on calcium deficiency applied to cancer as well.

Dr. Reich also reasoned that the minimum daily requirements of vitamins and minerals was way too low, and he was the first doctor in North America to prescribe "mega doses" of vitamin and mineral supplements. He figured out that a big factor behind why so many people showed signs of calcium deficiency was because they did not have enough vitamin D in their bodies. Even though calcium is one of the most important bioelements, it is also one of the more *difficult* elements for the body to assimilate. This is because, once calcium has been fully dissolved in the stomach, its absorption into the body is *completely dependent* on adequate levels of vitamin D in the intestinal tract. Thus, no matter how much dietary calcium a person ingests, without adequate vitamin D to aid in its absorption, most of this calcium will just pass through the body. Dr. Reich made the important discovery that many people who had enough calcium in their diets were actually not assimilating the calcium they were ingesting due to insufficient levels of vitamin D.

Unfortunately, vitamin D is quite rare in most foods. The only *common* food source with significant amounts of vitamin D is fish (and fish oils). Possibly one of the richest food sources of vitamin D is eel, a delicacy found in many sushi bars. A less common food source with significant amounts of vitamin D is Shiitake mushrooms, which may account for some of this mushroom's healing action. But, in general, food sources of vitamin D are rare. Luckily, Mother Nature has made up for this by providing our bodies with the ability to manufacture vitamin D at the surface of our skin when exposed to sunlight. This sunlight-induced vitamin D then gets relayed to our intestinal tracts. If the vitamin D receptors of the small intestine are saturated, a person's body can increase its absorption of calcium by a factor of 20.[10]

Vitamin D deficiency could be considered yet another nutritional deficiency of modern living because, before modern times, humans spent much more of their time outdoors exposed to sunlight. If they lived in cold climates, such as in the northern latitudes, and couldn't be exposed to a lot of sunlight, then they tended to subsist on large amounts of fish. (Mainly because very cold climates do not support agriculture or even sufficient game hunting.) In the old days, when people lived in warm climates, they generally had minimal clothing covering their skin and spent many hours every day exposed to sunlight while they did their hunting, gathering, farming, preparing of tools, and so forth.

Nowadays, many people spend most of their time *indoors* in artificial lighting, which does *not* provide the spectrum of light needed to produce vitamin D. And when people today are outdoors, they often have clothing covering most of their skin. For people wearing loincloths and spending most of their time outdoors, their bodies could produce between 1 million and 3 million IUs of vitamin D every day. This is quite a contrast to the ridiculously low recommended daily allowance (RDA) of vitamin D which is 400 IUs. To put this RDA amount in perspective, 400 IUs can easily be produced on the average person's skin surface in less than 18 seconds if that person's body is in full exposure to sunlight![11]

Dr. Reich eventually met and collaborated with the chemist, Robert Barefoot, to write *The Calcium Factor*. In this enlightening book, they make the following points:

- No mineral is involved in as many biological functions in the body as calcium.

- Calcium is the key "biological workhorse" that brings nutrients into all of our cells (helping to nourish all the cells of the body).

- None of calcium's jobs is more important than its role in helping to maintain proper pH levels in the body.

- One problem that can occur if the intracellular and extracellular fluids are too acid, is that cell walls can begin to disintegrate. When this happens, toxins and carcinogens are able to get inside the cell and possibly bind with the DNA's nucleotides. Some of these toxins and carcinogens can then cause the DNA to mutate with a result of cancer.[12]

In a sense, Dr. Reich actually considered cancer to be "'*tailor made*' to survive and to thrive in an ionic calcium deficient environment."[13]

It is interesting to look at the diet and lifestyles of the longest-lived and healthiest people in the world, because doing so supports the importance of a high assimilation of ionic calcium. For instance, the Hunzas in Pakistan; the Armenians, Azerbaijanians, and Georgians in Russia; the Vilcabamba Indians in Ecuador; the Titicacas Indians in Peru; the Bamas in China; and the Tibetans all are mountain-residing people and drink highly mineralized water from glaciers. This water is so full of minerals, including high levels of calcium, that it is "milky" color and is called "milk of the mountains." According to Barefoot and Reich, these long-lived people may ingest, on any given day, 100,000 milligrams of calcium. The Okinawans are another group of people who are incredibly healthy and long-lived and though they live at sea level, they do just as well by drinking water full of coral calcium. This water is a result of dissolved coral reefs, is also milky white in color, and is called "milk of the oceans."

All of the above groups of people are virtually disease-free and are not limited to our required daily amounts, or RDAs, of minerals. In fact, they consume about 70 times the RDA of calcium, 22 times the RDA of magnesium, and 18 times the RDA of potassium, to name just a few of their abundant dietary nutrients.[14] All of these minerals are highly alkalizing to the body and are therefore preventive to disease.

Barefoot and Reich suggest that a change in diet alone can, over time, bring a person's body back into correct pH balance. But if a person has cancer, they suggest that the person will want to bring about their pH re-balancing as quickly as possible—and that requires high doses of certain supplements. Calcium, magnesium, and vitamin D are very important for regaining pH balance, and in particular, many people find that supplementing with a coral calcium product helps immensely. Of the various coral calcium products on the market today, the "marine harvested" and "high-grade" versions are probably the best. Vitamin D is also added to coral calcium products.

In general, it is best to consult with your physician, nutritionist, or alternative cancer specialist about how to alkalize your body when you have cancer. This is to ensure that the alkalizng supplements and/or diet changes you choose are compatible with your cancer treatment approach and support your optimim recovery.

If you are *not* under the supervision of a knowledgeable practitioner who can advise you about diet and supplementation, then my research indicates that the *best* way to alkalize your body once you have cancer is *through the added use of mineral supplementation*, and not through diet alone. The two main reasons are:

1. Diet alone is often not a powerful enough way to regain acid/alkaline balance once a condition like cancer has developed.

2. People can fall into a trap of becoming deficient in certain nutrients by trying to alkalize just through diet alone. Common examples of this are when people avoid all meat because it is acid-forming, then suffer from a B_{12} deficiency. Or they avoid all fish because it is acid-forming, and then suffer from radically low essential fatty acids in their diets. Or they avoid acid-forming eggs, not realizing that the albumin in eggs can be extremely helpful to the healing process for cancer patients.

Well-chosen mineral supplements can replenish the body's reserves of alkalizing minerals much more quickly than diet alone can. As already mentioned, some of the most important supplements to focus on are calcium, magnesium, potassium, and vitamin D. Coral calcium products are very popular and are generally effective. Alkaline micro water can also be a good way to help alkalize the body. And a variety of other supplements can also be effective.

If you *also* wish to improve your diet for alkalizing purposes, then the best thing to focus on is probably the reduction of refined foods from your diet. Processed, refined foods such as chips, crackers, pastries, candy, white bread, white rice, and sodas are all acid forming and do not have any healing nutrition in them for your body to use. And, of course, while working on improving your alkaline/acid balance, saliva pH test strips are an easy way to regularly monitor your progress.

Resources:

Books

Robert R. Barefoot and Carl J. Reich, M.D. *The Calcium Factor: The Scientific Secret of Health and Youth.* Wickenburg, Arizona: Deonna Enterprises Publishing, 2001. (ISBN 0-9633703-3-2) (Can be ordered from Exxel Audio by calling: 800-443-9935.)

Herman Aihara. *Acid and Alkaline.* Oroville, California: George Ohsawa Macrobiotic Foundation, 1986. (ISBN 0-918860-44-X)

Websites

www.superior-coral.com (also can call 1-877-287-3263)

www.healthtreasures.com

www.cureamerica.net

www.hopeforcancer.com/OxyPlus.htm (Also contains information about Warburg's Oxygen Boosting and alkalizing formula, "Oxy Plus.")

www.alkalizeforhealth.net

www.cocoonnutrition.org

www.gethealthyagain.com

CHAPTER 19

What Women *Must* Know About Hormones

There can be many contributing factors to the development of cancer. But one particularly important factor for women is hormone imbalance. Many important hormones in our bodies work together and, when in balance, contribute to our overall health and well-being. Some of these important hormones are thyroid, DHEA, testosterone, and the cortisols. However, for women with cancer, the most important hormones to monitor closely are their estrogen and progesterone levels, and those are the hormones we will be focusing on in this chapter.

Estrogen, Progesterone, and Hormone Imbalance

Generally, hormone imbalance in women occurs when there is too much estrogen and too little progesterone in their bodies. In our discussion of women's hormones and cancer, two concepts need to be clarified up front. The first concept is that "estrogen" is really a *group* name because every woman actually has three different estrogen hormones in her body. These three types of estrogen are called: estradiol, estrone, and estriol. Whenever hormones are discussed, these three types tend to be *collectively* referred to as "estrogen."

The second concept is that, in discussing hormone imbalance, it is the *natural* estrogens and *natural* progesterone to which I am referring. So, if you are a woman and thinking something like, "Well, I am getting my hormones balanced right now because I am on hormone replacement therapy," then you may need to think again. The hormones provided in conventional hormone replacement therapy, such as those in "Premarin" and "Provera," are *not* natural, and do not rectify hormone imbalance in the body. Actually, most hormone replacement therapies prescribed by conventional doctors involve *synthetic* hormones. Also, the hormones in birth control pills are synthetic. The difference between synthetic and natural hormones will be discussed soon, but remember, it is only the *natural* forms of hormones that can bring about true hormone balance in a woman.

All hormones perform very important physiological functions. In doing so, hormones can be *so* powerful that nature has created checks and balances for them. The way that our bodies naturally keep the estrogen levels in check, for instance is by producing the hormone progesterone to *oppose* the estrogens. The opposing effects of progesterone keep the effects of the estrogens in balance, and this balance is necessary if the woman's body is to function normally and stay healthy. If a healthy balance is *not* maintained, and a woman has too much estrogen and too little progesterone functioning in her body over a significant period of time, then she is prone to many serious health problems. These health problems can even be life-threatening, and include stroke, heart attack, osteoporosis (or brittle bones), and yes, even cancer. The types of cancer in women that are most frequently caused by an estrogen/progesterone imbalance are the cancers of the sex organs. Thus, these tend to be breast cancer, endometrial (uterine) cancer, and ovarian cancer. But other cancers can result, in part, from hormone imbalance as well.

Estrogen/progesterone imbalances can also play a role in the development of cancer for men. The type of cancer most frequently caused by this type of hormone imbalance in men is prostate cancer. But there are reasons why an imbalance between estrogen and progesterone *can often be a much bigger cancer factor* for women than for men. One reason is that a woman's natural life cycle includes big changes in her hormone levels during her mid-life years. These changes are involved with the transition into menopause.

In general, a woman's progesterone production will begin to decrease 10 to 15 years before menopause begins, then will continue to drop even lower for several years afterward. Her estrogen levels, on the other hand, will not decrease much during her premenopausal years. Just before menopause her estrogen levels will, however, become more variable, with up and down surges. It is not until a woman is actually experiencing menopause and no longer having menstrual cycles that her estrogen levels have finally decreased a significant amount. Thus, hormone imbalance in women occurs partly because, during the pre-menopause phase, their estrogen and progesterone levels do not drop equally.

This gap between estrogen and progesterone is then widened even more by environmental and dietary factors that contribute to *increases* in a woman's estrogen levels. (These other factors will be discussed in more detail when we look at the causes of estrogen dominance.) Women in the modern western world suffer from these added environmental and dietary factors the most. This is why they tend to suffer more from menopausal symptoms than many women in third world or Asian countries.

Another *major* reason women are much more likely than men to suffer serious hormone imbalance is that they are so often recipients of some form of prescribed, synthetic hormones. These synthetic hormones are most often in the form of: (1) birth control pills, or (2) hormone replacement therapy (HRT). HRT is usually prescribed for symptoms of menopause, including the frequently occurring "surgically induced" menopause that is a result of hysterectomy. These two sources of prescribed hormones can cause many women to actually spend decades of their lives on a hormone regimen that can cause a very unhealthy imbalance in their bodies. And many of them are not told, and are thus not aware, that this imbalance can significantly increase their chance of developing cancer and other life-threatening conditions.

Estrogen Dominance

When women develop an imbalance between estrogen and progesterone, it is almost always the estrogen levels that are too high and the progesterone levels that are too low. It very rarely happens the other way. John R. Lee, M.D., has spent many years researching and writing books about the dangers of hormone imbalances in modern women. In discussing what causes these imbalances, Dr. Lee coined the term "estrogen dominance." Estrogen dominance refers to the *ratio* of estrogen to progesterone. In other words, before, during and after menopause, a woman may suffer from various menopause symptoms as a result of her estrogen levels being low. These symptoms of low estrogen might be hot flashes, dry skin, vaginal dryness, low sex drive, difficulty sleeping, and so forth. But even with low estrogen levels, she may *still* be estrogen dominant. This is because her progesterone level most likely is even *lower* than her estrogen, and the ratio of estrogen to progesterone in her body is still imbalanced in the direction of too much estrogen.

Breast cancer, which is now the second leading cause of cancer deaths among women (after lung cancer), is extremely sensitive to this type of hormone imbalance. Luckily, the good news is that the *correction* of hormone imbalance can not only help to *prevent* cancer in women, especially breast cancer, but can also significantly improve a woman's chances of recovery from cancer once she has it.

To understand how estrogen dominance contributes to cancer, we must first understand estrogen and progesterone a little better. The estrogens perform many functions in our bodies. But for women, one of the most important functions of the estrogens could be described in this simplified way: The estrogens prepare a woman for reproduction. (The word "estrogen" was coined originally when researchers first discovered its "estrus-producing" capabilities.) In other words, the estrogens bring on menses in teenage girls (or stimulate the proliferation of endometrial cells in preparation for pregnancy), and the estrogens stimulate the development of breast tissue in young women to prepare them for breast-feeding. Both of these important functions involve the stimulation of new cell growth.

On the other hand, one of the most important functions of progesterone in women could be described in this simplified way: Progesterone protects pregnancy once pregnancy has been initiated. (The word "progesterone" was coined originally to mean "pro-gestation.") In other words, there are many health benefits to the body that progesterone provides throughout the life of every woman, but it has a *particularly* important job during pregnancy. During pregnancy, a woman's progesterone production shoots sky high. This high level of progesterone in her body then protects the developing fetus by preventing ovulation and the ensuing sloughing off of the endometrial lining. In fact, women who have low levels of progesterone will sometimes experience repeated miscarriages because their bodies are not producing enough natural progesterone to safeguard the normal process of gestation.

Another thing to keep in mind is that estrogen is dominant in a woman's body throughout the first week of her menstruation, and progesterone is the dominant hormone in a woman's body right after ovulation and for the two weeks preceding her menstrual period. When a woman does not produce enough progesterone she will often experience symptoms of PMS. This is because the progesterone hormone is supposed to be dominant the two weeks before menstruation, and if there is insufficient progesterone at this time, a woman will feel noticeable symptoms. Thus, many women have reported great relief from their PMS symptoms after they started supplementing their bodies with natural progesterone.

So, it is a direct result of women being the child-bearing sex that initially sets them up for a roller-coaster ride with their hormones. Women's bodies must be able to switch between two drastically different modes—

gestation and non-gestation—and these different modes require different hormones being dominant at different times. Men don't have to switch between these different modes, and so their hormone balance is easier for their bodies to maintain. But normally, this roller-coaster ride should not be too difficult. Women's bodies have evolved to handle the changes in their hormones. It is largely because of modern living that these changes have instigated far more out-of-balance states in women than ever before.

Estrogen Dominance and Cancer

The cancer risk from estrogen dominance results from the fact that the estrogens tend to stimulate cell growth. Because of this simple factor, estrogen dominance puts a woman at serious risk for developing cancer. And if a woman *already* has cancer, the state of estrogen dominance can make it more difficult for her to achieve recovery. This cancer-promoting factor of estrogen is widely accepted by the medical community and is the reason most doctors will refuse to prescribe estrogen for menopausal symptoms to a woman who has cancer.

Exactly how does estrogen promote cell growth? It does this by activating an oncogene, or cancer-stimulating gene, in cells. The cancer-stimulating gene that responds to estrogen is called "Bcl-2." Progesterone, on the other hand, *down-regulates* this very same Bcl-2 gene, and up-regulates a tumor-suppressor gene in the same cells. This tumor-suppressor gene is called "p53." When p53 is activated, it slows cell reproduction and restores proper programmed cell death. This programmed cell death is called "apoptosis" (pronounced with the second *p* silent), and is an integral function of all normal, healthy cells. Thus, estrogen tends to stimulate uncontrolled cell growth by activating the Bcl-2 gene, and progesterone tends to stop uncontrolled cell growth by activating the p53 gene, which slows reproduction and restores proper programmed cell death.

As we have seen so many times before, nature tends to provide checks and balances for all physiological processes. As long as a woman's estrogen and progesterone levels are balanced, she will not experience out-of-control cell growth. But once her estrogen level is "dominant," then the many different effects of her estrogen can go unchecked.

So far, we have been discussing the type of estrogen dominance that can occur in a woman's body with her own natural hormones. But even more of a cancer risk is when a woman is prescribed estrogen for menopause symptoms and *not* prescribed natural progesterone along with it. This is referred to as prescribing "unopposed estrogen," and it rarely happens anymore because doctors are now very aware that they should not prescribe unopposed estrogen. The dangers of doing this became all too clear after mainstream medical doctors had been prescribing unopposed estrogen for about 20 years to menopausal women and then found out that a high number of these women were developing endometrial cancer.

But what conventional doctors have not yet fully admitted is that this practice of prescribing unopposed estrogen for two decades not only caused uterine cancer, but it also caused many women to develop and die of breast cancer. In his book, *What Your Doctor May Not Tell You About Breast Cancer*, Dr. Lee comments on the rapid rise in breast cancer during the middle of the twentieth century:

> The probable cause of the rise in breast cancer deaths was the prescription of unopposed estrogen (not balanced with progesterone) to menopausal women, a common practice from the early 1950s to the mid-1970s. While the medical community acknowledged that this practice caused endometrial (uterine) cancer, it never admitted that it also caused breast cancer.[1]

Thus, using prescribed estrogen *without* also supplementing with natural progesterone is a *huge* cancer risk to women. As Dr. Lee stated, this practice not only can cause fatal breast cancer and uterine cancer, but as we shall see later on, it can also cause fatal ovarian cancer.

Natural Progesterone and Breast Cancer

Over the last decade, the mainstream medical community has focused a lot on genetic predisposition factors for breast cancer. Some conventional doctors are pushing the genetic origins of breast cancer so much that some women who do not even have cancer are actually deciding to get "preemptive" mastectomies just because there is a history of breast cancer in their family. But according to Dr. Lee and his colleagues, only about 10 percent of all breast cancer cases in this country can be attributed to "inherited" genetic causes. And these genetic causes only predispose some women to breast cancer—they don't guarantee that cancer will develop. On the other hand, Dr. Lee believes that something as controllable as estrogen dominance can be a powerful contributing factor to cancer in women.

Support for the link between estrogen dominance and breast cancer comes from a study that was done back in the early 1980s by L. D. Cowan and colleagues at Johns Hopkins University. These researchers discovered that women who had low levels of progesterone in their bodies ended up having a 540 percent higher incidence of cancer than women who had good progesterone levels.[2]

An even more interesting study was carried out from 1975 to the mid-1990s (over an 18-year period) in England. This study was conducted by P. E. Mohr, M.D., a British physician, and the results were published in a 1996 issue of the *British Journal of Cancer*. Dr. Mohr and his colleagues went to the top three surgical hospitals in London and asked them to measure a variety of hormone levels in women at the time of breast surgery for all breast cancer patients in those hospitals. This was done, and the results were fascinating. (Incidentally, all of the women in this study were node-positive cases, meaning their breast cancer had already metastasized.) What Dr. Mohr's study showed was that those women whose breast cancer surgery was performed in the *second half* of their menstrual cycle (which is when their own production of progesterone was at its highest) were *much less likely* to have their breast cancer recur later on.

This study showed that, of the women who had higher levels of progesterone in their bodies at the time of surgery, about 65 percent were still alive 18 years later. But of those women who had low levels of progesterone on the day of their surgery, only about 35 percent were still alive 18 years later.[3] In other words, if you are a woman preparing to undergo breast cancer surgery, Dr. Lee says, "You *double* your survival rate just by having your progesterone level satisfactory on the day of your surgery!"

Dr. Mohr's study looked at women whose progesterone levels were high or low on the day of surgery simply due to part of their menstrual cycle they were in. Dr. Lee believes that if these women had been *supplemented* with natural progesterone at ages when their own levels began to drop, it is possible that they would have done even better. One of the reasons he believes this is that, since 1978, Dr. Lee has put many of his own female patients on natural progesterone for osteoporosis. In cases where the woman had a history of cancer, no estrogen was prescribed along with the progesterone because of the cancer stimulating effects of estrogen. Over the next 20 years, Dr. Lee made a point of following these women who had a history of cancer that he had put on natural progesterone. Amazingly, he found that *not one* of them died of cancer in those 20 years.

Thus, both the 18-year study done by Dr. Mohr and Dr. Lee's own experience with his female patients showed that supplementing with therapeutic levels of natural progesterone can *significantly decrease the likelihood that a woman will have a recurrence of her breast cancer.*

Natural Versus Synthetic Hormones

Unfortunately, when the medical community was finally forced to accept that they could not safely prescribe unopposed estrogen to women, rather than add *natural* progesterone to their prescriptions, they chose to add *synthetic* progesterone. There are various forms of synthetic progesterone, and they are all technically referred to as progestins. (The most commonly prescribed progestin today is "Provera.") Most likely, this practice came about because pharmaceutical companies could not patent and make high profits from selling natural progesterone, but they *could* make high profits from selling synthetic progesterone.

But synthetic progestins do *not* protect against cancer as natural progesterone does. After years of prescribing synthetic progestins along with estrogen, the medical community finally began to see evidence that progestins did not control the cancer risk of unopposed estrogen. In fact, it made it worse.

The problem is that doctors do not tend to be aware of the very important differences between "synthetic" progestins and "natural" progesterone. Since they know that estrogen and progestins can contribute to cancer, doctors often wrongly assume that natural progesterone will contribute to cancer as well. If you have cancer, and your doctor is leery of supplementing you with natural progesterone, keep this in mind: Synthetic progestins contribute to cancer. Natural progesterone protects against cancer. It is terribly unfortunate for women that many doctors still do not understand this functional difference.

Understanding the structural difference between natural hormones and synthetic hormones is simple. In a nutshell, *natural* hormones are those hormones that occur naturally in our bodies, *or* are produced in a laboratory to have *exactly* the same biochemical structure as those in our bodies. Each hormone in our bodies has a specific chemical structure that is unique to that hormone. For example, there is only one specific molecule that is estradiol, one specific molecule that is estrone, one specific molecule that is estriol and one specific molecule that is progesterone. Because pharmaceutical companies cannot patent and thereby cannot make exorbitant profits on any natural substance, they prefer to modify the hormones they sell. They do this by changing the natural hormone molecule in some way so that it is no longer the exact same molecule (or hormone) that occurs naturally. Then, they have a substance they can patent. Whenever a hormone molecule is even one atom different from the natural hormone found in nature, it is referred to as "synthetic."

However, natural hormones can also be "synthesized" in laboratories. For example, natural progesterone is produced by our bodies, but it can also be synthesized in a laboratory from plant sources to be completely "bioidentical" to the progesterone we make in our bodies. These plant sources tend to be either wild yam extract or soy, and contain "diosgenin," which is similar to our own natural progesterone. In laboratories, diosgenin can easily be altered just a little bit to become exactly bioidentical to the progesterone found in our bodies. Thus, in the field of hormone research and prescription, the synthesized result is called "natural progesterone." It is synthesized from something that is natural to plants, and it only requires a minimal change to turn it into something that is natural to humans.

One way to look at this terminology is the following: to "synthesize" something just means putting something together from parts. But "synthetic" refers to any substance *not found in nature.*

As long as the natural progesterone, which is synthesized in laboratories to put into natural progesterone creams and pills, is exactly bioidentical to the progesterone in our bodies, then it is completely safe and will carry out all the same functions in our bodies as the progesterone we naturally produce. Synthetic hormones, on the other hand, are produced to have almost the same, *but not exactly the same,* chemical structure as those hormones that occur naturally in our bodies. Thus, they carry out some of the same functions in our bodies as our own natural hormones, but not all of them. This is not a good thing for women because *all* of the functions of our natural hormones are there for a reason. Also, synthetic hormones can bind to receptor sites for much longer periods of time than their corresponding natural hormones would, which means they can *block* the action of a woman's own natural hormones that her body may still be producing.

In the case of progesterone, the synthetic forms (called progestins) definitely do not have many of the protective and beneficial effects on the body as the natural, bioidentical form of progesterone. Progestins do *not* provide the protective effects against stroke, heart disease, osteoporosis, and cancer that natural progesterone does. And because they block a woman's own natural progesterone from binding to cell receptor sites, they actually make estrogen dominance *worse.* Plus, one of the key ways that natural progesterone helps to prevent cancer is by activating the p53 gene in cells—the tumor-suppressor gene that slows cell proliferation and stimulates normal cell death. However, according to Dr. Lee, most synthetic progestins do *not* activate the p53 gene. In fact, because progestins are so dangerous and promote so many serious health risks, Dr. Lee states, "Prescribing a progestin to a menopausal woman should be considered medical malpractice." Yet, synthetic progestins, are the progesterone-like hormones in all birth control pills as well as in conventional hormone replacement therapy for menopause!

The fact that synthetic hormones are not exactly the same in molecular structure as those hormones naturally found in our bodies turns out to be a *huge* distinction. In the world of chemical molecules, changing just one atom can sometimes turn a molecule into a completely different thing—such as a completely different hormone. Nowhere is the difference between natural and synthetic hormones so clear as in diagrams of their chemical structures. For example, here is a graphic representation of three different molecules. The first shows the chemical structure of the hormone "testosterone," the second shows the chemical structure of the hormone "progesterone," and the third shows the chemical structure of the synthetic progestin "Provera."

Testosterone
(natural form)

Progesterone
(natural form)

Provera
(Medroxyprogesterone Acetate)

As you can see, the two hormones—testosterone and progesterone—are extremely similar in chemical structure. Yet, virtually everybody knows there is a big difference in how these two hormones function in the body. Thus, a very small change in chemical structure can produce a large change in how the molecule functions in the body. Look at the drug Provera. It is obvious this molecule has quite a few differences in its chemical structure from that of natural progesterone. In fact, natural progesterone is actually *more* similar in structure to testosterone, a completely different hormone, than it is to Provera, its synthetic counterpart!

The most common hormone replacement therapy regimen being prescribed to menopausal women today is a combination of the two drugs Provera and Premarin. This is the regimen that is supposed to "replace" their insufficient levels of estrogen and progesterone. We have already seen how different Provera is from the natural progesterone women need. Now, let's look at Premarin to see how similar that is to the natural estrogen women need.

Plain and simple, Premarin is a strange source of estrogen for women because it is made up of "horse" hormones. Yes, that's right. Premarin is synthesized from horse urine taken from pregnant mares. Because horses are a different species and their hormones are thus different from ours, this drug puts estrogen hormones into women that may be natural to horses but are not bioidentical to human estrogens. Premarin, therefore, is considered a source of "synthetic" estrogen for women. Moreover, the process of producing Premarin is very cruel to the horses that are used. Pregnant horses are kept in inhumane conditions so their urine can be used to create this very profitable drug. If you have any doubt as to whether this is where the drug Premarin comes from, just look at the name: "Premarin" is short for *pregnant mare's urine*.

The point to remember is that *all* synthetic estrogens and *all* synthetic progestins are *un*-natural hormones. And they *all* create an imbalanced situation in a woman's body that can contribute to stroke, heart disease, brittle bones, and cancer. Yet, how many reasons are there for women to be prescribed synthetic hormones? Here are six common ones:

1. To alleviate menopause symptoms.

2. To supply hormones depleted by hysterectomy.

3. To avoid pregnancy through use of "the pill."

4. To treat osteoporosis.

5. To alleviate painful or irregular menstruation.

6. To reduce acne.

The cruel reality is that, ever since the development of synthetic hormones, modern women have been turning into stroke, heart disease, and cancer casualties in alarming numbers.

In its January 26, 2000, issue, the *Journal of the American Medical Association* published a study that was done on a whopping 46,000 women. This huge study concluded that the most commonly prescribed form of HRT (Premarin and Provera) produced a 40 percent higher risk of breast cancer in women who used it for five years as compared to women *not* using conventional HRT. This breast cancer risk factor was deemed to increase by 8 percent for each year of use, so women on Premarin and Provera for 10 years could be assumed to have an 80 percent higher risk, women on Premarin and Provera for 20 years could be assumed to have a 160 percent higher risk, and so forth. Yet, a combination of Premarin and Provera is *still* the most common form of hormone replacement therapy prescribed to women today.

Unfortunately, the truth of the above study has still not completely reached the public. This is partly because, when the above study results came out, newspapers and other media around the country (such as medical writers and TV commentators) reported the study inaccurately. They mistakenly used the term "progesterone" when they were referring to the synthetic "progestins" used in the study.[4]

It is critical that the public and doctors distinguish between progesterone and progestins. And it is critical that people realize there are *many* results from studies and statistics showing that progesterone in its natural form carries a protective effect against cancer and other health problems. For instance, its cancer-protective effect is evidenced by the fact that the most common age for women to start showing the beginning stages of breast cancer is about five years before menopause.[5] This is exactly when a woman's own progesterone level has dropped dramatically, yet well before her estrogen levels have fallen.

The cancer-protective effects of natural progesterone are also evidenced by the statistic that going through a full-term pregnancy by age 24 can *reduce* the risk of breast cancer for a woman by more than half.[6] During pregnancy a woman goes through many months where her progesterone level is extremely high as compared to those times when she is not pregnant. This high level of progesterone contributes to normal differentiation of breast tissue and can have a long-term protective effect against cancer developing later on in the breasts.

Since birth control pills are made with synthetic progestins, the use of birth control pills at young ages can contribute to breast cancer as well. Dr. Lee states,

> It has been well established that when girls between the ages of 13 and 18—and to a lesser but still significant effect, women up to the age

of 21—use birth control pills, their risk of breast cancer can increase by as much as 60 percent. The younger a girl begins to use contraceptive hormones, the greater her risk of breast cancer.[7]

Dr. Lee and his colleagues believe that this predisposition to breast cancer caused by birth control pill usage happens in two ways: (1) the synthetic progestins in the birth control pills block the beneficial and cancer-protecting activity of a woman's natural progesterone; and (2) because the pill blocks ovulation, it thereby blocks a certain amount of a woman's own supply of natural progesterone from being produced in the first place.

Other Causes of Estrogen Dominance

If hormone imbalance *only* occurred as a result of conventional HRT or birth control pills, then many women who had never taken either of these would be able to rest easy. However, this is not the case. There are other causes of hormone imbalance and estrogen dominance in modern women as well that do *not* involve prescribed hormones. For those women who have never undergone prescribed synthetic hormone use, the main factors contributing to estrogen dominance are: environmental xenoestrogens, diets high in refined carbohydrates and low in phytochemicals, and excess body fat.

Xenoestrogens

Xenoestrogens are petrochemically derived compounds that are "estrogen-like," which most people are exposed to on a regular basis. (The *x* in xenoestrogens is pronounced like a *z*, as in "xylophone.") The prefix "xeno" means "foreign" and indicates that xenoestrogens are not normally found in nature. These unnatural compounds are considered "estrogenic" because they produce estrogen activity in our bodies.

We are exposed to xenoestrogens in a variety of ways:

- We ingest xenoestrogens from pesticides used on crops whenever we eat nonorganic supermarket fruits and vegetables.

- We absorb xenoestrogens into our bodies through our skin whenever we come in contact with common lawn and garden sprays, as well as indoor insect sprays.

- We breathe in xenoestrogens from car exhaust and smog.

- We drink in xenoestrogens in areas where industrial waste dumps have contaminated the ground water supply.

- We eat xenoestrogens sometimes when ingest eat meat or dairy products from livestock fed estrogenic drugs to fatten them up.

- We are exposed to xenoestrogens through the use of common solvents, soaps, and plastics.

Xenoestrogens are everywhere. They are nonbiodegradable and accumulate in our bodies over time. Because they build up in our bodies and mimic our own estrogen, they dangerously contribute to the condition of estrogen dominance. According to Dr. Lee, all xenoestrogens (as well as other xenohormones) should be considered toxic.

There are two main ways that environmental xenoestrogens contribute to estrogen dominance. The first way is that they bind to estrogen receptors in our bodies and produce an increase in estrogenic activity. The second way that xenoestrogens contribute to estrogen dominance in women is that they can damage a woman's egg follicles and cause ovarian dysfunction.[8] Ovarian dysfunction can then result in the decrease of a woman's own progesterone production. Chronic xenohormone exposure to adult women can bring about this ovarian dysfunction and result in reduced progesterone production, but it can happen much earlier, too. It is now known that exposure to xenohormones as early as during embryo development can cause this functional loss of ovarian follicles.[9] This means that estrogen dominance for many of us women may be partly caused by the environmental xenohormones *our mothers were exposed to when they were pregnant with us.*

It is imperative that the public at large become more aware of the dangers of xenoestrogens in our environment. These dangerous, nonbiodegradable chemicals are already reducing the populations of many other species on our planet, and are seriously contributing to reduced fertility in women and men as well. In general, men in industrialized countries are already showing greatly reduced sperm counts (compared to their grandfathers) as a result of these xenohormones. Some researchers believe that humans may, at some point, become an endangered species because of the multitude of xenohormones in our environment.

Diet

It is well known that eating lots of fresh fruits and vegetables on a regular basis can protect against all kinds of cancer. This is in large part due to the cancer-fighting vitamins and minerals, as well as the natural fiber that these healthful foods provide. However, few people know that diets high in fresh fruits and vegetables also protect against the cancer-prone condition of estrogen dominance. One of the ways they do this is by providing our bodies with what are called "phytoestrogens."

Phytoestrogens, or plant estrogens, are natural compounds found in plants that have weak estrogen-like activity in humans. They are part of the larger family of compounds known as "phytochemicals," and are a natural and important part of any healthy diet. There are presently 18 different phytochemicals known to be estrogenic in humans. These phytoestrogens bind to estrogen receptors in the body and convey many of the health benefits of human estrogen to men and women alike. And because they bind to estrogen receptors, they compete with our own estrogen hormones for the same receptors.

This is particularly helpful for women battling estrogen dominance because the weaker plant estrogens block some of the activity of the excess, stronger human estrogens. They do not cling to the receptors for long and are easily processed out of the body.

The seven subgroups of phytoestrogens are: isoflavones, coumestans, flavanones, flavones, flavanols, lignans, and chalcones. The isoflavones and coumestans are the most powerful of the phytoestrogens, with about a 10-fold stronger estrogenic effect than the others. Virtually all plants, including vegetables, fruits, seeds, legumes, and grains, have some form of phytoestrogen in them. Flavanones are primarily concentrated in citrus fruits, lignans are found in all fruits, vegetables, and cereals, and the stronger isoflavones and coumestans are mostly found in legumes.

Because of so much processed food in our diets, Americans generally don't eat as many "whole" foods as people in other countries do. There are many other populations around the world where a higher percentage of the daily diet consists of various forms of whole vegetables, grains, seeds, legumes and fruits than in the United States. In those populations, women generally don't have to deal with as much estrogen dominance because they haven't spent a lifetime eating processed and refined foods virtually devoid of phytochemicals.

The isoflavones are some of the most potent phytoestrogens to humans, yet, ironically, they are the most lacking in the modern western diet. This is because when most Westerners eat a phytochemical-containing plant, it is usually in the form of a piece of fruit or a salad vegetable. It is not usually in the form of some type of legume (or bean). Yet, in countries where women suffer the *least* from symptoms of PMS and menopause, legumes are part of their staple diet. In the orient, this staple legume tends to be the soybean, and in Central and South America, this staple tends to be made up of more than one legume, including chickpeas and lentils.

The important isoflavone category of phytoestrogens can be broken down into four *specific* isoflavones. These are: genistein, biochanin, daidzein, and formononetin. Every time we eat a legume, we are consuming at least one of these four beneficial isoflavones. A great deal of research has been done on the effects of isoflavones. Besides helping to alleviate the many uncomfortable symptoms of estrogen dominance, isoflavones have also been shown to have potent anti-cancer properties. They fight cancer in a variety of ways, including by inducing apoptosis (normal cell death) and inhibiting angiogenesis (new blood vessel growth to cancer cells). In addition to their direct anti-cancer properties, isoflavones are also known to be diuretics, have anti-inflammatory properties, are antioxidants, and can stimulate the immune system and improve cardiovascular health.

Thus, women who have diets low in fresh fruits, vegetables, and legumes, are deprived of many of the hormone-balancing nutrients these foods can supply. Soy products are becoming a more and more common way for women to naturally treat their health issues, but there is some controversy around soy as well. Unfermented soy products actually contain some anti-nutritive agents in them that are somewhat harmful to the body. Therefore, the healthiest way to get isoflavones is by eating fermented soy products, such as miso, tofu, and tempeh, as well as a variety of other legumes, such as various beans, chickpeas, and lentils.

In this discussion of diet, it is also important to note that the consumption of excess alcohol can contribute to estrogen dominance. This is because estrogen is processed out of our bodies through the liver. If a woman regularly consumes alcohol, she may be compromising the functioning of her liver and thereby not as able to process out the excess estrogen from her body as well as she should.[10] Excess ingestion of prescription drugs can also have the same effect on the liver as alcohol. Over time, the continued excess intake of alcoholic drinks and/or prescription drugs can compromise the functioning of a person's liver, which compromises the processing out of excess estrogen and thereby contributes to excess buildup of estrogen in the body and to estrogen dominance.

Body Fat

Yet another reason women in the modern western world have more problems with hormone imbalance than others is that they tend to be more overweight. Easy access to processed and fast foods, overly generous restaurant meal proportions, abundant candy and snacks, and less than optimum exercise levels have all taken a toll on both men and women. Little do most women know, however, that fat cells produce estrogen. In general, the more fat a woman has, the more estrogen she is likely to be making in her body, even *after* menopause.[11] These extra fat cells, each making estrogen, complicate the problem by being storage cells for xenoestrogens as well. It is no wonder that a largely overweight country like the United States is also a largely estrogen-dominant country.

So, when it comes to estrogen dominance, there are four main causes:

1. Synthetic hormones from HRT and birth control pills

2. Xenoestrogens from pesticides and other environmental sources

3. Diets low in phytochemicals and high in refined carbohydrates

4. Excess body fat

For more information on estrogen dominance, and how to correct female hormone imbalance, I highly recommend *any* of Dr. John R. Lee's books, videos, and audiotapes. According to Dr. Lee, one of the quickest and easiest ways to start correcting this imbalance, if you have it, is by using natural progesterone.

Pesticides and Breast Cancer

In examining direct causes of breast cancer, xenoestrogens, and other toxins from pesticides need to be looked at closely. These dangerous chemicals may promote a high risk of developing breast cancer in women for two main reasons. One reason is that toxins from pesticides and industrial waste tend to be stored in the body in fatty tissues and women's breast tissue is made up of about one-third fat. As long as these toxins sit in the fatty tissue, they pose a risk of genetic damage to cells. Moreover, these and other toxins can *accumulate* in breast tissue over time, posing a greater and greater threat to each woman as she grows older. Corporations that cause pollution often refer to the small amount of toxins that people are exposed to at *any given time* as being safe, without ever addressing the fact that these toxins can accumulate and concentrate in the body and have a *cumulative* effect over time.[12] This is an example of how science can be misused and facts can be presented in a misleading way.

If you think that pesticides are safely controlled by laws, you may not know that many of the pesticide chemicals used today are *exempt* from current laws. For instance, in 1970 the EPA set certain safe pesticide limits. But within this legislation, congress allowed "the continued use of all pesticides approved before 1970." (This is a curious way to enforce environmental protection regulations.) Similarly, in 1978, more accurate measures of testing pesticides for safety were enacted, but this legislation once again *exempted all pesticides that had been approved prior to 1978.*[13]

One of the most telling studies about the relationship between pesticides and breast cancer involved the entire country of Israel. After breast cancer deaths had been rising in Israel for about 25 years, they dropped sharply between the years of 1976 and 1986. The only apparent reason was a strict ban of three organochlorine pesticides that had been enacted in the early 1970s. (These pesticides were DDT, BHC, and lindane).[14] Organochlorines are considered to be "complete" carcinogens, which means that they both *initiate cancer as well as promote cancer once it has gotten started.*[15] Moreover, along with the decrease in breast cancer cases in women after this ban, it was noted that there was also a corresponding decrease of these pesticides in cow's milk and in *Israeli women's breast milk. Breast milk, therefore, is one way that infants can receive concentrated doses of pesticide xenohormones.*

It is important that we, the public, exercise more control over what pesticides we are exposed to. And it is not just those pesticides that are used on crops that we must think about, but also those used in public buildings, on lawns, gardens, and in our own homes.

Breast Cancer Statistics

The number of women getting breast cancer has been steadily increasing over the past century, and this increase appears to be accelerating. According to the National Cancer Institute, the incidence of breast cancer rose by a whopping 40 percent between 1973 and 1988. Breast cancer is now the most common cause of death from cancer in women between the ages of 18 and 54, and the *leading* cause of death for *any* reason in women aged 45 to 50.

It is not easy to come across accurate figures of what the "cure rates" for breast cancer through conventional medicine really are. This is because all "official" statistics are based on the definition of "cure" as being "alive five years after diagnosis." Keeping a woman with breast cancer alive for five years is often achievable through surgery, radiation, and chemotherapy. But it also often involves the woman going in and out of remission, feeling frequently ill, being surgically mutilated, and never becoming cancer-free.

This bogus way of defining "cure" is one of the biggest ways that official statistics are misleading and directly give women "false hope."

There is another way organized medicine has made "official" breast cancer cure rates misleading. It is by including something called "DCIS" in their breast cancer statistics. DCIS stands for "ductal carcinoma in situ," and is classified as a form of breast cancer within the duct. But many experts debate whether DCIS should even be classified as a cancer at all. When a woman is diagnosed with DCIS, it means she has abnormal cells scattered here and there, *not* clustered together into a tumor, which are *contained within* the duct and are *not* penetrating or infiltrating the deeper layer of cells in the breast.[16] The bottom line is that DCIS is essentially known to be a *benign* condition. If the abnormal cells begin to invade the deeper tissue, then it is no longer considered DCIS. The critical thing to understand is that only a very small fraction of DCIS cases go on to become actual cancer, and therefore it is really more of a "pre-cancerous" state.[17]

According to many experts, DCIS is 99 percent curable.[18] This makes it similar to many skin cancers in that it is not generally a life-threatening condition. But the cancer industry includes this easily curable, mostly benign condition in their official breast cancer cure-rate statistics, and thereby makes the overall cure rate for *all* breast cancers look considerably better. Over the past 20 years, DCIS diagnoses have comprised approximately 30 percent of all breast cancer diagnoses.

Conventional Breast Cancer Treatments

Surgery

For virtually all breast cancer cases, surgery is the primary treatment used. Following that, radiation, chemotherapy and hormone-blocking drugs are the treatments of choice. Whether a lumpectomy (removal of the lump and surrounding tissue) or a mastectomy (removal of the entire breast and surrounding tissue) is recommended, depends on the type and stage of the breast cancer. For women whose cancer has not yet metastasized, so that they only need surgery with *no* follow-up radiation or chemo, their chances of long-term recovery are the greatest in conventional medicine. In fact, Ralph Moss reports in his book *Questioning Chemotherapy* that for cases of non-metastasized breast cancer (lymph node-negative), surgery alone will cause about 90 percent of these cases to *not have a recurrence of the disease*.[19] Many women have survived their breast cancer under these conditions and gone on to live long, normal lives.

But surgery for breast cancer is generally only curative when the cancer has not yet metastasized. Once metastasis has occurred to *any* other location, including the lymph glands, the surgery may be considered only "palliative,"[20] or simply a procedure that is not expected to bring about long-term cure but merely to buy the patient time.

Unfortunately, when metastasis has occurred and follow-up treatments after surgery are required, long-term life expectancy drops dramatically for a woman with breast cancer using conventional approaches. Here are some comments on those follow-up treatments.

Radiation

The benefits of radiation treatment for breast cancer are questionable, yet radiation is still the most commonly used treatment for breast cancer after surgery. A recent article in the British medical journal, *The Lancet*, showed that, according to one study, the use of radiation on breast cancer patients *did* reduce deaths from breast cancer by 13.2 percent. However, these same radiation treatments *increased* deaths from other causes by 21.2 percent.[21] These "other cause" deaths were largely from heart disease as a result of the radiation administered right around the heart area. As Dr. Lee puts it, the only conclusion that can be made from this study on the use of radiation for breast cancer is that "the treatment was a success but the patient died."

Chemotherapy

After surgery and radiation, chemotherapy is the next most often prescribed treatment for breast cancer. However, it is *also* debatable as to how effective this type of treatment for breast cancer is. Ralph Moss reports that there is literally *no evidence* that chemotherapy can bring about long-term survival in cases of breast cancers that have already metastasized. Yet, over two dozen chemotherapy drugs have been approved for use in metastasized breast cancer. In these cases, it is apparently hoped that the chemotherapy treatments may be able to *extend* the life of the patient somewhat.[22] Once again, we are looking at a *palliative* treatment, with the doctor hoping to buy the patient time but not necessarily expecting a cure.

As mentioned earlier, surgery alone can prevent recurrence for about 90 percent of the women surgically treated for non-metastasized breast cancer. Of those 10 percent who do have a recurrence, it has been estimated that only about 3 percent could benefit in any long-term way from chemotherapy.[23] If Ralph Moss's research and the above statistics are accurate, we must conclude that *no* patient with metastasized breast cancer will benefit in a long-term way by the use of chemotherapy, and only about 3 percent of those patients with very early stage, non-metastasized breast cancer will benefit in a long-term way from chemotherapy.

By the early 1980s, the medical community was so discouraged with their lack of long-term success in treating breast cancer, that they tried something radical. For a period of about 10 years, from the mid-1980s to the mid-1990s, a new regimen of extremely high doses of chemotherapy (about 10 times the normal amount) followed by a bone marrow transplant was tried. For a while, this highly risky combination treatment was thought by many doctors to be a woman's best chance of surviving advanced breast cancer. The high-dose chemotherapy was the cancer treatment. The bone marrow transplant was the follow-up treatment used to save the woman's life after the chemo had destroyed her bone marrow and her body's ability to produce new red blood cells.

Before the mid-1980s, about a hundred of these treatments each year were performed for breast cancer. By 1994, this number had grown considerably with about 4,000 high-dose chemotherapy/bone marrow transplant procedures being performed each year in the United States for breast cancer. This type of combination treatment is truly barbaric. It might not be out of line to say that it is the most horrendous type of treatment for any patient to undergo. The high-dose chemotherapy seriously damages the intestinal lining from mouth to anus, causing patients to endure great pain whenever they swallow or defecate. Making this unbearable are the alternating bouts of nausea, vomiting, and diarrhea the chemo causes. On top of this, the patient has to undergo extreme loneliness by being kept in an isolation room for weeks while their bone marrow recovers. This isolation is necessary because their immune system has been so damaged that they are highly susceptible to infection at this time. Thus, it is too risky for even their family members to approach them.

In the early years, one out of every five women died directly from this treatment. In later years, after the procedure had been perfected considerably, the death rate directly caused by this treatment "improved" to one out of every 10 women it was used on. Those who survived the treatment often sustained *permanent* damage to their heart, kidneys, lungs, liver, and nerves.

Finally, after many years, the medical community realized that the long-term survival gain for patients who received this type of treatment for breast cancer was debatable. One revealing article in the August 2002 issue of *Discover* magazine summed it up as follows:

> Most oncologists now agree that high-dose chemotherapy is simply the wrong treatment for breast cancer. Chemotherapy works by killing cells when they're dividing, so the faster cancer cells divide, the harder they're hit. Blood cancers—some leukemias and lymphomas—grow rapidly and so are acutely vulnerable. But breast cancer cells reproduce more slowly and tend to be far more resistant to cancer drugs. No matter how many breast cancer cells are killed, at least a few survive, and they keep dividing after the chemotherapy ends.
>
> The slow pace of most breast cancers also helps explain why transplanters were so optimistic. Breast tumors can take years to reappear after treatment, but the transplanters were used to leukemia, which tends to come roaring back in a matter of months. If they found no evidence of breast cancer after a year and a half—the usual waiting period for blood cancers—they assumed a patient was cured, or at least in long-term remission. Yet the cancer was often lurking in the background, gathering its forces for another, more devastating appearance.
>
> From the moment [Dr.] Peters first administered high-dose chemotherapy until the first clinical trials were concluded, nearly 20 years passed. During that time, hundreds of physicians practiced the unproven treatment. An estimated 30,000 breast cancer patients suffered through high-dose chemotherapy, only a fraction of them as part of a clinical trial. All told, the nation spent around $3 billion paying for it, while an estimated 4,000 to 9,000 women died not from their cancer but from the treatment.[24]

According to the above article, doctors initially talked about high-dose chemotherapy/bone marrow transplant procedures as the "long-sought cure" for breast cancer they had been waiting for. Even many insurance companies were finally persuaded to pay for this expensive treatment.

But after longer-term studies were concluded, the medical community was forced to realize that any survival advantage the treatment may have provided for patients was actually wiped out by the fact that so many patients *died from the treatment itself.* One of these long-term studies was performed by the National Cancer Institute over almost 10 years and the results were presented to the public in 1999. This randomized NCI study only included patients whose breast cancer had not yet metastasized, but even in these cases of early breast cancer the survival benefits of high-dose chemotherapy followed by bone marrow transplant were negated by the number of women who died from the treatment. Thus, even for breast cancer that had been caught early, the high-dose chemotherapy/bone marrow transplant procedure was deemed ineffective.

It seems that if normal doses of chemotherapy had been saving the lives of women with breast cancer and having worthwhile long-term results, then the medical community would never have spent so much time and money on such a risky procedure — one where the treatment itself killed from 10 to 20 percent of the patients it was used on.

Tamoxifen

Tamoxifen is a nonsteroidal, estrogen-blocking drug that has become the most common conventional treatment for breast cancer after surgery, radiation, and chemotherapy. The reasoning behind the use of this drug is that Tamoxifen is actually a synthetic form of estrogen, but it is a *weaker* estrogen than estradiol (every woman's *strongest* natural estrogen in her body). By binding to the estrogen receptors of the breast, Tamoxifen blocks a woman's own more powerful estrogen from binding to those same sites and doing their work. Thus, in breast tissue, Tamoxifen is considered an "anti-estrogen."

However, what doctors don't generally tell their female patients is that Tamoxifen acts as a *stronger* estrogen in the uterus and is actually classified as a "cancer-causing" drug because it can *cause* endometrial cancer.[25] Moreover, according to Dr. Lee, the endometrial cancer caused by Tamoxifen is far more aggressive and more lethal than endometrial cancer caused by unopposed estradiol.

The following are five major downsides to using Tamoxifen:

1. About 20 to 30 percent of all breast cancers are not estrogen-driven, and therefore are not affected by Tamoxifen at all.

2. Even for estrogen-driven breast cancers, there is evidence that Tamoxifen is *not* effective once the cancer has metastasized to the lymph nodes.[26]

3. Research has now shown that Tamoxifen does not *permanently* stop cancer cells from growing, but rather puts them into a sort of "deep sleep." Once the Tamoxifen is removed from the body and a woman's own estrogen is again allowed access to those receptors, the cancer cells, if still there, will begin to grow again. For this reason, Tamoxifen is called a "cytostatic" drug rather than a "cytotoxic" one.[27]

4. There are many serious side effects that may accompany the use of Tamoxifen, some of which can be life-threatening. For instance, a woman's risk of developing a potentially fatal blood clot in the lung is *tripled* on Tamoxifen, and her risks of suffering a stroke, blindness, and liver dysfunction are also significantly increased.[28] Less serious side effects that this drug can induce are hot flashes, night sweats, depression, nausea, and vomiting.

5. As already mentioned, Tamoxifen can actually cause aggressive endometrial cancer in the very women who are taking it to recover from their breast cancer.

Short-term studies on the use of Tamoxifen for breast cancer in the United States have made the drug look a lot more successful than the long-term studies that have been performed in Europe on the same drug. For instance, Dr. Lee comments,

> The only large U.S. study was cut short, supposedly because the incidence of breast cancer dropped so much in the Tamoxifen group that they couldn't justify withholding this treatment from the placebo group. It's worth noting, however, that the trial was stopped at about the same time that breast cancer began to reappear, despite the Tamoxifen, in the two European studies.[29]

Thus, it appears that a number of European studies have concluded there is no long-term life extension gain for women with breast cancer who use Tamoxifen. One article in the *Lancet* suggested that the different conclusions from the American versus the European studies may have resulted from the fact that Tamoxifen only *temporarily suppresses* tumors, and that if the American studies had followed the women for a longer period of time, their conclusions would have been more like the European conclusions.[30]

Yet, despite the fact that European studies showed no long-term life extension through the use of Tamoxifen, despite the fact that Tamoxifen is not effective for lymph-node positive cases of breast cancer, and despite the life-threatening side effects that may be caused by this drug, approximately 60 percent of the women with breast cancer in the United States are being treated with Tamoxifen right now.[31] Surely, if women were made fully aware of all Tamoxifen's drawbacks, there would be a lot fewer women willing to use it.

Another estrogen-blocking drug currently being considered by the FDA for use on breast cancer is "Raloxifene." It apparently does not tend to cause uterine cancer the way Tamoxifen does; however, it *does* also carry with it some very dangerous side effects. Like Tamoxifen, Raloxifene tends to cause blood clots in the veins, and if one of these blood clots travels to the lungs, it can threaten the life of the patient.[32]

It seems odd that most conventional doctors are so willing to prescribe very expensive, very dangerous, and not very effective estrogen-blocking drugs to women with breast cancer, yet they so rarely consider prescribing low-cost, entirely safe natural progesterone. Natural progesterone safely opposes the effects of estrogen in the body, including normalizing cell growth, while at the same time providing other great health benefits to the body as well.

Estrogen Dominance and Other Cancers

Earlier, I referred to a study done at Johns Hopkins that showed women with low progesterone levels (estrogen dominance) to have a 540 percent *greater* risk of developing breast cancer. But that same study also showed that women with low progesterone levels had a *10-fold higher incidence* of *all types of cancer* compared to women with good progesterone levels.[33] In other words, women with insufficient progesterone carry a 1,000 percent higher risk of developing cancer *of any type* when compared to women with good progesterone levels. This study clearly indicated that breast cancer is not the only type of cancer that can result from estrogen dominance.

Evidence has been available for many years that proves the prescription of unopposed estrogen can cause uterine cancer. There is also evidence that the prescription of unopposed estrogen can cause ovarian cancer. One large study, done at Emory University, looked at 249,000 women over a period of seven years to find out more about which factors might be linked to fatal ovarian cancer. (The researchers had to study such a large group of women in order to be able to have a significant number of cases of fatal ovarian cancer naturally occur.) A computer was then used to analyze and compare common characteristics of those women who developed fatal ovarian cancer. What it came up with was this: *every one* of the women in this very large group who developed fatal ovarian cancer *was on prescribed, unopposed estrogen.*[34]

Also, Dr. Lee believes that estrogen dominance may be a contributing factor to prostate cancer in men. As we have discussed, estrogen dominance is not usually as serious a problem for men as it is for women, but men's progesterone levels do decline as they get older, and men are also subjected to many xenoestrogens from the environment which can make them estrogen dominant. Dr. Lee claims he has also had very good results supplementing his prostate cancer patents with natural progesterone.

Testing for Hormones—Blood or Saliva Test?

Let's say you are a woman who wants to know whether or not you are balanced or imbalanced in your estrogen and progesterone. Most *conventional* doctors will have you do a blood test to find out, and most *alternative* doctors will recommend a saliva test. What is the difference and which type of test is more accurate?

The answer to this question is somewhat controversial, but Dr. Lee makes a very good case for why the saliva test for these particular hormones is much more accurate and reliable than the blood test. His reasoning is that saliva testing is much more useful because it measures the amounts of bioavailable (or "free") hormones in the blood, whereas blood testing measures a lot of "bound up" hormones that will never be available to the cells in the body. According to Dr. Lee:

> Saliva tests are more useful than blood tests because they measure the bioavailable (free) hormone in the blood. After steroid hormones (progesterone, cortisols, estrogens, DHEA, testosterone) are manufactured by the ovaries, adrenal glands, or testes, they're released into the bloodstream, where they attach or bind to very specific hormone carrier proteins and, to a lesser extent, to red blood cells. Progesterone and cortisol bind to cortisol binding globulin (CBG). The estrogens (estradiol, estrone, estriol) and testosterone bind to sex hormone binding globulin (SHBG). All of the steroids also bind to albumin, which is a protein present in very high concentrations in the blood. For every 100 steroid mol-

ecules bound to these carrier proteins, only about 1 to 5 percent escape the binding proteins and make it into the cells during circulation through the blood. The small 1 to 5 percent of steroids that escape the binding proteins are considered the free or bioavailable hormones, and these are what you want to measure, because they represent the amount of hormone that the tissue actually receives and responds to.

Some of the steroids also bind to red blood cells. The more fat-loving a steroid hormone is, the more likely it is to hitch a ride on a red blood cell. Steroids hang on less tightly to red blood cells than they do to carrier proteins. This means that steroids bound to red blood cells will dissociate more easily and therefore are more bioavailable for use by your cells. Studies have shown that when red blood cells pass through the capillaries of tissues, the steroids bound to them can dissociate and enter tissues within milliseconds.[35]

The two problems associated with using blood tests to measure estrogen and progesterone levels are: (1) blood tests measure hormones that are bound to carrier proteins, only a small percentage of which will be available for use by the body; and (2) because blood tests generally measure the serum or plasma of the blood (meaning the blood cells have been removed), these tests are not able to measure those hormones bound to the fatty membranes of red blood cells which are largely available to the body because they tend to dissociate from the blood cells when they pass through the capillaries.

Progesterone is more likely to bind to red blood cells than other hormones. Dr. Lee refers to the research of one of his colleagues when he explains:

According to hormone researcher David Zava, Ph.D., progesterone is by far the most lipophilic, or fat loving, of the steroid hormones. It circulates in the blood, carried by fat-soluble substances such as red blood cell membranes. Some 70 to 80 percent of ovary-made progesterone is carried on red blood cells and thus is not measured by serum or plasma blood tests. This progesterone is available to the body for use and readily filters through the saliva glands into saliva where it can be measured accurately. The remaining 20 to 30 percent of progesterone in the body is protein bound and is found in the watery blood plasma where it can be measured by serum or plasma blood tests. However, only 1 to 9 percent of this progesterone is available to the body for use. That is why saliva testing is a far more accurate and relevant test than blood tests in measuring bioavailable progesterone.[36]

If you consult with a naturopathic or holistic physician who uses saliva testing, they will generally have a laboratory with which they work. However, you can order your own saliva tests *without* a doctor's prescription if you'd like to assess your hormone balance yourself. One very competent laboratory you can contact to do this is:

ZRT Lab, (503) 466-2445, http://www.salivatest.com.

If you live in any state of the United States *other than* California or New York, you can order your own saliva test from ZRT Lab without a doctor's prescription. If you live in California, however, you will need a doctor's prescription, and if you live in New York, you will not be able to order from this lab even *with* a prescription. You can also access more detailed information about saliva tests and hormone balancing on ZRT's website (www.salivatest.com).

Cream Versus Oral Progesterone

Once a woman has determined through testing that she needs to supplement her body with natural progesterone, there are two main ways she can do this. One way is by using a non-prescription natural progesterone cream that is rubbed onto various areas of the body. Another way is by getting a doctor's prescription for pharmaceutically compounded natural progesterone in pill form, and taking it orally.

Both ways can be successful, but evidence indicates that the cream, or transdermal route, is the most efficient way. Since natural progesterone is so lipophilic (fat-loving), it is easily absorbed through the skin. When taken in pill form, on the other hand, as much as 90 percent of the natural progesterone is destroyed in the gastrointestinal track within 15 minutes, and thus no longer available to the body.[37] This means that a much higher dose of progesterone must be taken when used orally as opposed to transdermally.

The important thing to remember if you decide to use a cream, however, is that not all natural progesterone creams are alike. It is critical to choose a cream with the correct amount of progesterone in it. Dr. Lee states that women should always use a cream that has at least 400 milligrams of progesterone per ounce. Most of the good progesterone creams provide about 480 milligrams of progesterone per ounce. Since the levels of progesterone in creams are not regulated, some progesterone creams on the market have carried as little as 10 mg of progesterone per ounce. (What a difference!) So looking into which creams have the right amount of natural hormone in them and are best to use is very important.

Also, some creams are sold as hormone-balancing creams when they only have wild yam extract in them. It is true that progesterone is often synthesized from wild yam extract, but that does *not* mean that the wild-yam extract itself is going to be the same as progesterone. If a cream boasts its wild yam extract content, but does not claim to have progesterone in it, then it will not do a woman any good.

There are many good natural progesterone creams on the market today, and I do not wish to recommend any particular one. But as a general help, I will mention some of the progesterone creams that I have heard are good hormone balancing creams. These are just *some* of the creams that have been independently tested and assessed as having about 400 to 600 milligrams of progesterone per ounce.

Natural Progesterone Creams

ProGest	by Emerita	(800) 648-8211 www.progest.com
Natural Prog. Cream	by Heartland Products	(888) 772-2345 www.heartlandnatural.com
Awakening Woman	by Alt. Med. Network	(877) 753-5424 www.altmednetwork.com
Balance Cream	by Vitality Lifechoice	(800) 423-8365
Gentle Changes	by Easy Way, Internat'l.	(800) 267-4522
Renewed Balance	by AIM Internat'l	(208) 465-5116
FemGest	by Bio-Nutr. Formulas	(800) 950-8484
Woman	by Nature's Garden	(909) 898-1466 www.progesteronecreme.net
Eternal Woman	by Mind/Body Solutions	(818) 879-1203 www.eternalwoman.com
Natural Prog. Cream	by Young Again Nutr.	(877) 205-0040 www.youngagain.com
Kokoro Balance	by Kokoro, LLC	(800) 599-9412 www.kokorohealth.com
ProBalance	by Springboard	(866)882-6868 www.springboard4health.com
Natural Prog. Cream	by Source Naturals	(800) 815-2333 www.sourcenaturals.com
Woman To Woman	by Woman To Woman	(888) 267-5032 www.womantowomanco.com
ProgestaCare	by Life-flo	(888) 999-7440 www.life-flo.com

There are many more good balancing creams on the market, and the creams listed here should not be seen as the *only* ones to choose from. There is a great deal of information on the Internet about natural progesterone creams, and visiting various sites can give you more information about each cream's specific number of milligrams of natural progesterone, as well as other ingredients that might be included.

For women who do not have cancer, or who are in remission from cancer, supplementing with natural progesterone is easy and safe. Instructions on how and when to apply the cream are provided with each product, as well as in Dr. Lee's and other books on natural progesterone. However, for women who are dealing with active cancer (especially those with large and aggressive tumors), seeking the guidance of a physician or holistic practitioner is recommended. This is because the first few weeks on natural progesterone *may* temporarily sensitize the estrogen receptors in a woman's body and initially cause mild symptoms of estrogen dominance. Thus, depending on your particular case, your practitioner may suggest you add natural progesterone supplementation very gradually, or may even suggest that you wait until the alternative approach you are using has your cancer growth under control first, before adding natural progesterone to your program.

What Can Women With Cancer Do for Their Hot Flashes?

For decades, menopause was thought of as an estrogen-deficient condition only. The reason for this is that, even though a woman's estrogen levels are proportionately *greater* than her progesterone levels at this time, her estrogen does nevertheless drop to new lows. When a woman's estrogen levels drop, there are various symptoms of low estrogen she will tend to experience. These symptoms do not tend to be life-threatening, as the low progesterone symptoms may be, but the low estrogen symptoms can be much more noticeable and annoying. This is because some of the main symptoms of low estrogen are hot flashes, low sex drive, dry skin, vaginal dryness, and difficulty sleeping. These very obvious symptoms were why modern medicine first focused so much on the low-estrogen aspect of menopause, rather than the even more dangerous low-progesterone aspect.

Most women who are diagnosed with cancer will be at an age where they are either a few years before, into, or after menopause, and these tend to be low estrogen years. Their doctors will *not* prescribe estrogen to them because of estrogen's ability to promote cancer. So, what does a woman with cancer do if she is having hot flashes during the day, night sweats during the night, and may be having severe difficulty sleeping? This can become a very challenging situation for someone who is trying to recover from a serious illness. Women who do *not* have cancer can supplement with natural estrogens or phytoestrogens to help them maintain their ability to sleep and to minimize their hot flashes and other symptoms. But if estrogen supplementation is a "no-no" for anyone with cancer, then what does a woman with cancer do when she has these symptoms?

Luckily, there are safe solutions. So far, I have talked about the estrogens promoting cell growth, and in general this is the commonly held position in the medical community. However, this is not exactly accurate. The truth is that estradiol and estrone *can* dangerously promote cell growth, but, according to Dr. Lee, the weaker estriol does *not* promote cell growth to any significant degree. So there is one form of estrogen that is actually safe for women with cancer to use, especially when they make sure they balance it with natural progesterone.

Let's look at the details of this issue. Estradiol is the strongest of the three estrogens and estriol is the weakest. By comparison, estradiol is about a thousand times more powerful at stimulating cell growth than estriol is. And there is scientific evidence that estriol is the one estrogen in our bodies that is actually *cancer-protective*. Dr. Henry Lemon, a University of Nebraska professor, did some very interesting research on estriol. He performed animal studies on breast cancer and found that when rats were given estriol prior to being exposed to cancer-causing substances, their development of breast cancer was significantly reduced as compared to the rats that were not given estriol. This protective effect, however, was *not* seen when estradiol or estrone were given to rats.[38]

Moreover, Dr. Lemon found that estriol did *not* stimulate breast cells or cells of the uterus when administered to either animals or humans. In fact, in one clinical trial, when a dose of estriol that was between 2.5 and 5 milligrams per day was given to 28 pre- and post-menopausal women with breast cancer, the results were extremely favorable. This clinical trial showed that supplementing with estriol alone induced remission or arrest of metastatic tumors in 37 percent of the women studied.[39] This same dosage of estriol (of about 2 to 5 milligrams per day) has also been shown in European clinical trials to be a sufficient amount to alleviate hot flashes and other menopausal symptoms.[40]

If you choose to use estriol, there is one obstacle. No pharmaceutical company in the United States sells it commercially. But there are some compounding pharmacists that can prepare it for you. If you find a way to get estriol in pill form, Dr. Lee claims that 2 to 5 milligrams per day should be sufficient. However, if you can find an estriol cream to use, then you can get along on a much smaller dose because the hormone is assimilated much more efficiently through the skin. In Europe, clinicians have been studying and administering estriol for more than 60 years and they have found that, when used transdermally (in cream form), a mere 0.5 milligrams of estriol every other day is usually sufficient to alleviate menopause symptoms.[41] This amount does *not* stimulate cell growth in the breasts or uterus.

Resources:

Books

John R. Lee, M.D., David Zava, Ph.D., and Virginia Hopkins. *What Your Doctor May Not Tell You About Breast Cancer.* New York: Warner Books, 2002. (ISBN 0-446-52686-X)

John R. Lee, M.D., with Virginia Hopkins. *What Your Doctor May Not Tell You About Menopause.* New York: Warner Books, 1996. (ISBN 0-446-67144-4)

John R. Lee, M.D., Jesse Hanley, M.D. and Virginia Hopkins. *What Your Doctor May Not Tell You About Premenopause.* New York: Warner Books, 1999. (ISBN 0-446-67380-3)

Websites

www.johnleemd.com (All of Dr. Lee's books, videotapes, and audiotapes can be ordered from this site.)

www.salivatest.com (For saliva testing.)

www.johnleemd.com/resfornatpro.html (For more sources of natural progesterone creams.)

www.natural-success.com/Progesterone_FactSheet.html (For more information on natural progesterone vs. synthetic progestins.)

www.rx2u.com/natural percent20hormones.htm (A site about natural hormones and how to obtain them.)

CHAPTER 20

Toxic Teeth

S ome of the most disturbing information to discover about modern living factors that can contribute to cancer involves common dental practices. However, on the bright side, dealing with some of these dental issues can be a very powerful step to overcoming cancer in certain cases. Although not everyone with cancer has toxic teeth, the information in this chapter may provide *some* people with an important key that could contribute to whether or not the treatment they use for "outsmarting" their cancer is successful or not!

There are three main sources of toxic teeth in dental practice today that can contribute to cancer. They are: (1) silver fillings, (2) nickel-alloyed porcelain crowns, and (3) root canals. People who have any of these in their mouths may be carrying around an extra load on their immune systems. Many people are healthy enough to be able to handle this extra load without serious problems. But others, especially those people who are fighting serious illnesses, may not be.

Silver Fillings

First, let's look at the most common of these three practices—that of installing silver fillings. This type of cavity-filling material is not quite as prevalent today as it used to be, but is still being administered widely. For those of us in our mid-life years, this was the *only* type of filling that was ever offered to us as children or young adults. The truth we were not told, however, is that silver fillings are only half silver. Technically, they are silver "amalgams" because they are always combined with another material to make them more pliable. That pliable material, which comprises the other half of the silver filling, is mercury.

Mercury is one of the most deadly substances found on earth, if ingested. Even the *vapor* from mercury is extremely toxic. Most of us have heard the term "mad as a hatter," which was popularized with the mad hatter character in Lewis Carroll's tale of *Alice in Wonderland*. The mad hatter syndrome was prevalent in the 1800s and may have continued into the early 1900s because mercury was used extensively in the hat-making process. A mercury compound called mercury nitrate was commonly used to remove fur from pelts and to produce felt for hats more easily. (Abraham Lincoln's big stovepipe hats were made this way.) The hat-makers themselves were exposed to large amounts of vaporized mercury and began to display symptoms of brain damage. Doctors who did autopsies on hatters sometimes reported seeing large holes inside their brains. Although the use of mercury in hat-making has been banned, the use of mercury in dental fillings has not. Mercury still comprises about 50 percent of all silver (amalgam) fillings.

In some European countries, mercury amalgam fillings have been banned for decades. However, in the United States, they continue to be standard practice, and many dentists are still telling their patients they are completely safe. The true toxic nature of silver-mercury amalgams has been played down by the American Dental Association and most dentists believe the standard line of the ADA. However, other American dentists began to wonder years ago how safe amalgams really are when the instructions they receives with the filling material include some alarming directives. These instructions on how to handle mercury amalgam fillings are still given with the material, and include warnings to dentists such as:

- Don't ever touch it with your fingers.
- Don't leave it lying around uncovered.
- Leftover amalgam material, or an extracted tooth with an amalgam filling still in it, *must* be disposed of under strict toxic waste protocols.

In other words, dentists are warned that the mercury for silver amalgams is too toxic to touch, breathe, or to just throw into the waste basket. (Yet, it's okay to put it into someone's mouth for many years.) As a result of instructions such as these, many thinking dentists often quietly stopped using amalgam fillings about 20 years ago and started using other materials whenever possible. This had to be done quietly, because dentists who were outspoken about the hazards of silver-mercury fillings often lost their licenses to practice.

One famous dentist who became probably the most outspoken against amalgam fillings was Dr. Hal Huggins. He wrote a controversial book about this issue and reported many illnesses such as multiple sclerosis, Parkinson's disease, and crippling arthritis that either cleared up or greatly improved when his patients' silver amalgam fillings were safely removed. Since so many of the side effects caused by silver amalgam fillings have been dismissed as "psychosomatic" complaints by doctors, Huggins aptly named his intriguing book *It's All in Your Head.*

Although the ADA still seems to hang onto the idea that the mercury in amalgams does not leak out once it is put into someone's mouth, there have been many scientific studies proving that it does indeed leak out. Included in these studies is proof that a significant amount of mercury can get into the brain and stay there. Some researchers believe this might be a contributing factor to Alzheimer's disease, since it is known that mercury in the brain can cause the sort of damage that is seen in Alzheimer patients' brains.

There are many ways that toxic mercury poisoning from dental work can bring about a gamut of illnesses. One of the ways this can happen is by weakening the immune system in general. Dr. David Eggleston of the University of Southern California measured T-lymphocyte levels in patients with mercury amalgam fillings. As an important contributor to health, T-lymphocytes normally comprise from 70 to 80 percent of the lymphocyte population in a healthy person's immune system. In one case, Eggleston found that a 21-year-old woman with amalgam fillings in her mouth had a T-lymphocyte level at only 47 percent of her total lymphocyte population. He removed her amalgams and replaced them with a plastic type of temporary filling. At that point, her T-lymphocyte levels rose from 47 percent to 73 percent. Next, he removed the plastic fillings and filled the teeth again with amalgam, and her T-lymphocytes fell back down to 55 percent. Finally, Eggleston removed this second set of amalgam fillings and filled the patient's teeth with safe gold inlays. At this point, her T-lymphocyte level went back up to a healthy 72 percent.[1]

It is very likely that a depressed immune system from mercury poisoning can also predispose a person to cancer, not to mention the fact that mercury is, itself, a directly carcinogenic substance. One cancer story involving mercury amalgams was reported by the son of a dentist named Dr. Pinto. Dr. Pinto first learned about the dangers of amalgams at a conference in the 1920s. According to the story, Dr. Pinto was asked to treat a child who was complaining that her gums hurt. The child was also dying of leukemia. To try to save the child, Dr. Pinto quietly removed all of her amalgam fillings. This child's condition dramatically re-sponded in just of few days and her doctors actually pronounced her as a case of "spontaneous remission".

Dr. Pinto then told the physician that he had removed her amalgams, but the physician and others in the medical profession wouldn't believe that had anything to do with the remission. To try to get through to them, Dr. Pinto re-inserted one amalgam filling in the little girl's mouth and told the doctor to look for a recurrence of the leukemia. There *was* a recurrence of symptoms, and Dr. Pinto then removed the amalgam fill-ing, which was followed again by the child's recovery.[2]

Dr. Pinto did further research into the historical occurrences of cer-tain types of diseases and found that Hodgkin's disease, another type of cancer, was virtually unheard of until 1832, shortly after amalgam fill-ings had been introduced into the very region where the first case of Hodgkin's disease was discovered. Unfortunately, no one in the dental profession listened to Dr. Pinto.

However, more recent research on amalgam fillings has been conclu-sive enough to cause some serious changes around the world. For in-stance, the government of Sweden performed its own research and con-cluded that 250,000 Swedes had immune system and other health disorders related to their amalgams. The Swedish government then put amalgam use on a schedule for complete phase-out. In 1994, a German company called Degussa, the world's largest producer of metals for use in dentistry, shut down its production of amalgam completely. Degussa apparently took the stance that it would reinstate the production of amalgam after mercury had been proved safe for the body. According to my research, there are four European countries that currently have ei-ther banned the use of amalgam fillings for children and women of child-bearing age, or have put amalgam use on a schedule toward com-plete phase-out.

Even though the United States has not banned amalgam use, one survey published in the December 1989, issue of *Dentist* magazine re-ported that over one-third of the dentists polled *did* believe that all silver amalgam fillings should be removed and replaced with composite fill-ings. Yet, dentists who feel this way in the United States are up against very powerful opposing forces that appear to control the policies of the ADA. As of 1994, the ADA "Code of Professional Conduct" stated:

> . . . the ADA has determined through the adoption of Resolution
> 42H-1986 that the removal of amalgam restoration from the non-allergic

patient for the alleged purpose of removing toxic substances from the body, when such treatment is performed solely at the recommendation or suggestion of the dentist, is improper and unethical.[3]

A CBS *60 Minutes* program aired a segment on the amalgam controversy in December 1990. Although it received one of the highest viewer responses ever, this segment was *not* repeated. Moreover, the Washington State Dental Association's response to this program was to immediately inform its dentist members that their patients "did not have a right to know that their 'silver fillings' contained mercury."[4]

The difficulty with this controversial issue is that not everybody with amalgam fillings has cancer or some other obvious illness. This is because many people's immune systems are strong enough to withstand the damage that the mercury does to the body. However, if you *are already* dealing with a serious illness, you may want to consider having your amalgam fillings safely replaced with another material.

What is *critical* to understand, however, is that there are safe ways to do this and unsafe ways. If you rush out and have your amalgams removed quickly by a dentist who does not understand the safety precautions required, you may be risking *even more damage to your health.* Sloppy removal of amalgam fillings can release even more mercury into your system than was leaking out before. You should definitely understand this issue thoroughly if you are fighting a terminal illness and you opt for amalgam replacement. In fact, you may want to seek out the services of a "biological dentist." (This is a more and more common description of dentists who specialize in understanding toxic teeth issues.)

When planning to get your silver amalgams replaced, two safety precautions to discuss with your dentist are the following:

1. Request a rubber dam. This is a piece of rubber designed to stretch between the lower right and left teeth with only the tooth being worked on uncovered. Its purpose is to keep any small pieces of amalgam filling material from falling onto your tongue or down your throat.

2. Request oxygen during the procedure. When amalgam fillings are removed, they must be drilled out. This can release mercury vapor into the air. The patient's nose, being closest to this vapor, is the first to breathe it in. Your dentist can provide an oxygen tube directly to your nose so that you breathe in clean oxygen rather than toxic substance.

Once your amalgams are removed and replaced with a safe material, you may also want to opt for chelation. This is not always necessary, but is a way to get rid of any remaining mercury that may have gotten into your body. The most important thing to remember, however, is that the amalgams need to be removed *safely* in the first place.

Nickel-Alloyed Porcelain Crowns

Although the toxicity of mercury in silver amalgam fillings is becoming more and more accepted, the toxicity of certain types of porcelain crowns and their possible link to cancer is not so widely accepted. Yet, about 75 percent of *all* crowns, including porcelain crowns, contain nickel, which is an incredibly toxic substance and a powerful carcinogen. The way that porcelain crowns contain nickel is not in the white porcelain covering itself, but in the stainless steel inner metal band that the porcelain is bonded to for strength. What we aren't generally told is this stainless steel is usually alloyed with nickel. The old-fashioned metal braces (used for straightening teeth) were also generally a stainless steel nickel alloy, and partial dentures often employ this form of alloy as well.

According to Dr. Eggleston, "Nickel is not nearly as active as mercury, however, it corrodes and is far more carcinogenic."[5] In fact, Dr. Eggleston states that the nickel alloys being used in dental practices today are actually quite similar to a form of nickel that is commonly used by cancer research centers around the country to *induce* cancer in lab animals.

Two cases involving nickel-alloyed porcelain crowns are particularly disturbing. The first one involves kidney disease, and the other involves breast cancer. The first story was a case of Dr. Eggleston's and is described by him. It involved a female patient who was admitted to Long Beach Memorial Hospital with kidney disease. However, the doctors attempting to treat her could not find the cause of her kidney problem. Her family physician then suggested special tests, which ended up showing she was highly reactive to nickel. The patient's doctor then asked her if she'd had any dental work done in the past seven years. She replied that she *did* have three porcelain crowns put in by her dentist. The doctor, knowing that porcelain crowns often have nickel-alloyed metal jackets underneath, suggested she get the crowns removed right away. The patient did this, and all of her kidney failure symptoms went away.

The other story involved breast cancer and was presented on one Internet site as told by Dr. Hal Huggins. According to Dr. Huggins, he came across a woman who had undergone a lumpectomy for breast cancer. While attending a support group for cancer in her area, she brought up the subject of the possible link between nickel crowns and breast cancer, since her husband had heard something about this from another source. One of the other women in the group replied that she had gone to a particular dentist down the street who had put nickel crowns in her mouth, and a couple of years later she developed the same type of breast tumor the first woman had undergone a lumpectomy for. It turned out that they both had gone to the *same* dentist, and both had gotten crowns put in. And then, these women found a third woman who had gone to the same dentist, gotten a crown, and later came down with the same type of breast tumor. Amazingly, with a little more investigation, these women found a fourth woman, a fifth, and then a sixth—all who had gone to the same dentist, had one or more crowns put in, and who later came down with the same type of breast tumor.[6]

Coincidence? Possibly. (It could also be that toxins or pesticides in that geographical region were contributing to this type of breast cancer.) But the fact that there are thousands of articles that refer to nickel as a carcinogen make this sort of situation definitely worth investigating. How many other women, or men, have *paid dentists or orthodontists big money to promote cancer in their bodies?*

As already pointed out, approximately 75 percent of the crowns placed currently in peoples' mouths in America contain nickel, which means that about 25 percent of them don't contain nickel. This is partly because gold alloys not containing nickel are also used sometimes as a metal base for crowns. It is also partly because, in recent years, the hardening process for porcelain used in dental applications has gotten better so that some crowns now do not use any metal at all and, instead, are 100 percent porcelain.

So there *is* a chance that, if you have a porcelain crown in your mouth, it might not contain nickel. But this could be worth calling your dental office to verify, since when nickel based crowns are used the patient is generally not told this. And when asked directly, a common response from your dentist or orthodontist might be that what you're getting is "stainless steel." This certainly *sounds* good, but if you want to be sure, you must make it clear that you know stainless steel for dental work is generally alloyed with some other metal and that you want to know *specifically* if the stainless steel in your mouth is alloyed with nickel.

If you are told that the crown in your mouth is gold-based, then you are most likely better off. Gold in itself is not toxic or carcinogenic. However, gold is way too soft to be used by itself in dental procedures and is always alloyed with a stiffer metal for dental work. Therefore, you must also be sure that you know what the gold in your mouth has been al-loyed with if you want to know whether it may be causing you illness, or not. As far as I know, gold alloyed with platinum is a safe metal combina-tion.

If you are unsure about the materials in your dental crown or crowns, you might look into being tested for levels of nickel in your body as an indicator. One way this can be done is through a hair analysis procedure.

Root Canals

So far, we have discussed silver-mercury amalgam fillings and nickel-alloyed crowns. Now, we come to the dental practice of administering "root canal" procedures. The very common practice of administering root canals may unfortunately be one of the biggest dental problems to-day because so many current dentists don't even know about the dangers that can follow after this type of treatment. In other words, many intelli-gent dentists will refuse to put mercury or nickel in people's mouths, but they will go right ahead and happily perform any number of root canals on their patients without any idea of the damage these procedures can cause.

Basically, a root canal is a procedure that is done when tooth decay, or infection, has advanced so far that the nerve in the root area of the tooth has become infected. The root canal is a narrow canal that runs from about the middle of the tooth down to the tips, or roots, of the tooth which are firmly buried in the jawbone. Front teeth have a single root into the jawbone and back teeth have two.

A healthy tooth contains a root canal that is lined with pink living tis-sue filled with tiny blood vessels, all of which surround a main nerve running down the center of the root and eventually connecting to other nerves in the surrounding jaw. Once this nerve is infected, the patient generally comes into the dentist's office in some degree of pain. This is in contrast to the more common dental decay that is confined to the hard shell of the tooth and is usually not painful because it does not in-volve nerves. When the nerve area in the tooth is infected, the most common procedure is for the dentist to perform a "root canal." In doing this, the dentist removes the nerve and cleans out the entire root canal area, which is usually infected as well to some degree. Then, the inside of the tooth is disinfected, filled with some form of filling material, and sealed up again, usually with a crown on top.

The positive side of the root canal procedure is that the tooth re-mains in your mouth and does not have to be extracted. This allows the tooth to remain functional for eating purposes, as well as to look good when you smile. On the negative side, the root canal-filled tooth is now a "dead" tooth because the inside living tissue and the tiny blood vessels that would normally bring nourishment to the tooth have been removed. Almost all root canal procedures appear, on the surface, to be wonderful solutions because rarely does the patient have any *noticeable* problem with the tooth itself after the procedure is done. Most dentists enjoy the fact that they rarely have a patient come back with complaints about a root canal-filled tooth.

The big problem, however, lies in the fact that the damage done by the root canal procedure is almost *never* noticeable at the location of the tooth. This of course is similar to the toxic effects of mercury from amalgams and nickel from crowns. But at least we know that mercury and nickel are extremely toxic substances, and we can test for those substances in the body with hair analyses and other procedures. Side effects from a root canal-filled tooth are much more difficult to pinpoint. The irony of the situation is that there may actually be more definitive research on the dangers of the root canal procedure than there is on any other type of toxic dental practice. But there is far less awareness of this research because it has been largely ignored by the dental profession for over 75 years.

The bulk of the research on root canal procedures was done from about 1900 to 1925 by a respected dentist named Dr. Weston A. Price. Dr. Price was a dedicated and thorough researcher who conducted meticulous laboratory research with a 60-man team. Over a 25-year period he conducted experiments on 5,000 lab animals after which he recorded and published his results in a two-volume report totaling 1,174 pages. Dr. Price also published 220 articles and two additional books, which can be found in the dental and medical literature.

It is extremely unfortunate for all of us that few dentists today have even heard of Dr. Weston Price and his research. In an effort to remedy this lack of awareness a noted dentist, Dr. George E. Meinig, recently undertook the mission of carefully reading all 1,174 pages of Dr. Price's two-volume report. Dr. Meinig then condensed Price's findings about the dangers of root canals into a much smaller and very readable contemporary book called, *The Root Canal Cover-Up*. Dr. Meinig had the perfect background and experience to do this because he, himself, had practiced and taught root canal therapy, and was one of the founding members of the American Association of Endodontists (root canal practitioners).

According to Dr. Meinig, what Price and other researchers have been able to prove is that there is an unavoidable problem with the root canal procedure. The problem is that, no matter how much a dentist tries to disinfect the inside of the tooth after the root area has been cleaned out, there is really no way that *all of the infection can be reached.* This is because teeth contain microscopically small tubules that run through the dentin like a huge lattice of caverns in a mountain. The purpose of these tubules when the tooth is alive is to transport nourishment-carrying fluid and oxygen throughout the tooth. (Thus, a healthy tooth is very much alive.) To give you an idea of just how extensive this lattice of tubules is, it is estimated that if you were able to string all the tubules in just one average front tooth together, end-to-end, they would reach about 3 miles long. And since back teeth are much larger than front teeth, their tubules put end-to-end would reach considerably farther.

Once infection has progressed into the depths of these microscopically small tubules in any tooth, there will inevitably be a certain number of bacteria that have roamed so deep there is no way any type of disinfectant can reach them. So there will invariably be some number of bacteria that are still left alive in the tubules of the dentin after the root canal procedure is done and the tooth is filled and closed back up again!

But the root canal-filled tooth is now dead. There is no longer a supply of nourishment going in and out of the tooth, and there is no longer any fluid flowing into and out of the tubules. Without fluid flowing through the tubules, there is no mechanism for transporting antibiotics to the trapped bacteria. But more importantly, there is no longer any transport of *oxygen* throughout the intricate maze of tubules. So the bacteria, which started out as normal "aerobic" bacteria, may now mutate to survive and become "anaerobic" bacteria. Unfortunately, the *anaerobic forms* of these bacteria can be much more dangerous than the aerobic form originally was. Dr. Price discovered that the entombed anaerobic bacteria are capable of creating powerful toxins that can then leak into the tissue surrounding the tooth. Once these toxins leak out of the tooth, they can get into a person's bloodstream and travel throughout the entire body.

Back in the early 1900s, after suspecting that some of the chronic illnesses of his patients were linked to root canal-filled teeth, Dr. Price started extracting those teeth. Then, by simply taking a piece of the extracted root canal-filled tooth and embedding this piece of tooth under the skin of a rabbit, he found that the rabbit would develop the same type of illness the person had!

For instance, Dr. Price found if he took a small piece of a root canal-filled tooth that had been extracted from a person who'd had a heart attack and placed it under the skin of a rabbit, that rabbit would die of a heart attack in about 10 days. He could then take that same piece of tooth *out* of the dead rabbit and put it under the skin of another rabbit, and in about 10 days, *that* rabbit would also die of a heart attack. Price found he could do this over and over with the same piece of tooth and get the same result for up to about 30 rabbits.

Moreover, heart disease only occurred in Price's lab animals when the person the root canal-filled tooth had come from had suffered from heart disease. If the person had suffered from another illness, *that* would be the illness that would show up in the rabbit. For instance, if the patient from whom the tooth was taken was suffering from kidney disease, then the rabbit with the piece of that person's tooth embedded in it would also develop kidney disease.

Dr. Price's first clinical case involved arthritis. In that case, he removed a root canal-filled tooth from a woman with severe arthritis and implanted the extracted tooth under the skin of a rabbit. Within 48 hours, the rabbit had developed crippling arthritis. Furthermore, after extraction of this tooth, the woman's arthritis improved dramatically. Dr. Price performed these types of experiments over and over, and kept getting the same results. Very rarely, did the rabbit *not* come down with the very illness the human patient was suffering from.

Price was a thorough researcher and he, of course, tested the possibility that just putting part of a human tooth into an animal was the problem. But he found that if he did the same procedure using a perfectly healthy, non-root canal-filled tooth, then the rabbit would suffer no ill effects whatsoever. He also found that if he sterilized the piece of tooth first by using a powerful procedure involving steam heat, then the rabbit would suffer no ill effects, either.

Dr. Price found a high number of chronic degenerative diseases to be linked to root canal-filled teeth. The most common appeared to be various forms of heart and circulatory diseases, presumably because the toxins from anaerobic bacteria in the teeth leaked into and circulated throughout the bloodstream. Other chronic conditions that his research linked to root canal-filled teeth were various forms of arthritis, nervous system disorders, and even digestive disorders. For more detailed information about Price's discoveries regarding the toxic nature of root canal-filled teeth, I highly recommend Meinig's book, *Root Canal Cover-Up.*

A very potent description of root canal therapy was given by Dr. Hal Huggins in a lecture he gave to the Cancer Control Society in 1993. Huggins stated, in his usual colorful way,

> ... Then we get into the root canal business, and that is the most tragic of all. Isn't there something you can put in the center of the canal that is safe? Yeah, there probably is, but that is not where the problem is. The problem with a root canal is that it is dead. Let's equate that. Let's say you have got a ruptured appendix, so you go to the phone book, and who do you look up? Let' see, we have a surgeon and a taxidermist, who do you call? You going to get it bronzed? That is all we do to a dead tooth. We put a gold crown on it, looks like it has been bronzed. It doesn't really matter what you embalm the dead tooth with, it is still dead, and within that dead tooth we have bacteria, and these bacteria are in the absence of oxygen. In the absence of oxygen most things die except bacteria. They undergo something called a pleomorphic change—like a mutation. They learn to live in the absence of oxygen (and) now produce thioethers, some of the strongest poisons on the planet that are not radioactive.[7]

Huggins went on to say in this lecture that the thioethers do escape into the body's bloodstream and he points out a correlation between the increase in the rate of heart attacks in the United States since the early 1900s, and the corresponding increase in the practice of performing root canals. This would be consistent with what Dr. Price found in his research, which was that the predominant damage caused by root canals was to the cardiovascular system of the body since the mode of travel for the toxins is through the bloodstream.

The main problem in accepting the dangers of root canals over the years has been centered around a debate over the "focal infection" theory. This is the theoretical idea that an infection focused in one part of the body can have a detrimental effect on a distant part of the body. Even though this debate continues, there are some transplant surgeons today who require root canal-filled teeth to be extracted before they will perform an organ transplant in a patient. This is because these surgeons believe there is a risk that focal infections in teeth might affect the new organ.

Josef Issels, M.D., of Germany, a world-famous cancer specialist, took the dangers of root-filled teeth very seriously. Dr. Issels was probably the first physician to require all of his cancer patients to have their dead teeth extracted as a part of his normal cancer treatment protocol. Over a

40-year period of working with more than 16,000 cancer patients, Issels had one of the highest total remission rates with late stage terminal cancer patients of any cancer practitioner. He also found that a survey of his cancer patients showed over 90 percent of them to have between two and 10 dead teeth in their mouths when they first arrived at his clinic for treatment.

In his well-written, in-depth book, *Cancer—A Second Opinion*, Dr. Issels talks about his research with root canals in his Chapter 8, titled "Focus on Foci." Issels found that dead teeth left in the mouth can become "toxin factories" and do, in fact, produce thioethers. Moreover, he presents very convincing evidence why thioethers have all of the qualifications of a substance capable of causing spontaneous cancer in humans.

Dr. Issels's writing is often highly technical, and he uses medical terminology that is often difficult for the layperson to understand. But one simple experiment he reports is quite clear and impressive. Issels found that he could use an infrared-sensitive instrument to measure the level of infrared emission anywhere in a person's body. In doing so, he found that the infrared emission on the outer skin next to a root canal-filled tooth was elevated slightly higher than the area around healthy teeth. He could also monitor the infrared emission around a cancerous tumor area.

What Dr. Issels found was that, when a dead tooth in a cancer patient was treated (presumably by extraction), the corresponding infrared emission of that area of the mouth decreased, *and the infrared emission of the person's tumor area also decreased at the same time.*[8] Thus, he proved a definite interrelationship between the dead tooth and the cancer.

Yet another possible relationship between root canal-filled teeth and cancer may have to do with a different mechanism than toxins. This mechanism involves acupuncture meridians. Although little research has been done on this subject, one alternative cancer practitioner, Dr. John Diamond of Reno, Nevada, has said, "I have a number of patients with breast cancer, all of whom had root canals on the tooth related to the breast area on the associated energy meridian."[9] This is certainly something to think about for anyone with any type of cancer.

Of course, we all know people who have root canal-filled teeth in their mouths and appear to be perfectly healthy. This seems to confuse the issue, and one alternative doctor I asked about this clarified the issue in the following way. He said, "Root canals are like mortgages. As long as you can make enough money to pay the payment every month, everything is fine. But once you *can't* make the payment, then you're in big trouble!"[10] In other words, it is the strength of the immune system and the body in general that determines whether or not a root canal-filled tooth is going to bring about obvious health problems in any individual. This could be applied to the effects of mercury amalgam fillings and nickel-alloyed crowns as well. With diet, stress levels, and other factors varying greatly from person to person, the effects of these dental practices are necessarily going to vary from person to person also.

As with amalgam removal, having your root canal-filled teeth removed *safely* is of utmost importance. If your dentist or oral surgeon does not fully understand the issues of toxicity, there could be a danger that after the dead tooth is removed, toxic infection still remains in the surrounding bone socket. Once more, seeking out a competent "biological dentist" who knows how to safely extract root canal-filled teeth is a good idea. On pages 193–194 of his book, *The Root Canal Cover-Up*, Dr. Meinig details how a root canal-filled tooth should be removed to ensure none of the infection is left behind, and it might be a good idea to make sure your dentist or oral surgeon is familiar with the instructions in Meinig's book.

Although it is common practice for endodontists to leave behind the periodontal ligament when a tooth is extracted, Dr. Meinig and Dr. Hal Huggins both believe it is likely for root canal infections to have infected this ligament as well. They both recommend total removal of this ligament along with approximately 1 millimeter of surrounding jawbone following extractions. This procedure usually causes any residual infection from the root canal-filled tooth to be removed.

One last word of caution is warranted. Some alternative cancer specialists recommend that people who are in a weakened state from cancer may not be strong enough to have all of their toxic teeth dealt with at once. For some people, it might be best to have toxic teeth addressed slowly, over time. Again, consulting with a knowledgeable alternative cancer specialist, if possible, is a good idea.

Resources:

Books

Hal A. Huggins, D.D.S. *It's All in Your Head: The Link Between Mercury Amalgams and Illness*. Garden City Park, New York: Avery Publishing Group, 1993. (ISBN 0-89529-550-4)

George E. Meinig, D.D.S, F.A.C.D. *The Root-Canal Cover-Up.* Ojai, California: Bion Publishing:, 1998. (ISBN 0-945196-19-9)

Josef Issels, M.D. *Cancer—A Second Opinion.* Garden City Park, New York: Avery Publishing Group, 1999. (ISBN 0-89529-992-5)

Websites

www.curezone.com/diseases/cancer_dental_risk.html

www.curezone.com/dental/root_canal.html

www.price-pottenger.org/Articles/Rootcanal.html

www.dairylanedental.com/root_canals.htm

www.whale.to/d/cancer.html

www.yourhealthbase.com/amalgams.html

SECTION IV

Deciding for Yourself

CHAPTER 21

Evaluating
Conventional Methods

A re conventional cancer treatments *ever* warranted? Yes, they are. In particular, surgery alone may sometimes be a curative approach. Beyond that, if a person's tumor is so large that it is restricting vital organ functioning, or if the cancer is so advanced that there is not enough time left for an alternative treatment to have a chance to work, then immediate surgery, chemotherapy, radiation, or other conventional method may be used to one's advantage. However, this is often simply short-term damage control. When it comes to *long-term recovery*, the efficacy of toxic conventional treatments is a different story.

The current medical establishment would like us to believe that *most* cancers, if caught early, are curable with standard medical techniques. Impressive-sounding conventional cure-rate statistics are advertised. But these statistics are achievable only after *gross* statistical manipulations have been done, and after key terms like "cure" have been re-defined. To review from Chapter 1, the following are six major ways that official cancer cure-rate statistics are often "fudged" so that conventional methods for treating cancer can look better than they really are:

1. By re-defining "cure" as "alive five years after diagnosis," instead of using the word's real meaning, which is "cancer-free."

2. By simply omitting certain groups of people, such as African Americans, or by omitting certain types of cancer, such as all lung cancer patients, from their statistical calculations.

3. By including types of cancer that are *not* life-threatening and are easily curable, such as skin cancers and DCIS.

4. By allowing earlier detection to erroneously imply longer survival.

5. By deleting patients from cancer treatment studies who die too soon, even if that is on day 89 of a 90-day chemotherapy protocol.

6. By using a questionable adjustment called "relative survival rate."

The problem is that if you or someone you care about are dealing with life-threatening cancer, the misleading "official" statistics are the numbers that will be offered to you as representative of your chances of survival, should you choose conventional treatment. It is critical that you understand how to *accurately* evaluate conventional cancer treatment methods because your life literally depends on the treatment decisions you make.

The Big Three—Surgery, Chemotherapy, and Radiation

What *are* the real statistics on conventional medicine's "big three" cancer treatments today? Unfortunately, nobody knows. Nobody *can* know when there are no data in mainstream medicine that reflect real cures. The only data we have to work with are figures that reflect the phony re-definition of the term "cure," that talk about short-term results, and that are recorded selectively in the first place in ways that defy correct statistical methodology. Thus, trying to figure out the *true* cure-rate statistics for conventional cancer treatments is a lot like trying to figure out which cup the magician's red ball is under.

Having said that, there are a number of things you *can* learn about conventional cancer treatment efficacy. For instance, out of all the conventional cancer treatments available today, it is probably safe to say that surgery alone has the best track record. Cancer researcher, Dr. Ralph Moss, claims that *most* of the conventional cancer cures today can be attributed to surgery alone.[1] However, the types of cases where surgery can be effective in a long-term way apply to only a small percentage of cancer patients. For instance, everyone agrees that surgery is virtually helpless as a curative procedure in any case where the cancer has already metastasized, and unfortunately, the *majority* of cancer patients are told they have metastasized cancer at the time they are first diagnosed.

Thus, for most people with cancer, surgery is no more than a "palliative" treatment (meaning it cannot save the patient, but is merely performed in the hope that it will buy the patient some time). For surgery to have a chance at actually being curative, it must be performed at a very early stage, before the cancer has spread past the primary site. Even for many of *these* cases, surgery cannot guarantee recovery. Some medical experts believe that there are early cancer situations where surgery may even cause the cancer to spread throughout the body by releasing free-floating cancer cells into the bloodstream or lymph system. But overall, the use of surgery alone probably still accounts for the largest number of long-term survival cases in conventional cancer treatment.

After surgery, we have radiation and chemotherapy. Unfortunately, the true long-term effectiveness of these methods can only be said to be "dismal." Some studies have even produced evidence that cancer patients may be able to live longer *without* these treatments. For example, a *Science News* article, published August 1, 1998, presented a review of data about radiation treatment after surgery for lung cancer. The immense amount of data, which was collected from nine studies over a 30-year period, actually showed the two-year survival rate after lung cancer surgery to be 48 percent for patients who got post-surgical radiation treatments, and 55 percent for patients who underwent surgery alone. In other words, more patients who did *not* receive radiation treatments after surgery lived to the two-year mark than those who *did* receive radiation after surgery.

When it comes to chemotherapy, which is prescribed to about four out of five people with cancer in the United States today, Ralph Moss states in his book, *Questioning Chemotherapy*:

> A close look at chemotherapy yields some major surprises. Few would dispute its usefulness in acute lymphocytic leukemia, Hodgkin's disease, testicular and ovarian cancer, and a handful of rare tumors, mainly of childhood. But evidence for the life-prolonging effect in other common malignancies is weak, even for those cancers in which almost certainly it has some marginal success. And proof is simply non-existent for the majority of cancers, especially the advanced carcinomas.
>
> Even for the common cancers in which chemotherapy "works," such as small-cell lung cancer, the actual survival benefit is reckoned in weeks or months, not in years. And during this time, the patient is likely to experience major, even life-threatening side effects from the treatment. Thus, the overall advantage to the patient is moot.[2]

Thus, the official claims of success for toxic treatments such as radiation and chemotherapy often refer to "short-term" effectiveness only. We will be going into more detail on radiation and chemotherapy in the

next few pages, but first, let's look at the very important difference between "short-term" and "long-term" effectiveness.

Short-Term Versus Long-Term Effectiveness

Studying and quoting short-term effectiveness is just one tactic of a
medical establishment that is *not* having success with long-term effectiveness. Since mainstream medicine is losing its war on cancer, it is very
beneficial for those in charge to only study short-term effectiveness. This
way, the actual long-term effectiveness (or "real" effectiveness) of conventional treatment does not have to be considered. Better yet, long-term
side effects of treatment (which may take the patient's life a few years
down the line) do not have to be considered.

For example, in Chapter 19, we saw that many European studies
showed the use of Tamoxifen for breast cancer to have no overall long-
term survival benefit at all. According to Dr. Lee, Tamoxifen can temporarily suppress tumors, and that is why the short-term studies done in
the United States made Tamoxifen look so good. However, the long-
term studies done on Tamoxifen in Europe showed breast tumors *coming back* at just about the period of time when the studies in the United
States were being cut short. The short-term U.S. studies did not show all
the deaths caused by Tamoxifen's side effects later, such as from fatal
blood clots in the lungs, from stroke, from liver dysfunction, or from
uterine cancer, all of which can be caused by the Tamoxifen drug
treatment.

But the most ludicrous aspect of short-term attention to conventional
treatments is represented by how the term "cure" is re-defined. By re-
defining the meaning of "cure" as *alive five years after diagnosis*, our current conventional cancer establishment is basically saying that the medical establishment considers five-year survival to be the best they can
aspire to. Make no mistake—by labeling anyone with cancer who
reaches the five-year mark as "cured," conventional medicine is pro-
claiming that once you have lived five years after diagnosis, they have
done a great job—even if you still have cancer and have been miserably
sick the whole five years. This official tactic of re-defining "cure" also
frequently creates the ironic situation where a cancer patient can be
listed as a "cure" in the official statistics data base, yet *die from their
cancer.*

Maybe for some people, living another five years is a great thing. For
instance, it may be wonderful for those who are quite elderly when they

are diagnosed with cancer, and they just want to live a few more years. But what if you are 25 or 40 years old, or 50 or 60? Living only five more years is not so good at all! Or maybe you are one of many people raising small children when you are diagnosed with cancer. Most parents do not just want to see their children become teenagers—they also want to see them become adults, go to college, get married, have their own children, and so forth. And if it is your *child* who has been diagnosed with cancer, then to aspire to your child living just five more years is simply unacceptable.

The bottom line is that, when you are considering treatment for cancer, you should know whether or not the statistics your oncologist presents to you reflect "long-term" or "short-term" effectiveness. After all, you obviously want a long-term, not a short-term, recovery!

Response Rates

Another way that short-term results are used by mainstream medicine to imply long-term effectiveness is by the common conventional practice of studying and quoting cancer treatment "response rates." In mainstream medicine, the "response rate" of a particular treatment is often quoted as if it means *recovery rate*, or *cure rate*. But this is just another way that people seeking cancer treatment are misled by meaningless numbers. The term "response rate" is *not* synonymous to "recovery rate," or "cure rate." Quite the contrary. Common conventional cancer studies define a "response" as simply meaning a 50 percent reduction in tumor size for a particular period of time (usually about 28 days).

Because chemotherapy and radiation are "cytotoxic" (toxic to cells), it is common for malignant tumors to shrink for a time when bombarded with these types of toxic treatments. However, that merely means that the tumor has died a little after being poisoned or burned. If there are any cancer cells left alive *after* the treatment, which there virtually always are, then the tumor will start growing again as soon as there is a break in the treatment. Since toxic treatments generally involve time breaks in their administration to let the patient's overall body recover, cancerous tumors often have a chance to grow back.

Thus, when tumor response rates are quoted, these rates do *not* indicate that patients regained their good health or their cancers were overcome. Response rates are just a convenient way for conventional cancer researchers to report the short-term, often *partial* effectiveness of a particular treatment. As Ralph Moss states,

It is one of the central fallacies of chemotherapy that shrinkages or "response rates" have been proven to correlate with increased survival time. Yet, in answer to a patient's inevitable question, "What are my chances?" the doctor may give impressive-sounding "response rates" of, say, 60 percent.[3]

In other words, if your doctor tells you that the cancer treatment he or she is recommending to you has a response rate of 60 percent, you should know that what that *really* means is this: 60 percent of the time, that particular treatment protocol will cause tumors to "shrink" by at least half for at least a month. It does not mean that 60 percent of the cancer patients who get that treatment will become cancer-free.

Since toxic cancer treatments can often damage vital organs and suppress the immune system, the use of toxic treatments that are unable to effect a long-term cure must always beg the question as to whether or not the patient might have lived longer *without* the treatment. W. John Diamond, M.D., and W. Lee Cowden, M.D., report on this issue in their book, *An Alternative Medicine Definitive Guide to Cancer*. In it, they write:

> Virtually all the FDA-approved anticancer drugs are markedly *immunosuppressive*, because they ruin a person's natural resistance to disease, including cancer. Ulrich Abel, Ph.D., of the Heidelberg Tumor Center in Germany, conducted a comprehensive review of the world literature on survival among cancer patients receiving chemotherapy. He found that chemotherapy can help only 3 percent of the patients with epithelial cancers (e.g., cancers of the breast, lung, prostate, and colon). These cancers account for about 80 percent of all cancer deaths. In a study of chemotherapy-treated breast cancer patients, the researchers concluded, 'Survival may even have been shortened in some [breast cancer] patients given chemotherapy'.[4]

A few pages later, Dr. Diamond and Dr. Cowden follow with:

> German cancer researcher Ulrich Abel, Ph.D., observes that the temporary shrinking of a tumor mass—defined as either a partial or complete remission—is not necessarily a good sign, because the remaining tumor cells often grow much faster and more virulently after the first series of chemotherapy treatments. Highly aggressive chemotherapy actually shortens survival times compared with patients in whom

chemotherapy was delayed or administered less aggressively, says Dr. Abel. Paradoxically, patients whose tumors showed no response to chemotherapy actually survived longer than patients who did respond.[5]

Dr. Diamond and Dr. Cowden also report on evidence that some men with prostate cancer may survive longer without radiation treatments. They write:

> Radiation therapy—implanting radiation seeds in the prostate gland—routinely given for early signs of prostate cancer can actually hasten the development of that cancer. Prostate cells can double in as little as 1.2 months after radiation treatment while unradiated prostate cancer cells may take an average of 4 years to double.[6]

It is extremely misleading for doctors to allow cancer patients to believe that quoted "response rates" are the same as "recovery rates." It may be that many doctors who quote response rates don't know, themselves, the real meaning of what they are quoting. But for you, the person trying to get well, knowing the real meaning of response rate statistics will help you to more correctly evaluate conventional cancer treatment methods you may be considering.

Damage to the Heart

There are many ways that short-term effectiveness of conventional cancer treatments can look very good for a while, yet long-term effectiveness turns out to be *not* good at all. For instance, radiation to the chest area for either lung cancer or breast cancer can cause damage to the heart severe enough to precipitate a fatal heart attack at some time in the near future. If the heart attack does not occur until the patient has been pronounced in remission, then the radiation treatment will look like it was successful. Deaths from subsequent heart attacks caused by cancer treatment do *not* have to be folded into the cancer treatment statistics. As mentioned in Chapter 19, one study on radiation treatment given to women with breast cancer showed that the use of radiation *did* reduce deaths from breast cancer by 13.2 percent, and this was most likely the figure that was publicly advertised. However, this same radiation increased deaths from *other* causes (mostly heart disease) by 21.2 percent!

Can Radiation or Chemotherapy Cause Cancer?

One fact that is often difficult for many people to believe is that many of the conventional treatments for cancer commonly used today are actually carcinogenic. This means they *can cause a secondary cancer to develop* a few years later, provided that the patient is lucky enough to survive their first cancer that long. This is just another way that short-term effectiveness of conventional cancer treatments may look good, while the long-term effectiveness may not look good at all.

Radiation-Induced Cancer

Evidence that radiation treatments can cause cancer goes back to the early days of X-ray technology. In *The Cancer Industry*, Ralph Moss reports:

> In 1902 a German doctor recorded the first case of human cancer caused by radiation: the tumor had appeared on the site of a chronic ulceration caused by X-ray exposure. Experimental studies performed in 1906 suggested that leukemia (cancer of the blood) could be caused by exposure to the radioactive element radium. By 1911, 94 cases of radiation-induced cancer had been reported, more than half of them (54) in doctors or technicians. By 1922, over 100 radiologists had died from X-ray-induced cancer, and many other research workers, laboratory assistants, and technicians had also succumbed . . . .[7]

More and more cases of people developing cancer due to X-ray technology were reported over the decades, and when radiation began to be used as a treatment for cancer, secondary radiation-induced cancers began to be reported. Today, it is *well-known* that radiation treatments for cancer may also cause secondary cancers.

In her video, *Cancer Doesn't Scare Me Anymore*, Dr. Lorraine Day shows medical manuals that list the possibility of secondary cancers due to radiation treatment. She also talks about the many *other* very serious and life-threatening side effects that can be caused by radiation treatments for cancer. Dr. Day makes the point that the ACS, AMA, and FDA refer to radiation treatments as "safe and effective" for cancer patients, yet radiation technicians, doctors, and nurses are all urged to protect themselves against much lower, indirect doses of the same radiation by wearing lead vests and carrying out other protective procedures. In other words, it is quite ironic that radiation is considered safe for anyone with cancer, yet extremely dangerous for a healthy person!

Chemotherapy-Induced Cancer

Many people are already aware that some sources of radiation can cause cancer because they have heard reports of cancer being caused by nuclear fallout, radiation accidents, and so forth. But it seems counter-intuitive that a carcinogenic drug would be intentionally given to someone trying to recover from cancer. A brief look at the history of chemotherapy will help to shed light on this.

The roots of modern chemotherapy go back to the early 1940s when poisonous "mustard gas" was being developed for chemical warfare. (A potent form of mustard gas had already been used during World War I, and in 1942, the U.S. government contracted with various research centers to further investigate possible war-time chemical agents.) Researchers at Yale University experimented with substituting a nitrogen atom for a sulfur atom in mustard gas, which, at the time, was called "nitrogen mustard."[8] A Yale anatomist then came up with the idea that it would be interesting to inject this nitrogen mustard into mice with cancer to see what would happen.

As luck would have it, the first such mouse experimented on showed impressive tumor regression. Although the mouse's cancer never completely went away, the mouse lived about four times longer than it was expected to live with no treatment at all, and this got people's attention. Researchers followed with more experiments and, though they could not achieve similarly good results on subsequent mice, it was decided to try the nitrogen mustard treatment on a human cancer patient.

The man experimented on had late-stage lymphosarcoma, and showed dramatic tumor regression within the first few days of receiving nitrogen mustard. Researchers were ecstatic. But as with the mice, the man's cancer was never "cured." Within the first month of treatment, his white blood cell count fell dismally low. Then his cancer regenerated in his bone marrow and he died.[9] But because the man's tumor had regressed within the first few days, his case was considered in some ways to have been a "success." One-hundred-sixty more patients were then administered experimental chemotherapy. The results showed that *not one* of these patients recovered from their cancer. In other words, *all* the evidence from early chemotherapy experiments indicated that it was an unqualified failure!

But in the early 1940s nitrogen mustard was the only "synthesized chemical agent" that had *ever* shown anti-tumor activity, and some people in positions of power were too excited by this to let it go. Chief of the U.S. Army Chemical Warfare Service, Cornelius "Dusty" Rhoads, was one of these people. Rhoads became a powerful advocate of chemotherapy when World War II ended and he became head of the Memorial Sloan-Kettering Institute for Cancer Research. He initiated tests on more than 1,500 different types of nitrogen mustard, and by 1955, about 20,000 of these types of chemicals were being looked at every year.[10]

Because chemotherapy was developed out of poisonous chemical warfare agents (and is still poisonous), there has always been a fine line in its administration between giving a therapeutic dose and killing the patient. In his outstanding book, *When Healing Becomes a Crime*, author Kenny Ausubel notes that in one clinical trial on the chemotherapy drug called "ICE," 8 percent of the patients died from the drug treatment directly, and in another trial on a chemotherapy drug studied for leukemia, 42 percent of the patients died from the drug treatment directly.[11]

From the days when chemotherapy was first used to the current day, this mode of treating cancer has *never* shown significant long-term effectiveness. Dr. Dean Burk was a chemist at the National Cancer Institute from 1939 to 1974. He also taught biochemistry at Cornell University Medical School from 1939 to 1941. When he retired from NCI in 1974, Dr. Burk retired from the position of "chief chemist" at the National Cancer Institute. The year before he retired, Dr. Burk wrote a letter to Dr. Frank Rauscher, a higher-up member in the NCI. In it, Burk wrote:

> Ironically, virtually all of the chemotherapeutic anti-cancer agents now approved by the Food and Drug Administration for use or testing in human cancer patients are (1) highly or variously *toxic* at applied dosages; (2) markedly *immunosuppressive*, that is, destructive of the patient's native resistance to a variety of diseases, including cancer; and (3) usually highly *carcinogenic* [cancer-causing] . . . These now well established facts have been reported in numerous publications from the National Cancer Institute itself, as well as from throughout the United States and, indeed, the world . . . .
>
> In your answer to my discussion of March 19, you readily acknowledged that the FDA-approved anti-cancer drugs were indeed toxic, immunosuppressive, and carcinogenic, as indicated. But then, even in the face of the evidence, including your own White House statement of

May 5, 1972, all pointing to the pitifully small effectiveness of such drugs, you went on to say quite paradoxically it seems to me, "I think the Cancer Chemotherapy program is one of the best program components that the NCI has ever had."...One may ask, parenthetically, surely this does not speak well of the "other program areas?" [12]

Ralph Moss clarifies the subject of chemotherapy being carcinogenic even further in his book, *Questioning Chemotherapy*, when he writes:

Perhaps the strangest thing about chemotherapy is that many of these drugs themselves are carcinogenic. This may seem astonishing to the average reader—that cancer-fighting drugs themselves cause cancer. Yet this is an undeniable fact.

It is sometimes said that only the alkylating agents, such as busulfan, carmustine, and melphalan, are carcinogenic. But this is not true. The authoritative International Agency for Research on Cancer (IARC) has identified 20 single agents or regimens which cause cancer in humans, and about 50 more in which such effects are suspected (236,248). Many, but not all, of these are alkylating agents. The offending drugs include doxorubicin and streptozocin (toxic antibiotics used as cytotoxic agents), BCNU (a nitrosourea), as well as the various hormone-like products. Perhaps the distinction between alkylating agents and other drugs in this regard is moot, since alkylating agents are predominantly included in most of the regimens commonly used in cancer.

To give just one example of carcinogenicity, doctors looked at one-year survivors of ovarian cancer from five randomized trials. The incidence rates for acute nonlymphocytic leukemia and for pre-leukemia were about 100 times more common in women who got the drug melphalan than in those who received no chemotherapy.

"The magnitude of these risks suggests that the drugs are causally related to leukemia," NCI epidemiologists cautiously concluded. However, they add, characteristically, that "the identification of a carcinogenic effect does not preclude its use for treatment in patients." In other words, the fact that these drugs cause cancer is immaterial in the doctor's decision to administer these cytotoxic agents. [13]

Using my home copy of *The PDR Family Guide to Prescription Drugs* (New Second Edition, copyright 1994), I looked up one commonly used chemotherapy drug called "Cyclophosphamide," also called "Cytoxan." On page 167 of the Physician's Desk Reference, where side effects of Cytoxan are listed, I found this statement: "One possible Cytoxan side effect is the development of a secondary cancer, typically of the bladder, lymph nodes, or bone marrow. A secondary cancer may occur up to several years after the drug is given."

Cyclophosphamide, or Cytoxan, is an alkylating agent. It is also an integral part of the following commonly used chemotherapy protocols:

BACOP	CHOP	COMLA	MACC
CA	CHOP-B	COP	M-BACOD
CAMP	CISCA	COP-BLAM	Pro-MACE
CAP	CMF	CVP	Pro-MaACE-cytaBOM
CAV	CMFP	CyVADIC	
CFPT	CMFVP	FAC	
COAP	Hexa-CAF	VAC	

Cyclophosphamide is also known as "Neosar" in the United States and "Endoxan" in Germany. According to Dr. W. John Diamond,

> A study of over 10,000 patients shows clearly that chemo's supposedly strong track record with Hodgkin's disease (lymphoma) is actually a lie. Patients who underwent chemo were 14 times more likely to develop leukemia and 6 times more likely to develop cancers of the bones, joints, and soft tissues than those patients who did not undergo chemotherapy.[14]

And, the March 21, 1996, issue of the distinguished *New England Journal of Medicine*, reported:

> Children who are successfully treated for Hodgkin's disease are 18 times more likely later to develop secondary malignant tumors. Girls face a 35 percent chance of developing breast cancer by the time they are 40—which is 75 times greater than the average. The risk of leukemia increased markedly four years after the ending of successful treatment, and reached a plateau after 14 years, but the risk of developing solid tumors remained high and approached 30 percent at 30 years.[15]

Some people may be willing to take the risk of getting secondary cancer from the treatment they receive to rid themselves of their current cancer. But other people might not like the idea of seeing their cancer go into remission only to have to go once again into battle a few years later against a secondary treatment-induced cancer. (Especially when there are non-toxic, *non-carcinogenic* treatments they could choose from.) And the fact that so many chemotherapy drugs actually cause cancer is a very real threat to the public at large as well as to the environment. When cancer patients receive chemotherapy, much of their drug treatment gets passed into the public sewage systems through their urine. It thereby becomes an environmental carcinogen that may eventually cause cancer in other humans or animals.

False Hope?

How many times are doctors prescribing chemotherapy or radiation when there is very little evidence that this type of treatment will improve long-term life expectancy? About 80 percent of all cancer patients today are given chemotherapy, yet some researchers believe that chemotherapy may only show long-term effectiveness in as little as 2 to 3 percent of all cancer cases. And how often are radiation treatments prescribed to cancer patients when there is little evidence that doing so will help achieve long-term recovery for their particular type of cancer situation?

I know of a woman whose elderly father-in-law was prescribed radiation treatments for his late-stage, metastasized prostate cancer. When this woman called her father-in-law's oncologist directly to find out what his life-expectancy was, she was told by the oncologist that he had only about six months to live. The woman, being a clear thinker, then asked the oncologist if that prognosis for her father-in-law was "with" radiation treatments, or "without." The unbelievable answer she got was "either way". Yet her father-in-law had been prescribed radiation treatments and was *not* told that his chances were *exactly the same* whether he did the treatment or not. I happen to know that both this elderly man and his wife thought the radiation treatments could cure him. These people were never told the truth, but instead were given "false hope" by their conventional oncologist.

I believe that the following statements are accurate: It is *false hope* when patients are prescribed a conventional cancer treatment and not told that the treatment is only considered to be palliative (not expected to cure the patient). It is *false hope* when response rates are quoted and presented in a way that implies long-term recovery. And it is *false hope* when any official cancer cure-rate statistic that has been "fudged" is presented to a cancer patient as representative of his or her chances for real recovery and survival.

Does Newer Mean Better?

It is wrong for the mainstream medical establishment to mislead patients about the actual long-term effectiveness of conventional cancer treatments. But one thing that plays into this problem is the readiness of the public to think that anything "newer" is "better." One of the most distressing patterns I have come across when talking to people who have recently been diagnosed with cancer, is their frequent willingness to overlook the long-term effectiveness of many alternative, non-toxic cancer treatments—and to eagerly look for the *most recent* conventional cancer drugs or procedures for their healing, instead. I have heard people say things like, "There is a *new* cancer drug that is showing great results in clinical trials. I'm going to talk to my doctor about that."

Moreover, the media supports this type of frenzy, even when some of the new cancer drugs have not been tested for more than a few months. They often are given all kinds of acclaim as possible "magic bullets" in newspaper or magazine articles. Ever since antibiotics were developed, and ever since strides in technology helped to make medical accomplishments soar, people in the modern world have come to think that anything *new* in medicine must be *better*. But cancer is not a simple bacterium that can be targeted by a simple antibiotic, nor is it a type of wound that can easily be addressed by modern technology and hardware. Therefore, the "newer is better" stance does not necessarily apply to cancer.

Doctors play a role in the "newer is better" syndrome, as well, whenever they actively recommend that a cancer patient take part in a "phase I" clinical trial. You, yourself, may have been recommended this and possibly are still considering it. But what all cancer patients should know about phase I clinical trials is that they are little more than *toxicity tests*. They are clinical trials used to establish "safe" doses of new drugs. In any phase I trial, the medical establishment does not know the safe dose of that particular treatment for humans yet, so they put a bunch of patients through various doses of the new treatment and watch for side effects. Sometimes the doctors recommending phase I trials don't even believe that the patient they are referring will be likely to benefit from the trial. But they hope that, in the long run, patients in the future may benefit from the trial. Basically, in phase I clinical trials, you are just a guinea pig used for determining dosage levels.

Of course, some new drugs may actually show promise. They might put a certain percentage of people into temporary remission. But remission does not always equate to long-term cure. Basically, if a treatment has only been tested for a short time, then the *only* results available on it are short-term. In looking for *long-term* recovery, it makes more sense to go with a treatment that already has a good long-term track record. Again, it all boils down to a simple question: Are you interested in surviving your cancer short-term or long-term?

When an oncologist says to a patient, "I'd like you to try this new treatment that clinical trials are just starting on," one has to wonder if this isn't just a little bit like a pilot saying to you, "Well, I don't have a plane available right now that I *know* can get you to where you want to go—but over here, on this other runway, is a brand-new type of plane we are just trying out. It's never been flown successfully before, but the pre-flight tests show it to be very promising." If it were me, looking for a plane to get me somewhere, I'd much rather walk a block down the road to another airport that has a tried-and-true plane that has already successfully made the trip many times. This is often what you can do when you avoid the "newer is better" syndrome and look into what treatments (conventional or alternative) have actually worked in a long-term way for many people before you.

The Double Standard

One of the things I have heard over and over from people who are dealing with a cancer diagnosis is, "What formal, large-scale studies have been done on this or that alternative cancer treatment?" When the person then hears that no large-scale studies have been done, they often figure the treatment approach must be bogus and no longer consider looking into it.

The first thing to understand is that the developers of most of the alternative treatments mentioned in this book *did* try for many years to get formal, large-scale studies done on their innovative cancer treatments. If these approaches had been fairly evaluated by mainstream medicine, as they should have been, there *would* be large-scale formal studies to quote from. But only the richly funded mainstream research organizations (backed by pharmaceutical or government money) can afford to do these types of studies. So, if a treatment approach is not considered by pharmaceutical companies to be something that could be extremely profitable to them, large-scale formal studies will not be done.

The second thing to understand is that, in many cases, small but significant studies *have been done* on many alternative cancer treatments, but they have not been responded to. Examples of these types of studies that have been done are the following:

- A team of 10 reputable doctors studied the clinical records of patients using the Hoxsey therapy and recommended it as an effective cancer treatment.

- A congressional committee looked into the Gerson therapy and concluded it was an effective cancer treatment.

- A scientifically sound clinical study of Dr. Kelley's enzyme therapy showed it to be significantly better than conventional methods for pancreatic cancer.

- Studies on Burzynski's antineoplaston therapy showed it to be significantly better than conventional methods for numerous types of cancer.

- In vitro studies done by the NCI on Jim Sheridan's formula now called Protocel showed results that were much better than chemotherapy results for a variety of different cancer cell lines.

Generally, the public is *not* aware that these studies have been done and have shown significant positive results for alternative cancer treatments.

But more importantly, people expect there to be unbiased, third-party, large-scale studies done on everything, without realizing that *these types of studies have not even been done on conventional cancer treatments.* In other words, cancer patients rarely say to their oncologist, "Doctor, I can't consider this particular type of chemotherapy or radiation treatment unless you are able to show me positive results from unbiased, large-scale studies showing that people who underwent this protocol got well—really got well, not just lived with their cancer for five years after diagnosis." This is largely because patients *assume* that the studies for conventional treatments have already been done.

What is so ludicrous about this double standard is that radiation and chemotherapy agents are still officially listed as "unproven" cures and are required in many cases to be classified as "experimental." The fact is that many doctors, and most of the public, erroneously assume that anything approved by the FDA has been rigorously proven in scientific studies. In his June 6, 2003, newsletter, Dr. Moss enlightens us about the process of officially approving a new cancer drug:

The FDA has approved the drug Iressa (gefitinib) for the treatment of non-small cell lung cancer, despite evidence that it does not prolong the lives of patients. Approval came after an FDA panel heard testimony from patients, one of whom claimed to feel much better after taking the little brown pill. Her moving story helped convince members of the Oncologic Drug Advisory Committee to give final approval.

. . . Some critics are beginning to wake up to the fact that the FDA is now approving drugs that emerge from "Big Pharma" without requiring the rigorous proof once considered necessary. In fact, when proof is offered that the drugs in question do *not* work it seems that the FDA is quite willing to throw out the studies and revert to anecdotal accounts.[16]

When extremely high standards of study results are required for under-funded alternative treatments, but are *not* required for richly funded conventional treatments, then we are dealing with a deadly double-standard.

But it is not only the Big Pharma that is biased toward their types of conventional treatments. There is also often a strong personal bias among conventional doctors against alternative treatments for cancer. Here is one story to illustrate some problems people face when they discuss treatment options with their doctors. I spoke to a man whose wife was suffering from late-stage cancer, most of which was in her brain and growing fast. So, she didn't have much time. This man claimed he had looked into many alternative treatments for his wife, but said, "The problem with those is that so many of them turn out to be bogus." I found out later from him that the way he had decided they were bogus was by asking his doctors what they thought of the alternative treatment every time he heard of one. Since his doctors looked at *all* alternative cancer treatment approaches as bogus, that is what they replied in every case, without having any knowledge of the specifics of the therapy.

This man's wife died of her brain cancer a few months later. Her doctors had nothing effective to offer her, and yet they were quite effective in keeping her from trying any alternative treatments — treatments they were totally uninformed about, but adamantly claimed were ineffective.

Unfortunately, most conventional doctors are completely uninformed or worse, *misinformed*, about any treatment that is not conventional. By this I mean that they usually know very little about anything not endorsed by pharmaceutical companies (or by medical organizations that are influenced by pharmaceutical companies). Thus, there is a very real problem in thinking that your doctors are going to know the truth about alternative cancer treatments. And doctors are not motivated to find out more about alternative cancer treatments because, in most U.S. states, it is illegal to prescribe any treatment for cancer *other* than what is specifically approved by the FDA.

We have been brought up to regard doctors and medical organizations as experts. We have been brought up to think that if we don't get our doctor's approval on some treatment approach we are interested in, then we are being irresponsible, maybe even "killing ourselves." We have *not* been brought up to believe that big industries, and not true science, are affecting which medical treatments are available to us.

New Cancer Drugs Are Big Business

It is understandably difficult to fathom why the most effective nontoxic approaches to treating cancer are *not* being used by oncologists and cancer clinics everywhere—and why toxic treatments that do not show significant effectiveness *are* being used. The only answer to this is that cancer treatments are "big business." In particular, new cancer *drugs* are big business. And the effectiveness of new drugs can easily be exaggerated and promoted in press releases by drug companies. Ralph Moss shows us how this can happen in his June 13, 2003, newsletter. Moss first states that,

> On July 30, 2001, Erbitux was hailed in a *Business Week* cover story, "The Birth of a Cancer Drug." The drug, then called IMC-225, was celebrated as a "blockbuster" that "halts the spread of cancer." In an editorial entitled "The Dawn of a New Era," the magazine claimed that Erbitux "seems effective against cancers of the colon, pancreas, head and neck and lungs." It suggested that victory might be within sight in the war on cancer.[17]

Then, Moss goes on to explain that the Associated Press, CNN, and Wall Street all joined in with incredible excitement about this amazing new cancer drug. But what these news organizations *never* did was to look at the studies themselves. If they had, they would have found that, on average, the studies done on Erbitux showed the overall response rate to be only about 10 percent. (And we know that response rate is not equivalent to recovery—it just means that a 50 percent reduction in tumor size was achieved for a short while.) Plus, the studies on Erbitux showed an average of just 45 days to progression. This means that the common length of time that Erbitux could *slow* the cancer was only about one-and-one-half months before the cancer would progress again. Moreover, about 50 percent of the patients given Erbitux in the studies suffered what were considered "severe" side effects.

Yet, with so little effectiveness to boast, Erbitux went into clinical trials to get approval by the FDA as a cancer drug. If approved, Erbitux could be worth billions of dollars a year in sales to drug companies.

Apparently, FDA approval of cancer drugs like Erbitux does not require studies that show significant long-term effectiveness. For example, another highly touted cancer drug, "Iressa," has already achieved FDA approval. But according to Moss, "The approval came despite the fact that Iressa has been shown in rigorous studies not to prolong overall survival."[18]

The FDA itself appears to operate in ways that involve huge conflicts of interest. This organization is supposed to protect public safety where drugs are concerned, yet many of its personnel, including heads of departments, either have had, or will move on to, highly paid jobs in pharmaceutical companies. The FDA personnel are not unbiased! Not only are they not unbiased, they are practically autonomous because much of what they do is *not* under direct control of Congress. Unbelievably, congressional hearings that uncover problems in the FDA are only allowed to "make suggestions" to the FDA where they think change is warranted. It appears that the FDA does not have to do anything Congress says!

Questions to Ask Your Oncologist

What can you do to protect yourself? At the very least, cancer patients have the right to know what the long-term efficacy of a treatment being offered them is, as well as what side effects they might experience. In other words, *they have a right to make a truly informed decision*. To make sure that *you* are able to make a truly informed decision for yourself, you can start by asking your doctor the right questions. Some questions I highly recommend that you ask your oncologist regarding the conventional treatment he or she is recommending to you are:

1. "What kind of *long-term* efficacy does this type of treatment offer for my type of cancer? In other words, what are my chances of living longer than five years *and becoming cancer-free?*"

2. If your oncologist quotes "response rates" to you, you might want to say, "I am not interested in hearing about tumor response rates

because I know that they only refer to short-term tumor shrinkage. What are the long-term, cancer-free statistics on this treatment?"

3. If you have a child who has been diagnosed with cancer, you might want to ask your pediatric oncologist, "What are the chances that my child will recover using this treatment and grow up to be a healthy adult? Have you seen any children fully recover with this treatment and go on to live totally normal lives?"

4. "Is the treatment you suggest considered to be a *curative* treatment in this case, or just a *palliative* treatment?" (Remember, a palliative treatment is considered to be one that is *not* expected to save the patient's life, but is simply administered in the hope that it will prolong the patient's life. Sometimes this expectation for longer survival is only a few months.)

5. "What will this treatment do to my quality of life?"

6. "How long do you think I will live if I do not undergo any treatment at all? And how long do you think I will live if I follow your treatment sugestion?"

7. "Can you give me any phone numbers of other patients you have successfully treated with the type of treatment you are suggesting to me? Or, if you can't give out phone numbers, can you at least *describe* to me any cases of people who fully recovered from their cancer using the method you want to prescribe to me?"

8. "If I go through this treatment, what are all the serious, or even life-threatening, side effects I might experience? For example, is it possible this treatment could cause me to die from heart failure or a blood clot? Is it possible this treatment could cause me to develop a secondary life-threatening cancer within a few years?"

Do not be shy about asking these direct questions. This is information you have a right to know. Depending on your type of cancer, you may be making a decision that your life depends on. Also, if your oncologist is not comfortable with these types of questions, then you should consider seeking out another oncologist who *will* answer them honestly for you. Remember, you are paying your doctor—he or she is working for you. Your doctor is supposed to be on your side, trying to help you save your life.

Hopefully, the information in this chapter will help you to be able to make a truly informed decision about your cancer treatment. I suggest you be just as open and objective about considering the treatments your conventional oncologist recommends to you as you are when you consider any alternative treatment for your cancer. However, do not fall prey to a double standard. Do not let yourself be "rushed" into treatment before you have considered your options. Understand the terminology and statistics that are presented to you by your doctor. Be aware of short-term versus long-term effectiveness. Be aware of all possible side effects for any treatment you are considering, whether it is a conventional or alternative approach. And try to find out if other cancer patients have used that approach successfully to become cancer-free (not to just live 5 years after diagnosis). Speak with some of these patients, if possible. Never forget that your goal is to *recover* from your cancer and regain a normal, cancer-free life!

Resources:

Books

Ralph W. Moss, Ph.D. *The Cancer Industry*. New York: Equinox Press, 1999. (ISBN 1-881025-09-8)

Ralph W. Moss, Ph.D. *Questioning Chemotherapy*. New York: Equinox Press, 2000. (ISBN 1-881025-25-X)

Kenny Ausubel. *When Healing Becomes a Crime: The Amazing Story of the Hoxsey Cancer Clinics and the Return of Alternative Therapies*. Rochester, Vermont: Healing Arts Press, 2000. (ISBN 0-89281-925-1)

Video

Cancer Doesn't Scare Me Anymore, by Dr. Lorraine Day. To order, call (800) 574-2437, or visit Dr. Day's website: www.drday.com.

Newsletter

For the free weekly newsletter put out by Ralph W. Moss, Ph.D., go to www.cancerdecisions.com.

CHAPTER 22

Choosing an Alternative Treatment Plan

After reading the previous chapters of this book, I hope you have gained an understanding of some of the *many* options you can choose from to "outsmart" your cancer. However, if you make the decision for yourself to go with an alternative, non-toxic approach, you may also feel somewhat overwhelmed by all the possible options. This chapter will give you some important tips to help you more effectively choose an alternative treatment plan that is right for you. These tips address narrowing down your choices, contacting practitioners for more information, dealing with conventional doctors, prioritizing your overall treatment program, and monitoring your progress.

Narrowing Down Your Choices

How does one narrow down the choices? The best way to start is by evaluating four main treatment factors and how they apply to your particular situation. They are:

1. Efficacy of treatment

2. Difficulty of treatment

3. Cost of treatment

4. Level of supervision

In other words, considering these factors in the very beginning to see if there are some treatment options you may want to rule out may help you to more easily zero in on the approaches you want to consider.

Efficacy of Treatment

Efficacy of treatment is, of course, going to be foremost in importance. But it is really impossible, without comprehensive comparative studies, to say that any particular alternative cancer approach is more effective than another. And no cancer treatment, whether conventional or alternative, is 100 percent effective for 100 percent of the people that use it. This is because cancer is such a complex condition that often occurs when people's bodies are already extremely toxic, out-of-balance, or weakened in many ways.

When trying to ascertain for yourself the "overall" effectiveness of any alternative cancer approach, there are some important issues to understand. For example, you may be concerned about some people you know about for whom that approach did *not* work. One thing to remember is that most of the people who use alternative approaches start them at a much later stage in their disease than is optimal. Because most people are not initially aware of the benefits of non-toxic treatments, they generally use conventional treatments first. It is only after these conventional treatments have failed that many people turn to alternative approaches. This tends to bring down the success rates of the alternative treatments because these people are often already seriously damaged by the chemotherapy and/or radiation they have been given, or possibly already seriously damaged by the cancer that may have spread more extensively throughout their body. The general rule is that, the sooner after diagnosis that you start *any* treatment (whether alternative or conventional), the better your chances for recovery will be.

Another thing to remember is that, because alternative approaches are much more self-administered than conventional approaches, there will always be a certain number of people who do not use them correctly. I have heard more than once about someone who claimed that a particular approach did not work for them, but then I also heard that they either did not give the treatment enough time, or there were things they were doing that interfered with the treatment.

One issue for some types of alternative approaches, such as the herbal therapies, is that it may be important to find sources that provide these treatments in as close to their original form as possible. Herbs are "nature's medicine," but they must be grown, harvested, and used in optimal ways to be effective. The Hoxsey herbal formula, as well as Essiac, were both originally harvested from wild-crafted herbs grown in healthy, virgin soils. They were administered shortly after preparation and did not have to be prepared for "mass" marketing and long-term storage. Even though the Hoxsey therapy and Essiac are still achieving cancer recoveries for many people (especially in early stages of cancer), their overall effectiveness, particularly for late-stage cancer, may not be quite as good as when they were originally used.

Thus, if you are planning to use any herbal approach, I suggest you research that treatment as much as you can and try to find the best possible source to get the herbs from. If you decide to use the Hoxsey herbal approach, you may want to go *directly* to the clinic in Mexico that Mildred Nelson established to obtain good quality herbs and guidance on how to use them. For good quality Essiac, you may want to search out an independent herbal source that has high standards for the quality of herbs they sell rather than use a mass-produced herbal formula. Many small herb providers carry the Essiac herbs and can sell them to you shortly after harvesting, with instructions on how to mix and prepare them in your own home.

In a similar way, the diet-based approaches which focus primarily on high amounts of fresh vegetables and fruits, such as the Gerson therapy or wheatgrass therapy, may not be as effective as they were decades ago. This may be partly because it is difficult in this modern world to find fruits and vegetables grown in truly balanced, healthy soils. Even organically grown fruits and vegetables are likely to come from soil that has been overused. Artificial fertilization techniques are helpful, but may not be able to produce crops that are as abundant in nutrients as virgin soils can. Also, people are more toxic these days than they used to be, in general. So the approaches that place a large focus on detoxification may have further to go in today's world than they did earlier in the 20th century.

However, we can learn from *all* of the successful non-toxic approaches and can often use parts of each. For instance, pancreatic enzymes (Kelley), Laetrile (Krebs), herbs (Hoxsey or Essiac), diet (Gerson or Budwig), or coffee enemas (Gerson and Kelley) can often be combined to optimize one's chances for recovery. Just make sure, whenever combining approaches, that the aspects you use from different approaches do *not* conflict with each other.

In general, alternative non-toxic cancer approaches tend to work well for *most* types of cancer, and they are *not* focused on treating specific cancers the way conventional treatments are. This is because they address the common characteristics of all cancers. Thus, the efficacy of any particular alternative approach will usually not be limited to a specific type of cancer. Having said that, some alternative approaches may boast that they are *particularly* good at dealing with particular systems of the body. For example, Dr. Burzynski's antineoplaston therapy is particularly effective for brain cancer and lymphomas, and Dr. Kelley's enzyme approach is particularly effective for pancreatic cancer. But both of these approaches have also achieved great results for cancers in other locations of the body, and there are other non-toxic approaches, such as Protocel or flaxseed oil and cottage cheese that are effective for brain cancer and lymphomas as well.

The most important way to ensure effectiveness of any alternative, non-toxic approach is by acquainting yourself with it enough to make sure you are doing it optimally, and/or by finding a qualified practitioner or support group to help guide you through it. Along with that, taking care of yourself in other ways may also be important to your healing process. Some people may have to continue going to work while they are trying to recover from their cancer because of their financial needs. But if possible, it might be best to stay home and reduce stress while recovering. Some key aspects of taking care of yourself may involve getting the sleep you need, eating a nutritional and balanced diet, drinking lots of good water for hydration and detoxification, reducing unnecessary stress, and dealing with your emotions.

Difficulty of Treatment

In some cases, difficulty of treatment may be the biggest factor of all to consider when choosing a treatment approach. For instance, this factor particularly comes into play when treating very young children or elderly people with cancer. In terms of "sheer volume" of work, the Gerson therapy is considered by many to be the most difficult alternative cancer treatment available. It requires the juicing of fresh, organic vegetables and fruits about 13 times every day, along with performing multiple coffee enemas every day, along with carrying out other specific daily requirements. Even some strong, young adults have found it necessary, when doing the Gerson therapy, to actually *hire* outside help in order to carry out the juicing required. And the daily coffee enemas may just not be "do-able" for young children, some older people, and even some middle-aged adults who may not have the energy or mobility to carry out the protocol. (However, for those people who want to use a strictly nutrition-based approach and *have* the energy or help required to do it, the Gerson therapy may be their best choice.)

Another issue to consider is the number of pills required by the approach you are considering. For example, the Gonzalez-Isaacs enzyme therapy requires an extremely high number of pills to be taken every day (possibly up to 150). This can also be difficult for young children or the elderly. There may be ways to work around this, such as opening the pills up and putting the powdered contents into a drink, but it is certainly a factor to consider when prioritizing one's treatment options.

Overall, the *easiest* approaches to administer to young children or elderly adults are probably the following: Protocel, cesium high pH therapy, flaxseed oil and cottage cheese, the Hoxsey therapy, or Essiac. (Remember, however, Protocel should *not* be done with Hoxsey or Essiac, and it is unknown at this time as to whether flaxseed oil and cottage cheese or cesium can be done together with Protocel without conflicting on the cellular level. So, it is probably safest not to combine Protocel with the others listed here.) Burzynski's antineoplaston therapy has *also* been successfully administered many times to young children, and should always be considered when brain cancer is involved.

Thus, ruling out those approaches that may be too difficult to administer for your particular case can help to narrow down your choices.

Cost of Treatment

Considering the cost of approaches you may be looking into is sometimes another way to narrow down your choices. The ideal situation would be for each person to have unlimited money and unlimited time, but this is not usually the case. Fortunately, alternative treatments are much less expensive than conventional treatments for cancer. However, health insurance policies rarely cover alternative approaches, even if the alternative doctor you are working with is a fully accredited M.D. Therefore, when it comes to using some of the more expensive alternative approaches, it might be important to find out ahead of time if your insurance company will pay for any part of it, or not.

There is a wide range of costs for alternative cancer approaches, so it is a good idea to consider the different costs listed at the back of each treatment chapter. These will at least give you a general idea of the expenses required. Besides the cost of treatment, one must also consider possible time away from work. If you start an effective treatment soon after diagnosis, you may have a very good chance of being able to carry on with your life normally while you recover. But many cancer patients may not feel well enough to work at all for at least some period of time. Or if you choose a very time-consuming method, then just carrying out the treatment may rule out time to go to work and bring home a paycheck. This means that when you consider treatment expenses, you may also need to factor in a certain reduction of income occurring at the same time.

The important thing to remember is that, when considering your treatment options, *more expensive* does not necessarily mean *more effective*. One of the more expensive approaches may turn out to be the best choice for some people, while one of the less expensive approaches may turn out to be the best choice for other people. The good news is that, if you are particularly challenged financially, there are still excellent options available in the alternative cancer treatment world. Protocel, the flaxseed oil and cottage cheese diet, 714X, cesium high pH therapy, the Hoxsey therapy, and Essiac tea, are all relatively inexpensive approaches.

I believe that a good rule for anyone looking into alternative cancer treatments is to *first* try to decide which form of treatment you would choose if money were not an issue. In other words, put aside all of the money considerations you have, just at first, and try to evaluate what approach you think will give you the best chance for recovery. Once you have sorted out which treatment you would *like* to try, then see if there is any way you can come up with the money.

Think carefully before choosing a treatment approach that is not your first choice just because you can't afford your first choice approach. In some cases, it may be that there is no way around this. But whenever possible, it is a good idea to try to pursue the treatment approach you feel you can most fully commit to and have confidence in.

Level of Supervision

Another factor to consider is the type or amount of guidance or supervision you require to feel comfortable with your treatment approach. If you are the type of person who can feel comfortable primarily self-administering your own treatment after obtaining initial guidance, then there are certain approaches that can be considered. These include the Gerson method (once you have received guidance from the Gerson Institute), 714-X, cesium high pH therapy, Protocel, Dr. Budwig's flaxseed oil and cottage cheese diet, and the Hoxsey therapy. Some of these have Internet-based user support forums available. For example, many people using Protocel or flaxseed oil and cottage cheese are not seeing practitioners for guidance, but they *are* involved with large private support groups where they can learn from other's experiences and also get emotional support for what they are going through.

If you are the type of person who would be *most* comfortable with on-going supervision and guidance from a medical practitioner, then some professionally supervised approaches to consider might be: Burzynski's Antineoplastons (Texas), Hospital Santa Monica (Mexico), Dr. Brodie's Laetrile/Integrative approach (Nevada), or Dr. Gonzalez and Dr. Isaacs's Enzyme Therapy (New York).

Preferably, geographical location will *not* be a deciding factor for most people, because airline flights are not that difficult to take. But for some, choosing a treatment approach with a supervising doctor or clinic might also involve finding one that is geographically close to where they live. Some people may want to search in their own area for practitioners who are using one or more of the approaches listed in this book.

Contacting Practitioners for More Information

If you decide to try an alternative cancer approach, you may want to quickly call each place of treatment you are considering. This could be to verify that they are still in operation as well as to ask some detailed questions about their treatment program. Feel free to ask what kind of success they have had dealing with your particular type of cancer, but don't expect hard numbers or studies. The best type of answer you will probably get is a comment based on their own experience with their patients. This information is valuable, especially since they sometimes may be able to give you the phone number or email address of one or more of those patients. If they have not yet treated your particular type of cancer, this does *not* necessarily mean you should stop considering them for treatment. After all, there are many different manifestations of cancer, and yours may be one of the more rare types. If any of their patients have given them permission to give out their phone number, then you may be able to quickly phone someone who has been through the treatment and who can tell you more details about the approach, the doctor, or the process of recovery that they experienced.

If your preliminary research looks promising, you may want to either start treatment immediately or consider making a consultation appointment first to discuss your particular case. (Refer to the contact information listed at the back of each treatment chapter.) This will use up some of your valuable time and money, but it can be an important step in choosing the treatment that will be best for you. Even if you have to go to several different treatment center consultations before you decide, it could be worth your efforts in the long run. Yes, it is important for you to start treatment as soon as possible, but it is also important to be able to make a *well-informed* decision as to which treatment you choose.

Most alternative doctors will want you to come in for a consultation with all of your diagnostic test results. These include biopsy reports, X-rays, CT scan results, blood tests, and whatever else you have been able to get from your conventional physicians so far. Ask first over the phone what types of records they want you to bring, and ask how much the consultation will cost.

Often, an in-person consultation with an alternative practitioner or clinic can be of great help in determining which approach you want to follow. It not only will give you an idea as to whether you would feel comfortable with that practitioner or clinic, it also may give you a better idea as to the likelihood of that approach working well for you, and even possibly how long it may take.

Another way to get this sort of information is to ask for an informational packet to be mailed to you. There is a $10 video about 714X you can request, Hospital Santa Monica in Mexico offers a free videotape describing their services, and Dr. Gonzalez and Dr. Isaacs offer a set of lecture tapes describing their program.

Time is obviously *always* of the essence when dealing with cancer. But spending a little more time in the beginning can sometimes save time later on. It may be hard to take a few extra days for research or a consultation appointment in the beginning, when your doctor and family members are urging you to rush into surgery, radiation or chemotherapy. But just remember that a well-spent number of days doing research in the very beginning can sometimes make the difference between life and death. Getting onto a cancer treatment plan as fast as possible is always a priority, but getting started on treatment that will give you a good chance for long-term recovery is also of utmost importance.

Dealing With Conventional Doctors

Every person who chooses to use an alternative treatment approach to "outsmart" his or her cancer will be going against the grain of modern conventional medicine. One difficulty that can arise as a result of this is the difficulty involved with declining the modern treatment your conventional doctor thinks you should get. Most people with cancer are first diagnosed by a conventional doctor. If you are one of these people, you may have seen an oncologist who is very committed to the mainstream "accepted" approaches. It is no easy task to turn down a medical specialist's recommendation—especially when you may be told that, in doing so, you will be killing yourself. One thing to remember in this situation is that, specialist or not, *your doctor works for you.* You are paying your doctor for his or her expertise and professional service. It is important to listen to and consider any recommendation for treatment your conventional doctor gives you. But when it comes to the final decision you make, that is up to you.

If you choose to follow an alternative approach, you may be in a situation where you still want to see your conventional doctor at certain intervals for diagnostic monitoring. Even people using alternative methods will want to have blood tests, CT scans, MRIs, or other tests done regularly to ascertain their progress. Also, having these performed by a conventional doctor will generally allow these tests to be covered by your health insurance policy. Or there may be side complications of your cancer that you will want to go to a conventional doctor for help with at times.

I recommend being as open as possible with your conventional doctor. I believe it is best to be honest and to give your doctor the opportunity of deciding to follow your progress while you use an alternative approach. You may be surprised to find that your doctor is more open-minded than you expected. If, however, your doctor takes a stance against alternative approaches and will *not* prescribe diagnostic tests to you unless you undergo conventional treatments, then you have the option of finding another doctor or oncologist who will. If you phone different doctors' offices, you may be able to find another doctor in your area who *is* willing to monitor your progress even though you are not using a conventional approach. I recommend that you make an effort to find a doctor with whom you can work openly. In doing so, you are also emotionally standing up for yourself and your right to choose your own treatment.

But if you do employ a conventional doctor to prescribe diagnostic tests for you, remember that, in some cases, your doctor may *not* know how to interpret the results of the tests. A good example is, when using Protocel, cancer marker levels may rise as the cancer cells lyse and fall apart. Conventional doctors may not interpret these results correctly, since they are trained to see any rise in cancer markers as indications that the cancer is growing or spreading. It is up to you to be informed about the particular approach you are using so that you can help your conventional doctor to interpret your diagnostic tests accurately.

Also, it is important for doctors to find out how many people choose alternative approaches and how well these approaches work. In this sense, you are helping to educate them.

Prioritizing Your Overall Treatment Program

Once you have decided on a primary approach to use, figure out your priorities. You may want to make a list on paper to help you keep your overall recovery plan in mind. I would suggest that you list the primary treatment approach you have chosen to use as "priority number 1." Secondary to that, you can list any adjunctive treatments you would like to add to your program. Then, lower on the priority list might be balancing hormones, alkalinity issues, dealing with toxic teeth, or working on emotional or psycho-spiritual issues. Different people will list their priorities in different order from other people.

Seeing the important issues prioritized and listed on paper can help to reduce some of the confusion that may arise when you think about what it is you need to do to "outsmart your cancer." As mentioned earlier, we can learn from *all* of the successful alternative approaches, and many of these can be combined effectively. For example, you may want to use Protocel as your primary treatment approach, but you would also like to supplement your program with pancreatic enzymes and foods high in B_{17}, work on balancing your alkalinity, and supplement with natural progesterone (if you are a woman). Or you may choose to use 714X as your primary treatment, but also want to use Essiac tea or the Hoxsey therapy as an adjunctive treatment, while you take care of your toxic teeth and deal with your psycho-spiritual issues. Another example might be that you choose to use cesium high pH therapy along with other supplements as your primary treatment, but at the same time follow the flaxseed oil and cottage cheese diet, balance your hormones, and perform daily coffee enemas.

Just be careful when choosing any adjunctive treatment to not combine aspects of different treatments that may conflict. Most alternative cancer treatment approaches have very specific guidelines, and these guidelines are there for good reasons. Although combining approaches can often be an excellent and powerful way to treat your cancer, you must be sure to do it knowledgeably and cautiously. Thus, a very important rule to remember is to *always* thoroughly research the approach you are using and make sure you follow it (or combine it with others) correctly.

Monitoring Your Progress

As already mentioned, most people using an alternative cancer approach will still want to have conventional diagnostic tests performed at regular intervals to help them monitor their progress. But one tricky situation that can arise for people using any self-administered type of approach is that there is a tendency to interpret every bit of discomfort, pain, or swelling as a sign that their cancer is getting "worse." This is where an experienced alternative practitioner or helpful support group for that particular approach can be invaluable. Often, some level of discomfort, pain, or swelling is normal on the path to recovery. But if you do not have an expert telling you that these symptoms are nothing to worry about, then they can be very scary.

Unfortunately, too many people stop using an alternative cancer treatment just when the treatment is effectively working, because they don't have a doctor telling them it is working. When you think about it, if chemotherapy were a self-administered cancer treatment approach, how many people would stay with it after their first bout of vomiting, hair loss, or other symptoms? I doubt any cancer patient would stay the course if chemotherapy were an alternative, self-administered approach. Patients only stay with treatments such as chemotherapy because their doctors tell them that the symptoms they are experiencing are necessary to go through in order to get well. So, too, must you be informed about possible discomforts you may experience with an alternative cancer treatment. Although these discomforts will generally be much less severe than those experienced with toxic conventional treatments, they still may occur at times.

The good news is that, when you *do* go against the grain and use an alternative approach to treating your cancer, you end up playing a much bigger role in your own recovery. You may need to do more of your own research and thinking than you would with a conventional approach, but taking a bigger role in your own healing can also be a very empowering process. Even if you have chosen an alternative medical practitioner to work with, you can still be very involved in your own healing. Be sure to ask your alternative practitioner lots of questions. If the approach you choose does *not* offer a practitioner, try to find a support group that can give you experienced advice. There will almost always be ways to find out what you need to know in order to achieve your optimum chance for recovery.

CHAPTER 23

Dealing With Fear and the Mind/Body Connection

I f you have just been diagnosed with cancer and have not yet chosen a treatment approach, then it may be too soon for you to be dealing with your emotions in any depth at this point. But at some point *after* you are securely established in your chosen treatment plan, this may be an important thing for you to consider as part of your recovery process. The two key aspects of your emotions that you may find most important to examine are those involving (1) fear, and (2) the mind/body connection. Actually, since fear comes into play from the very *first* moment after diagnosis, it is even worth thinking about to some extent right away. This is because you don't want overwhelming fear to influence your decisions about treatment any more than necessary.

Dealing With Fear

Very few things are better at generating fear than a cancer diagnosis. The challenge for the cancer patient is to not let your fear make your decisions for you when it comes to treatment. This can result in disaster. What I mean here is that *managing the fear* and *making a treatment decision* need to be two very separate processes.

From my years of working with clients in individual and family therapy settings, as well as in hypnotherapy sessions I conducted, I developed what I believe are some very helpful ways to look at and deal with the above-mentioned "F" word. The truth is that fear is something to be *highly respected*. Too often, we are afraid of fear and minimize it or try to push it away. But it is much more helpful to *not* minimize and push away fear. Instead, it is best to *acknowledge* fear and give it the respect it deserves as a very important "signal." In other words, it is just as important as your car's dashboard light which comes on when the oil is low.

Those of us who wish to drive safely and prolong the life of our car don't minimize this dashboard signal—we don't ignore it or push it away from our awareness by placing tape over the light so we can't see it. So, too, must we *not* minimize or ignore the emotional fear signal our bodies give us.

On the other hand, fear is just a signal. That's all it is. *You* are in control, *not* your fear—just as the light on the dashboard is not in control of your car, but you are.

The best way to deal with fear is to acknowledge it whenever it appears. Notice when it starts. Notice how strong it is, how it feels physically in your body. Notice the thoughts that go on in your head when you are feeling fear. Then say to yourself, "It's okay to feel this fear." You might even acknowledge to yourself what all the reasons are that you are feeling this fear. Many times people who acknowledge fear in this way will notice it quickly dissipate on its own. It may not always go away completely, but by acknowledging that it is an important signal, you are telling your subconscious mind that you have "noticed" the light on the dashboard. You thereby allow your subconscious mind to reply back, in effect, "Oh—all right . . . I guess I don't have to flash that signal so much anymore because I now have your attention."

Sometimes, when you acknowledge your fear, it may feel like you are more vulnerable and helpless than before. Tears may flow. This is also okay. It takes a lot of energy to suppress strong feelings, and if you allow them to come out, you can actually free up some extra energy for your body to use in healing itself. If you feel comfortable enough to share your fears with those close to you, this may also help. And, of course, whenever possible, asking close friends or family whom you trust and feel safe with to *help* you make decisions or help you start on treatment can be invaluable in relieving some of the fear that comes with facing an illness alone.

Here's the next step: Once you have acknowledged and felt your fear more clearly than before, then you can learn to remind yourself that you are *more* than your fear. Your fear may feel like the biggest and strongest part of you, but it is really just a very small part of you. You can take control of your own body and life with the decisions that you make. If you have already acknowledged your fear rather than suppressing it, you are less likely to have the fear subconsciously driving your decisions. Remember, acknowledging your fear does not mean you are letting it make your decisions for you. Quite the contrary. Acknowledging your fear actually undermines its power over you and places you firmly in control!

But remember, dealing with your fear and other emotions is a long-term process. It is not something you do just once or twice, and then you're done. Thus, you may notice the fear cropping up again at various times over the weeks or months. (Or maybe it never completely goes away.) When this happens, it will be helpful to just periodically acknowledge the fear and remind yourself that it is just a light on your "mental dashboard," that you are *more* than your fear, and that you *are* handling the problem and *are* in the process of adding the appropriate oil, so-to-speak.

Another helpful tip is that, whenever making important decisions for your recovery, it can be very constructive to ask yourself, "Is this decision based on fear? Or is it based on rationally weighing the information I have gathered?" Try to avoid going with choices that seem to be based mostly on fear.

The Mind/Body Connection

The mind/body connection is an amazing aspect of each of us that is very powerful, yet rarely consciously dealt with. It is the psycho-physical force behind the "placebo effect." When the mind speaks, the body listens and obeys on some level. In fact, the Latin word "placebo" simply means "I shall please." Because there can be a very real effect even on the cellular level from this force, it is widely accepted as an important force in any healing process.

What many people do not realize, however, is that the mind/body connection only remotely involves the rational, conscious mind. The biggest part of one's consciousness involved in this force is the deeper, subconscious and emotional mind. Only this deeper level of mind has the power to command the body on a deep, cellular level. Yes, we can command our bodies on a "surface level" quite easily with our rational mind. For instance, I can command my arm to lift my hand and reach over and pick up a coffee cup. Or I can think, "I want to slow my breathing and then hold my breath," and I can do that if I wish. But I cannot consciously, in a normal state of mind, command my blood flow to slow down or my white cell activity to speed up. This, however, *can* be done from a more meditative state that provides a connection to the subconscious mind.

It is well known that a person working with a hypnotherapist, or in a self-induced trance state, *can* effectively command changes in his or her body down to the cellular level. This is because these situations involve getting into a state where the conscious mind takes a back seat and the subconscious mind can be accessed. In this sort of situation, the conscious mind plays only a small role in communicating to the subconscious mind. Many emergency medical workers, such as 911 personnel or firemen, have even been trained in certain hypnosis techniques to help accident victims survive certain critical situations. For instance, they are sometimes trained to direct people who are bleeding to death to slow their blood flow or to reduce their awareness of pain. This can work very effectively since a traumatized person in shock is already in a sort of trance state.

Deep meditation also promotes a deep connection to the subconscious mind and is why yogis can often perform amazing physical feats, such as slowing their heart rates down to where they appear almost dead. Tibetan initiates into priesthood learn to control their body heat so effectively that they can crouch outside in winter snow with no more than a wet sheet wrapped around them. They have learned to make their own body heat rise so high that the sheets quickly dry and they can then spend the night in the snow in just a sheet without freezing to death.

Similarly, many people with cancer have experienced remarkably positive results in their recovery through meditation, hypnotherapy, or guided imagery. All of these examples simply show the power of the mind/body connection.

Working with your *own* mind/body connection can support and enhance your healing process. To do this, some people may want to seek out a therapist or guided imagery specialist who has experience working with cancer recovery. Part of working with your mind/body connection may involve dealing with your emotions, such as fear, part of it may involve active visualization of the cancer cells going away, and part of it may involve examining your own personality dynamics.

Examining Your Personality Dynamics

On a daily basis, our thoughts and behavior patterns can affect our physical bodies. To exemplify this, just think about how you would feel if you entered a dinner party and suddenly realized you didn't have your clothes on! Your muscles would probably immediately tense up, you would feel adrenaline running rampant, and you might even start to break out in a sweat. These are examples of how the body can very quickly respond to certain thoughts with certain physical responses.

Although you are not likely to find yourself in the above situation, you may be in many more similar situations on a regular basis than you realize. When you are attempting to pick up your child from after-school practice and you are stuck on the freeway starting to experience the physical effects of anxiety, you are in a similar situation. When you are panicking about getting something done at work before a deadline and you feel your blood pressure rise, you are in a similar situation. Anxiety in stressful situations *always* produces some type of physical response in the body. It is part of the mind/body connection.

But our bodies are designed to handle anxiety and physical stress reactions, as long as they don't occur too often. It is when these reactions occur chronically, or *habitually*, that our physical bodies run into trouble. Some types of personality characteristics can produce habitual physical stress responses that overstress the body. One way that chronic stress is hard on us physically is by causing the body to secrete stress hormones on a daily basis that deplete our bodies' stores of vitamin C. Another way that chronic stress is hard on us is by promoting the dehydration of healthy cells. This can happen as a result of the increased metabolic activity involved with hyper-vigilance, or worry.

Constantly worrying about what others think of you, how well you are performing at something, what you are going to do next week, and so forth, can produce constant triggering of the physical "fight or flight" mechanisms of the body, such as adrenaline and other responses. Holding emotions in for fear of expressing oneself can also deplete much-needed energy from the body. These are just a few of the examples of how personality dynamics can be one factor that plays a role in how well your body's immune system functions, or how well your body recovers from illness.

Although there is no one-to-one correlation, a number of studies appear to have validated the reality that personality dynamics can play a role in both the development of and recovery from illness. The most common finding in all the studies done on this subject was that people who tend to "suppress" their feelings are more likely to develop cancer than those who tend to "express" their feelings. In other words, your physical body will more often fare better if you do *not* hold your feelings in.

One of the longest studies to focus on the relationship between personality characteristics and cancer was begun in 1946. A group of 972 students at Johns Hopkins School of Medicine was divided into five subgroups based on various psychological measures, then followed for three decades. Results showed that those students initially characterized as people who suppressed their emotions behind a bland exterior of facial expression were actually 16 times more likely to develop cancer than those who generally expressed their feelings.[1]

Dr. Douglas Brodie of Nevada (mentioned in Chapter 6) supports the idea of a "cancer-prone personality." In fact, he has compiled seven common characteristics of people who develop cancer. On his website, Dr. Brodie lists these characteristics in the following way:[2]

In dealing with many thousands of cancer patients over the past 32 years, it has been my observation that there are certain personality traits which are rather consistently present in the cancer-susceptible individual. These characteristics are as follows:

1. Being highly conscientious, dutiful, responsible, caring, hardworking, and usually of above average intelligence.

2. Exhibiting a strong tendency toward carrying other people's burdens and toward taking on extra obligations, often "worrying for others."

3. Having a deep-seated need to make others happy, tending to be "people pleasers." Having a great need for approval.

4. Often having a history of lack of closeness with one or both parents, sometimes, later in life, resulting in lack of closeness with spouse or others who would normally be close.

5. Harboring long-suppressed toxic emotions, such as anger, resentment and/or hostility. Typically the cancer-susceptible individual internalizes such emotions and has great difficulty expressing them.

6. Reacting adversely to stress, often becoming unable to cope adequately with such stress. Usually experiencing an especially damaging event about two years before the onset of detectable cancer. The patient is unable to cope with this traumatic event or series of events, which comes as a "last straw" on top of years of suppressed reactions to stress.

7. Showing an inability to resolve deep-seated emotional problems and conflicts, usually arising in childhood, often even being unaware of their presence.

What can be very helpful in reducing the body's stress responses is learning to "let go" of worrying about unimportant things. In other words, "Don't sweat the small stuff!" I know of one woman who, while fighting breast cancer, made up a list of all the things she needed to do each day as part of her alternative treatment "program" for healing.

Then, whenever she felt a stress reaction triggered inside her due to outside time crunches, issues with her children, and so forth, she would simply say to herself, "Stress is not part of my program." This simple technique always reminded her to let go of the little worries and greatly helped her to keep her physical stress reactions down.

Another woman realized, while fighting spinal cord cancer, that she was undergoing too much anxiety and worry about the future. She had a type of cancer that her doctors claimed would take her life in just a few months, but she also had four small children who needed raising. The "what ifs" plagued her mercilessly. She finally developed an effective way to let her worry go while she was recovering from her cancer. Every morning when she woke up, she would say to herself, "I got through yesterday . . . I can get through today." Then, every night before bed, she would say to herself, "I got through today, I can get through tomorrow." (This woman *did* fully recover using an effective alternative approach and has been cancer-free for the past 14 years.)

When it comes to fears and worries, it is unrealistic to expect anyone with cancer to *not* be afraid or worry at all. But trying to suppress, or ignore the fears and worries is probably the most damaging thing an ill person can do. This is because the body feels and *responds to* the suppressed fears and worries anyway! In other words, you can suppress a thought or feeling so that it is no longer in your *conscious* awareness. But you cannot suppress a fear or worry so that it is no longer in your *subconscious* awareness and therefore in your physical body's awareness, too. So, acknowledging your fears or worries whenever they come up, and then learning ways to "let them go" or to deal with them more constructively is most often the best way to support your healing.

Along with resolving chronic stress, a person who has a history of always taking care of others to the exclusion of themselves, must learn to take care of himself or herself. This is sometimes one of the biggest challenges a person with cancer must face. One must learn to take care of one's physical needs of adequate sleep, nutrition, water, and emotional support. And through dealing with and changing some of one's personality characteristics or patterns, a person can often learn to take care of these needs much better than they did before.

Other than simple stress reactions, our thought patterns and emotional baggage can also create other types of damaging messages that get sent to our bodies' cells and physiological systems. Many alternative and conventional practitioners who work with cancer agree that a patient's attitude, level of hope, and active participation in their own healing are all very *real* factors in recovery. In fact, Dr. Nicholas Gonzalez of New

York has been quoted as saying, "I've had patients whose cancer didn't get better no matter how perfectly they did my program" . . . "until they resolved serious emotional issues in their lives."[3]

The physical body is accustomed to fulfilling instructions that emanate from the mind. Often, we are very aware of these mental thought instructions, such as when we decide to walk across a room, pick up a book, and sit down on a couch. However, we also have mental thoughts that we are not normally aware of. These are usually on a deeper, more subconscious level. (But they are not totally out of conscious access.) For instance, a person may be avoiding dealing with an important issue in his or her life—sweeping the problem under the rug, so to speak. The resultant suppression of feelings about this issue then leaves the person with the deep subconscious mental thought that the issue is "eating" him or her up on the inside. The mental concept of being eaten up inside can then possibly translate as a message to the *physical* body, which might result in the physical body fulfilling that message as if it were an instruction and creating a cancer that eats them up. Or, if a person feels on a mental/emotional level that they are "weak and falling apart," there is reason to believe that the cells and systems of the body may at times comply with these instructions, as well.

There are many ways to deal with one's emotions, personality dynamics, and subconscious thought messages. Seeking professional counseling is one way. Simply sharing one's fears and thoughts with other caring people is another way. Cancer treatment specialist, Dr. W. John Diamond, believes it is often important for his patients to address some very difficult psycho-spiritual questions. He even talks about the importance of cancer patients addressing whether they have a deep-seated will to live or not. This may seem an odd question to ask a person with a life-threatening illness, because the first reaction is usually, "Well, of course I want to live!" But the question is actually very pertinent when you consider that some cancer patients may have been struggling with extremely difficult issues or situations in their lives previous to their cancer diagnosis. They may have been suffering through problematic marriages, constant financial stress, working at jobs they hate, or possibly trying desperately to emotionally survive the death of a child or spouse. It is not uncommon for a person to put on a good face and just tough it out through hard times, while deep inside, they subconsciously wish their struggles were over.

In his book, *An Alternative Medicine Definitive Guide to Cancer*, Dr. Diamond states,

A rather hard question must be posed: Is it the patient's personal priority to eliminate the cancer? This may sound absurd at first glance, but it isn't. In some instances, people may not want treatment at all despite the fact that they are sitting in the physician's office. They may desire to pass on to another reality; they may wish to weather the storm using their own resources; they may be seeking encouragement and ways to reduce their pain and suffering.[4]

I agree with Dr. Diamond's emphasis on the importance of cancer patients looking at whether they truly want to live or not. But I would add one point to that. From a "mind-body" perspective, the desire to live is most effective in helping a person to recover from cancer if that person wants to live *for himself or for herself*. In other words, if you have cancer and you do get in touch with a deep desire to live, then you might ask yourself, "Do I want to live for *myself*? Or, do I want to live for my children, my spouse, or my parents?" Are you hoping to recover because someone else needs you and you want to be there for them? Is your reason to live based on the thought, "What would they do without me?" If so, your physical body may be getting "mixed" messages. Your conscious mind may be saying "I want to live" (for Joan or John), but your subconscious mind may be saying "I don't really want to live for myself; I just want to be there for someone else."

There is nothing wrong with wanting to be there for others. But when it comes to overcoming a difficult disease such as cancer, your body's power to heal and fully recover will be best supported if you can get in touch with a desire to live *for yourself*. This is because, in terms of the mind/body connection, the body only responds to messages for "self." It does *not* respond to altruistic messages on a higher philosophical plane.

Thus, if you find out that you are only trying to recover from your illness because you want to be there for your daughter and see her graduate college and get married, or because you want to help your son mature into a fine young man and give him the support and help you never had, or because your fragile parent would die if anything ever happened to you, and so forth, then you may have more introspection and psychological work to do. You will need to go deep inside and find reasons to live *for yourself*. Sometimes this may simply involve a little "re-framing." For example, you can realize that your interest in seeing your daughter get married is *for your own pleasure*, or that *you will be satisfied* if you can give your son the support and guidance you never got, or that *you want* to be there for your parents because you care about them and you also care about yourself.

In order for this process of re-framing to be effective on the mind/body level, however, it must be honest. You can't "fool" the mind/body connection by making ungenuine statements to yourself. The body only responds to what you *truly* feel or think.

Once you have gotten used to your daily cancer treatment regimen, making an effort to include fun in your day whenever possible, is also a good idea. If "fun" is too much to ask for, then just do something that gets your mind *off* your cancer every day. This, in itself, can be a helpful way to let go of the fears that having cancer has triggered. To a certain extent, just being active in your own healing process can also help to lessen those fears. This is one of the great aspects of all the alternative treatments—every one of them involves active participation on the patient's part, and thereby creates a message to the mind/body connection that the person is in control, not the illness

Last, but not least, participating in some form of meditative activity while you are following your alternative cancer treatment can greatly help you to relax on the emotional and mind/body level. Thus, if you do not already practice one of these, you might consider learning some form of meditation, gentle yoga, tai chi, or qi gong. The healing benefits of these mind-quieting activities cannot be overstated.

The Negative Placebo Effect

One aspect of the mind/body issue, which is too rarely addressed, is the "negative placebo effect." It is the flip side of the "positive placebo effect," which we have all heard about. The positive placebo effect occurs when someone heals because they *think* they are being given an effective treatment, and therefore they *think* themselves well. Countless studies have proven the positive placebo effect to be a powerful healing force. Yet, the positive placebo effect is simply the wondrous power of the mind/body connection. It is simply the physical body saying, "I shall please" as it responds to a person's genuine thoughts.

But the negative placebo effect is the exact same wondrous force. It occurs when a person thinks they are *not* going to recover, so they don't. This can happen when a doctor communicates in various ways to a patient that there is nothing more that medical science can do for them and that they, the patient, will soon die. Too often, doctors tell their patients they only have "X" number of months to live and often that is exactly how many months those patients *do* live.

When it comes to dealing with cancer, however, it is not only the doctors who can cause a negative placebo effect to take place. It is also friends, relatives, society, and even ourselves. This is because, on a societal level, cancer carries a high fear factor (or expectation of death). Unfortunately, with modern conventional medicine the way it is, most of the people we ever know or hear about with cancer *do* die from their disease. Many of us have witnessed cancer deaths among close friends or family members. This can cause us to be surrounded by negative expectations for recovery, and promotes in the cancer patient's mind a subconscious belief system full of negative expectations. In terms of the mind/body connection, it can be very helpful to the healing process if the cancer patient can counteract these negative thought patterns.

I am *not* saying that you cannot get well unless you have a positive attitude—that would simply be incorrect. But by maintaining a positive and *proactive* attitude about your own healing process, you can greatly counteract the negative messages that are all around you, that are bombarding you all the time. At the same time, you will be supporting your own healing process on the mind/body level.

The gist of this chapter is this: To enhance your own healing, you may want to practice dealing with your fear in constructive ways so that you make informed decisions for yourself and don't get caught in the trap of making decisions based on fear. You may want to look at any personality characteristics you have that could be causing chronic physical stress reactions in your body. You may want to stop holding in your feelings so much, which is tiring to your body, and learn to take care of yourself if you have had a pattern of not doing so. You may want to practice letting go of worry, or not sweating the small stuff, if this is an issue for you. And you may want to ask yourself the hard question of whether you really want to live *for yourself*. All of this may require some extra courage and honesty, but it is usually well worth it.

Having to fight cancer is never, in itself, a good thing. But many people who have done so and won have felt they received positive side benefits, or gifts, as a result of their battle. Sometimes these gifts include being more in touch with one's true self than before and having a deeper appreciation of life.

CHAPTER 24

Concluding Comments

The primary point of this book is to make it abundantly clear that you *do* have choices, even though all of these choices may not be sanctioned by "mainstream" medicine or paid for by your health insurance company. You are not limited to the big three conventional cancer treatments: chemotherapy, surgery, and radiation. (Or as some in the alternative cancer field call: *poison, slash, and burn.*)

You are also not limited to the alternative, non-toxic treatments listed in this book. Although I have presented those approaches I believe to have shown the *best* track records, there are still more non-toxic approaches to cancer worldwide. Some that have shown great merit and success for cancer, which I was not able to discuss due to lack of space, are: Immuno-augmentative therapy (IAT), Iscador, Poly-MVA, Wheatgrass therapy, Hansi, Cytoluminescent therapy (CLT), Dr. Rath's approach, Cancema, Ambrotose, Artimisinin, and traditional Chinese medicine (TCM). Any of these approaches may be well worth looking into.

How you decide to treat your cancer should be *your* choice, and you have a right to make that choice an "informed" one. If you are one of the many people whose doctors tell them, "There is no cure for your type of cancer," you now know that what they really mean is, "There is no cure that *conventional* medicine currently has to offer you." And you also now know there is very real hope in the world of alternative cancer approaches. Although, there is never a 100 percent guarantee for recovery, countless people have "outsmarted" their cancer with alternative, non-toxic treatments!

It is time that cancer treatments be prescribed by mainstream medicine based on what truly works. It is time that our FDA function as the protector of the American people (as it was designed to function), instead of as a protector of big corporations. If the many effective, non-toxic approaches to cancer known today were finally approved by the

379

FDA and supported by the ACS and NCI, there would be many more people starting to use these approaches in earlier stages of their illness. This factor alone could make recovery rates for non-toxic approaches soar to record highs, and cause cancer deaths to decrease dramatically.

Some people believe that if effective alternative treatments were to become mainstream, then millions of people would suddenly be out of work who are currently employed by the conventional cancer industry. I do not think this would have to happen. Quite the contrary; oncologists, nurses, technicians, and medical researchers would still be needed to help patients use the alternative approaches. Even with alternative, non-toxic approaches, patients still need medical care. They need frequent diagnostic tests to monitor their progress. They need qualified practitioners helping them to understand their treatment approach. And they often need side complications of their cancer to be dealt with by medical professionals and/or hospitalization. Plus, many of the conventional surgical techniques will still play an important role, as well as some of the conventional fast-acting toxic treatments (when fast-acting damage control is necessary).

The personnel in medical research laboratories could also remain employed. But instead of researching further toxic approaches that don't bring long-term recoveries, they could research non-toxic approaches and how to improve them or combine them for optimal results. (There is no doubt that these treatment approaches work, so proving they work need no longer be the focus.) And, with public opinion about cancer therapy changing, the first health insurance company to cover alternative cancer treatments would probably make a fortune!

Unfortunately, when a cancer treatment is denied mainstream acceptance and labeled "alternative," then the biggest obstacle to people being open to that approach is the *disbelief factor*. And this disbelief factor occurs in the minds of physicians as well as patients. Most medical experts know very little, if anything, about alternative, non-toxic cancer treatments because these approaches are *not* taught in medical schools or written about in medical journals. It is understandably difficult for physicians to believe that an approach to cancer can be more successful at achieving long-term recoveries than conventional methods and yet *not* be talked about in their medical circles.

But just because most conventional doctors don't know about them, that does not mean alternative approaches don't work. Aside from the many documented cases of politically suppressive events that have blocked alternative methods from mainstream medicine, there is also the fact that it is prohibitively expensive for most of these methods to become "accepted" approaches *without* pharmaceutical financial backing. (As things are set up now, it can cost around $800 million for a new cancer treatment to fully go through the institutionalized processes required for official approval.) Thus, the fact that alternative approaches are not FDA-approved says little about their effectiveness, but it says a lot about how much money the developers of that approach had.

One direct outcome of the disbelief factor is the common mistake of assuming that whenever anything unconventional *does* work, it must be the result of "spontaneous remission." It is medically inaccurate to assume that most or all of the recoveries using alternative approaches are attributable to spontaneous remission when the point in time that cancer patients start to recover virtually always coincides closely to the point in time they start the alternative treatment. As you probably noticed in the testimonials presented in this book, many recoveries happened to people whose cancer was getting *worse* while they were on conventional treatments. It was not until after these people started using an alternative approach, that they began to show signs of recovery, and then finally recovered.

Another outcome of the disbelief factor is the common mistake of assuming that alternative approaches must have been developed by "non-scientific people" in "non-scientific ways." However, just the opposite is true. For example, referring to the alternative treatments discussed in this book:

- The Hoxsey Therapy was clinically evaluated by an independent group of 10 physicians from various parts of the United States. These physicians formally concluded that the Hoxsey treatment was superior to any cancer treatment being used by the medical establishment at the time.

- Essiac tea not only resulted from Native Americans testing and using herbs for hundreds of years, but was also clinically proven by Canadian and American physicians. This included Dr. Charles A. Brusch who had been the personal physician to John F. Kennedy. After 10 years of studying Essiac, Dr. Brusch concluded that Essiac was "a cure for cancer, period."

- Dr. Gerson was a highly esteemed physician in his home country of Germany, whom the famous humanitarian doctor, Albert Schweitzer, called "one of the most eminent medical geniuses in the history of medicine." Known in New York as someone who could cure "incurables", Dr. Gerson's clinic showed astounding results, which he even presented to a sub-committee in Congress known as "the Pepper Commission."

- Dr. Krebs and his son, Dr. Ernst T. Krebs, Jr., (developers of Laetrile), were both prominent physicians and renowned medical researchers. Besides their own meticulous laboratory research, Laetrile was tested clinically on humans and shown to be successful by many physicians around the world.

- Dr. Kelley's metabolic therapy involving the powerful use of enzymes was independently evaluated and proven effective for many types of cancer. And for pancreatic cancer, it was proven to be "off-the-charts" better than any current conventional method.

- Dr. Stanislaw Burzynski gained recognition as one of the youngest people in the history of Poland to receive both an M.D. and Ph.D. diploma, and later scientifically researched his antineoplastons at the Baylor College of Medicine in Texas. Independent clinical evaluation has proven antineoplaston therapy to be more effective than current conventional medical approaches, especially for brain cancers and lymphomas.

- Jim Sheridan was a chemist who obtained a private grant to work at the Detroit Cancer Institute where he tested his early versions of Protocel in a formal, scientific laboratory environment. Later, Sheridan worked on his formula in the Biosciences Division of the Batelle Institute in Columbus, Ohio. There, he tested his formula using the same rigorous standards that were being used to test new chemotherapeutic agents for the National Cancer Institute. Finally, in 1990, the NCI tested Sheridan's formula in vitro on many different cancer cell lines and all the results were excellent.

- The mechanism of anaerobic functioning in cancer cells was scientifically proven by the famous biochemist, Otto Warburg, who received a Nobel Prize for his contributions to science.

- The effectiveness of oxygenation therapies (Hospital Santa Monica) against cancer has been well-proven and many countries around the world today are currently using various forms of these therapies with success.

- Dr. Johanna Budwig was a brilliant biochemist who was nominated for a Nobel Prize seven different times. Her impeccable laboratory research on essential fatty acids was a monumental contribution to science and her own clinical work reportedly demonstrated over 1,000 documented cases of cancer recoveries using her dietary approach.

- Aubrey Keith Brewer, Ph.D., was the pioneering physicist for cesium high pH therapy. He was highly qualified for his research that focused on the study of cell membranes and, for a time, was chief of the National Bureau of Standards Mass Spectrometer and Isotope section. Clinical trials later proved his approach using cesium to be effective at bringing about late-stage cancer recoveries in humans.

- Royal Rife and Gaston Naessens were considered by many to be the greatest geniuses of the 20th century. Their contributions to microbiology and the understanding of micro-organisms were immeasurable. Brilliant inventors, they even independently developed new types of microscopes to aid them in their work. Rife's "Universal Microscope" and Naessens's "Somatoscope" were far more powerful than any microscope being used at the time and both allowed observation of virus-size organisms in their alive state, something that still cannot be done today.

Thus, the belief that alternative cancer treatments are "non-scientific" is simply as wrong as it could be!

Some physicians *are* open to alternative approaches and to their patients using them. More and more oncologists and other doctors are overseeing patients using a non-toxic approach for their cancer. Many of these physicians are seeing the alternative approach work and are saying to their patients, "Keep doing what you're doing!" But a very real obstacle to any physician *prescribing* an alternative approach for cancer is that most states in the United States do not legally allow physicians to do this. Many doctors are in the unenviable position of having to say, "Keep doing what you are doing because it is working . . . but don't tell me the details of what you are doing because I can't prescribe it anyway."

As a result of state laws restricting doctors to only prescribing certain types of treatments, medical freedom is not yet secure for us in the United States. Moreover, medical freedom is not yet protected as a "right" in the Constitution. However, at least one signer of our Declaration of Independence had the foresight back in 1776 to proclaim that medical freedom should be a protected right, and should be in our Constitution. Benjamin Rush, M.D., was the Pennsylvania delegate to the Continental Congress as well as a prominent medical doctor of his day. Dr. Rush wisely stated:

> Unless we put medical freedom into the Constitution, the time will come when medicine will organize into an undercover dictatorship to restrict the art of healing to one class of men and deny equal privileges to others; the Constitution of this republic should make a special privilege for medical freedom as well as religious.

Hopefully, the day will come when *all* effective medical approaches are available to us. But until that day comes, how you choose to treat your cancer is still your decision. Don't let others push you into doing something you don't want to do, whether they happen to be doctors, friends, or family. And don't let your own fear push you either. Instead, take a deep breath and do your research as quickly as you can. Get someone you trust to help you, if possible. Listen to your heart. Once you have started treatment (whether conventional or alternative), *keep* doing research at a slower pace. There may be even more you can do for yourself as you start to recover.

Cancer is never easy, but many others have "outsmarted" their cancer with alternative, non-toxic treatments that work, and you can pursue the same methods, too!

Recommended Resources

Multiple Alternative Cancer Treatments

Options: The Alternative Cancer Therapy Book, by Richard Walters (Avery/Penquin Putnam, New York, 1993). ISBN 0-89529-510-5.

An Alternative Medicine Definitive Guide to Cancer, by W. John Diamond, M.D. and W. Lee Cowden, M.D., with Burton Goldberg (Future Medicine Publishing, Inc., Tiburon, California, 1997). ISBN 1-887299-01-7.

Cancer Therapy: The Independent Consumer's Guide to Non-Toxic Treatment and Prevention, by Ralph W. Moss, Ph.D. (Equinox Press, New York, 1996). ISBN 1-881025-06-3.

I Beat Cancer: 50 People Tell You How They Did It, by Zack Vaughan (Awareness Publishing, Oxnard, California 2003). ISBN 0972167803.

How to Fight Cancer and Win, by William L. Fischer (Agora Health Books, Baltimore, Maryland, 2000). ISBN 1-891434-01-2. (Contains one of the best descriptions of Dr. Budwig's cottage cheese and flaxseed oil approach.)

Alternatives in Cancer Therapy, by Ross Pelton, R.Ph., Ph.D., with Lee Overholser, Ph.D. (Simon and Schuster, New York, 1994). ISBN 0-671-79623-2.

Specific Alternative Cancer Treatments

Antineoplastons

The Burzynski Breakthrough, by Thomas D. Elias (Lexikos, Nevada City, California, 2001). ISBN 0-938530-66-6.

Cesium High pH Therapy

Cancer Cover-Up, by Kathleen Deoul (Cassandra Books, Baltimore, 2001). www.cassandrabooks.com.

Essiac Tea

The Essiac Report, by Richard Thomas (The Alternative Treatment Information Network, Los Angeles, 1993). ISBN 0-9639818-0-3.

Essiac Essentials, by Sheila Snow and Mali Klein (Kensington Books, New York, 1999). ISBN 1-57566-563-8.

Gerson Therapy

A Cancer Therapy: Results of Fifty Cases, by Max Gerson, M.D., (The Gerson Institute, Bonita, CA, 1999). ISBN 0-9611526-2-1.

Censured For Curing Cancer: The American Experience of Dr. Max Gerson, by S. J. Haught (The Gerson Institute [under the P.U.L.S.E. imprint], Bonita, California, 1991). ISBN 0-88268-109-5.

The Gerson Therapy, by Charlotte Gerson and Morton Walker, D.P.M. (Kensington Publishing, New York, 2001). ISBN 1-57566-628-6.

Hoxsey Therapy

When Healing Becomes a Crime: The Amazing Story of the Hoxsey Cancer Clinics and the Return of Alternative Therapies, by Kenny Ausubel (Healing Arts Press, Rochester, Vermont, 2000). ISBN 0-89281-925-1.

Issels's Approach

Cancer—A Second Opinion, by Josef Issels, M.D. (Avery Publishing Group, New York, 1999). ISBN 0-89529-992-5.

Kelley's Enzyme Approach

Cancer: Curing The Incurable Without Surgery, Chemotherapy, or Radiation, by Dr. William Donald Kelley, D.D.S., M.S., with Fred Rohe (New Century Promotions, Bonita, California, 2000). ISBN 09704290-0-2.

Laetrile

World Without Cancer: The Story of Vitamin B_{17}, revised edition, by G. Edward Griffin (American Media, Westlake Village, California, 1997). ISBN 0-912986-19-0.

Alive and Well: One Doctor's Experience with Nutrition in the Treatment of Cancer Patients, by Philip E. Binzel, Jr., M.D. (American Media, Westlake Village, California, 1994). ISBN 0-912986-17-4.

Rife Machine

The Cancer Cure That Worked! Fifty Years of Suppression, by Barry Lynes (Marcus Books, Ontario, Canada, 1987). ISBN 0-919951-30-9.

Video: "The Royal Rife Story: Historical Documentary." 1-888-486-4420.

Conventional Cancer Treatments and/or Politics

The Cancer Industry, by Ralph W. Moss (Equinox Press, Brooklyn, New York, 1999). ISBN 1-881025-09-8.

Questioning Chemotherapy, by Ralph W. Moss, Ph.D., (Equinox Press, Brooklyn, New York, 2000). ISBN 1-881025-25-X.

Racketeering in Medicine: The Suppression of Alternatives, by James P. Carter, M.D. (Hampton Roads Publishing Company, Inc., Charlottesville, PA, 1992). ISBN 1-878901-32-X.

Politics in Healing: Suppression and Manipulation in American Medicine, by Daniel Haley (Potomac Valley Press, Wash., D.C., 2000.) ISBN 0-9701150-0-8.

The Healing of Cancer: The Cures, the Cover-Ups, and the Solution Now!, by Barry Lynes (Marcus Books, Queensville, Ontario, Canada, 1989). ISBN 0-919951-44-9.

Video: "Cancer Doesn't Scare Me Anymore!" , by Lorraine Day, M.D. 1-800-574-2437, or www.drday.com. (Dr. Day also speaks about her own battle and approach.)

Other Medical Issues Relating to Cancer Recovery

Women's Hormones

What Your Doctor May Not Tell You About Breast Cancer, by John R. Lee, M.D., David Zava, Ph.D., and Virginia Hopkins (Warner Books, New York, 2002). ISBN 0-446-52686-X.

What Your Doctor May Not Tell You About Menopause, by John R. Lee, M.D., with Virginia Hopkins (Warner Books, New York, 1996). ISBN 0-446-67144-4.

Video: "Managing Your Hormones at Menopause and Beyond." Can be ordered from www.johnleemd.com.

Alkalizing the Body

The Calcium Factor: The Scientific Secret of Health and Youth, by Robert R. Barefoot and Carl J. Reich, M.D. (Deonna Enterprises Publishing, Wickenburg, AZ, 2001). ISBN 0-9633703-3-2.

Toxic Teeth

Root Canal Cover-Up, by George E. Meinig, D.D.S., F.A.C.D. (Bion Publishing, Ojai, California, 1998). ISBN 0-945196-19-9.

It's All in Your Head: The Link Between Mercury Amalgams and Illness, by Dr. Hal A. Huggins (Avery Publishing Group, Inc., Garden City Park, New York, 1993). ISBN 0-89529-550-4.

APPENDIX

Five Big Environmental Cancer Triggers

In Chapter 2, we looked at many cancer-causing factors of "modern living." Some of these factors involve insufficient or imbalanced dietary habits, others involve environmental pollutants, and still others occur as a result of life-style choices. This Appendix goes into extra detail about five big *environmental* cancer-causing factors that are extremely important today. They are:

1. Chlorine byproducts
2. Fluoride
3. Asbestos
4. Fiberglass
5. Nuclear radiation

Chlorine Byproducts

Right up there with pesticides and herbicides is another *huge* threat to public health in our modern world. However, unlike the issue of pesticides and herbicides, it happens to be an issue that most people are not the least bit aware of. It is the issue of chlorine byproducts. Since about 1908, chlorine has been used in the United States to treat public water supplies. For a long time, this was seen as a great advance in public welfare because chlorinating water greatly reduced the risk of disease from waterborne microbes that could cause cholera, typhoid fever, and other devastating illnesses. Dow Chemical Company was the leading producer of chlorine for water disinfecting, and Dow's business soared even more when the paper and plastics industries skyrocketed. Paper mills use chlorine for bleaching purposes and the plastics industry uses chlorine in their production of polyvinyl chloride (PVC plastics.)

For many years, chlorine was thought to be quite safe because under controlled laboratory conditions it harmlessly breaks down into salt and water. In truth, chlorine in its pure form does *not* cause cancer in laboratory animals. However, what was not being looked at, was a host of *unintentional byproducts* that resulted from the chlorine used in industry. It wasn't until about 1974 that scientists discovered the chlorine used to disinfect public water supplies was combining in the water with organic material from plant and animal sources to produce byproduct compounds in our drinking water. These byproduct compounds are called "organochlorines," or chlorine byproducts.

The problem is that when chlorine combines with organic material in water, the majority of the resulting organochlorine compounds are extremely toxic. These toxic compounds are a bigger problem in water supplies that come from surface water sources (such as reservoirs, lakes, and rivers) than they are from well-water sources. This is because the surface water sources tend to have more natural organic material (algae, leaves, and other plant materials) to which the chlorine can bind. The well water, or groundwater sources have much less organic material and therefore, when chlorinated, result in far fewer organochlorines than the surface water sources.

Organochlorine compounds are not found naturally anywhere in the world, but once formed as a byproduct of water chlorination, they are not only toxic, they also extremely stable. Most organochlorines don't break down in nature for hundreds of years. Yet, organochlorines are easily absorbed into the bodies of virtually *all* animals and tend to *accumulate* over time in fat cells. With enough exposure, they can produce birth defects, reproductive disorders, immune system breakdown, and cancer.

These toxic chlorine byproducts are a more and more alarming problem to authorities. One type of organochlorine that has been heavily studied in recent years is a group of compounds called "trihalomethanes." Epidemiological studies have shown that the number of years a person drinks water with certain levels of trihalomethanes directly correlates with an increased risk of bladder and rectal cancer. Yet, the first trihalomethane limits in public water were not set by the U.S. Environmental Protection Agency (EPA) until 1979. Since then, specific types of filters have been set up in many water supplies to finely filter out organic material before chlorine is added to the water. But not all water companies currently meet the standards and the EPA still has not regulated *other* chlorine byproducts in public water supplies that may also cause cancer.

If you think you have not been exposed to dangerous organochlorines because you only drink pristine well water, think again. We are exposed to organochlorines in other ways than through the water we drink. For instance, there are often high levels of organochlorines in swimming pools. Once again, the chlorine in the swimming pool water combines with organic material in the water. These organochlorines can enter the body through the skin. We can also inhale them from fumes near the surface levels of swimming pools and hot tubs. And it is not uncommon to breathe in organochlorines every time we open our dishwasher at home! In this case, the chlorine compounds that originate from both the dishwashing soap and the water are "volatized" and released with the steamy mist when the dishwasher door is opened. In the same way, organochlorines are also released into the air after chlorine from laundry detergents mixes with organic material from clothes in our washing machines!

Unfortunately, organochlorines are so persistent in our environment now, that probably every person on Earth, as well as almost all animal and marine life, have been contaminated with them. In fact, people considered to be average Americans have been shown to have 177 *different* organochlorines in their bodies when tested. These dangerous compounds are found in the fat cells, mother's milk, semen, blood, and breath of probably every person alive today. Because organochlorine molecules are shaped like some of our own hormone molecules, they can easily slip into our cells in place of hormones, and this is partly why there is an alarming increase of infertility in people these days. Some scientists are now relating the dramatic decrease in men's sperm counts to organochlorines. It is no small matter that the average man's sperm count has dropped by about 50 percent over the last 50 years. One has to wonder whether or not we will be able to reproduce naturally at all in within a few decades!

But the *most* toxic type of chlorine byproduct does not come from our public water systems. This most toxic type of compound is a family of organochlorines called "dioxins." The chemical category called "dioxin" *is the single most carcinogenic type of manmade chemical known to science.* The EPA considers dioxin to be 300,000 times more potent as a carcinogen than DDT. No level of dioxin is considered safe!

Most of the dioxin we are exposed to is released into our environment from the following three sources:

1. Industrial incinerators that burn chlorinated wastes

2. Industrial production of plastics

3. The paper production industry

Modern living involves lots of paper. Chlorine is used in the paper industry in two ways. Firstly, it is used to dissolve the lignan in the wood pulp before the pulp can be turned into paper. Secondly, after the paper is made, chlorine is used again to bleach the paper white. Dioxin results as a byproduct. Strangely, the most common way we are exposed to this sort of dioxin is through the food we eat. This is because the dioxin waste from paper mills and other industries is dumped into streams and waterways where it is easily absorbed into fish and food crops. It then bioaccummulates up the food chain into the beef, dairy products, chicken, pork, fish, and eggs that we buy at our supermarkets. The most concentrated amounts of dietary dioxin are found in beef and dairy products!

Some of the dioxin we are exposed to, however, comes from paper itself. Studies have shown that dioxin from paper milk cartons leaches into the milk we drink and that dioxin from bleached (white) coffee filters leaches into the coffee we drink. This is why many people choose to only use unbleached paper coffee filters. The deadly carcinogen, dioxin, even crosses the placental barrier into growing fetuses and is fed to infants through their mother's milk. This may be another reason so many children these days are developing cancer.

Of course we can't go back to drinking totally untreated water, but there *are* alternatives to the chlorination of public water supplies. For example, most of Europe is now using "ozonation" to purify their water, and some cities in the United States, such as Seattle, are already starting to use that procedure. Hydrogen peroxide is also a possible alternative to using chlorine in the paper industry. Although Europe is leading the way in this type of progress, millions of dollars are spent every year in the United States on federal lobbying by the chemical industry to keep chlorine in use. Unfortunately, chemical industries would prefer to avoid having to use safer alternatives that might be more expensive.

Fluoride

Another common health hazard in our environment, and primarily in our water, is fluoride. This is still a controversial issue, but it is well documented that fluoride is an extremely toxic and carcinogenic substance. It is added to many of our public water supplies which means that many people are drinking it in on a daily basis. It can also be found in countless common foods and dental products.

Just how water fluoridation in the United States got started is an interesting story. Our more than 50-year history of water fluoridation started with the atomic bomb industry during World War II. Developing atomic bombs required the processing of uranium. And the processing of uranium produced toxic fluoride waste. Initial problems of fluoride waste were evident early on when New Jersey chemical industries producing bomb-grade uranium allowed fluoride waste to escape into the air. This event resulted in severe damage to fruit trees and animal life downwind of the factories. The early chemical factories also allowed fluoride waste to run off into local waterways, which resulted in "dead" lakes (after the fluoride killed everything in the lakes).[1] Mistakes like these and their damages were covered up at the time, but it quickly became apparent to uranium manufacturers that toxic fluoride waste was going to be a serious problem to them.

Other industries that created fluoride waste were also developing in the mid-1900s. For example, steel-producing was becoming big business. The steel industry has historically produced fluoride waste and emitted fluoride air pollution. Zinc mills also produce fluoride waste. One well-known disaster occurred in Donora, Pennsylvania, in 1948 when a zinc mill emitted a fluoride-rich smog so deadly that about 6,000 people became ill, 20 people died, and numerous pets and livestock were adversely affected or killed over a five-day period.

In the mid-20th century, aluminum manufacturing was also developing. Aluminum manufacturing is a big producer of fluoride and, with the use of aluminum cans rapidly rising, the aluminum industry soon became a *huge* source of industrial fluoride waste. At the same time, aluminum manufacturers and other fluoride-producing industries (steel, zinc, aluminum, phosphate fertilizers, glass, and others) were facing extremely high costs involved with safely disposing of their fluoride waste.

Physician John R. Lee was chairman of a 1972 environmental health committee that was tasked with evaluating water fluoridation for an area in California. In the "John R. Lee, M.D. Medical Letter" of February 1999, Dr. Lee reports that it was the chief legal counsel for the Aluminum Company of America who got the concept of water fluoridation started. His name was Oscar Ewing. It was in 1947 that Ewing hatched an insidious plan to allow the aluminum industry to avoid high costs of safely disposing their deadly fluoride, and to actually *make money* on it instead. Apparently, it was such a good idea, the other fluoride-producing industries followed in the aluminum industry's footsteps. According to Dr. Lee, here is how it happened.

Oscar Ewing was named head of an organization that oversaw the governmental PHS (Public Health Safety) Department. This department is now called Health and Human Services. He then made it an official policy of the PHS to promote the concept of water fluoridation under the guise of reducing dental cavities. This was based on the understanding that a certain amount of dietary fluoride is important for the development of healthy teeth. Ewing then influenced changes in federal regulation to occur, which resulted in the establishment of all control of drinking water fluoride levels to be under the control of the PHS Department.

Ewing's idea was an ingenious profit-maker because, instead of paying high costs to dispose of their toxic waste, the aluminum manufacturers could now sell it to public water companies for a huge profit! With more and more industries developing that produced toxic fluoride waste, a big public campaign touting the benefits of fluoridated water was widely supported by big money interests, and scientific researchers soon found that it was career suicide to oppose water fluoridation. Soon, countless toothpaste companies jumped onto the bandwagon and became new markets to which industries could sell their toxic fluoride waste.

But there was a deadly bait and switch involving the *type* of fluoride studied for dental health versus the type of fluoride put into our water and toothpaste! The original tooth decay prevention tests were done using *calcium fluoride* (CaF_2), or dietary fluoride. Calcium fluoride is the type of fluoride found naturally in water and plants. Yet, the type of fluoride from industrial waste that got added to our public water supplies and dental products was *sodium fluoride* (NaF)! Sodium fluoride is highly toxic. To give an idea of just how toxic it is, back in the 1930s, before the big water fluoridation campaign was launched, the only way the aluminum industry could sell off its toxic fluoride waste (sodium fluoride) for a profit was by selling it to companies that made *rat poisons* and *cockroach poisons*! Sodium fluoride, in other words, does a great job of killing off rats and cockroaches.

So the public campaigners were putting one type of toxic fluoride into our country's water supplies as they were referring to research done on a totally different type of fluoride that has some benefit for teeth. And all of this to save the toxic fluoride-producing industries the expense of disposing of their toxic fluoride waste!

The public campaigners working for the fluoride waste-producing industries knew very well how toxic sodium fluoride was and still is, so they were not referring to calcium fluoride by mistake. Moreover, the toxic type of fluoride waste from industrial sources which is used in public water fluoridation and toothpaste (primarily sodium silicofluoride and fluosilicic acid) has *not* been tested in any widespread way as to general safety or benefit for teeth,

The fluoridation scam was so successful, it still thrives in the United States today in water supplies and dental products. You will be hard-pressed to find a brand of toothpaste at your local drug store that does *not* contain fluoride in it. And many children are still given fluoride washes in the dental chair and/or fluoride supplements to protect their teeth. Yet, large studies have shown there is *no* significant reduction in dental cavities through the use of this type of fluoride. In fact, it often causes damage to the teeth in the form of "dental fluorosis," which results in mottled, yellowish teeth for life.

Clinical toxicology organizations list sodium fluoride as more toxic than lead poisoning. Even Proctor and Gamble, the makers of Crest toothpaste, have admitted that the fluoride in a family-sized tube of Crest could, if ingested all at once, be enough *to kill a small child!* Of course, it is not likely that a small child is going to ingest a whole tube of toothpaste at once, but they do ingest much more than that amount of fluoride from fluoridated toothpaste *over time*. The accumulated effect can have a serious negative impact on health and can contribute to cancer.

It is truly amazing that fluoride supplements for children are still being marketed under the guise of helping their teeth when the companies selling these supplements have *never* been required to demonstrate that their supplements are safe. This is because fluoride supplements were developed and sold before 1962, which is the year that the FDA started requiring new drug applications to demonstrate safety and effectiveness. The FDA chose to *exempt* products marketed before 1962 from this safety requirement and continues to allow them to be sold.

We should at least learn from the many cases where children have actually died as a direct result from fluoride treatments done on their teeth. In 1979, a large settlement was awarded the parents of a three-year-old child who was unnecessarily killed this way. In this case, the court found the dentist and dental hygienist to be at fault but did *not* find the American Dental Association to be at fault. Apparently, the ADA took the following defensive stance:

> The ADA owes no legal duty of care to protect the public from allegedly dangerous products used by dentists . . . The information it disseminates is intended for the benefits of its membership only. Dissemination of information relating to the practice of dentistry does not create a duty of care to protect the public from potential injury.[2]

From the above statement, one must conclude that the ADA only feels obligated to protect its members (the dentists), and that any dental advertisements or products claiming the support of the American Dental Association are simply giving the public a false sense of security!

Not only does public water fluoridation *not* protect teeth, it has now been officially linked to dental fluorosis, skeletal fluorosis, increased hip fractures, increased infant mortalities, lowered IQ, increased hyperactivity in children, and cancer. Numerous studies have proven that fluoride can cause damage to chromosomes in concentrations as low as one part per million, and *one part per million is the average target level used in fluoridating public water supplies*. Various studies have linked sodium fluoride to bone cancer, bladder cancer, liver cancer, oral cancer, lung cancer, and other types of cancer.

One of the insidiously dangerous effects of fluoride on the body is its ability to interrupt, or interfere with the functioning of many different enzymes, thereby disrupting a variety of important processes in the body. The U.S. National Academy of Sciences and the World Health Organization have published lists of *over 100 enzymes* in the body that are inhibited at the fluoride levels common in our drinking water. Studies have also shown that fluoride adversely affects the migration rate of white blood cells in the human body and causes a breakdown in collagen, which is a protein that helps to hold every cell in our bodies together.

There have been *many* epidemiological studies linking water fluoridation with increased cancer incidences in various geographical areas. In fact, too many to report here. But in 1977, one top fluoride researcher told a congressional committee that unless something were done to stop the fluoridation of water in the United States, more than 500,000 people alive at the time of his speech could be expected to die from fluoridation-linked cancer!

It is also suspected by many researchers that fluoride may even be a contributing factor to the development Alzheimer's disease. This is because aluminum in the brain has been suspected to be a factor in this debilitating disease. The connection here is that elemental aluminum cannot pass the blood-brain barrier by itself. But elemental aluminum *can* interact with sodium fluoride in our bodies to form "aluminum fluoride." And aluminum fluoride *can* pass the blood-brain barrier!

The really scary part is that even in a country like the United States, where not all communities have fluoridated water, the effects of water fluoridation are nevertheless *everywhere*. In other words, you may not live in an area that has fluoridated water for drinking purposes, but many of the fruits and vegetables you buy at the grocery store have been grown using fluoridated water. These fruits and vegetables absorb the fluoride from the water through their roots. The amount of toxic fluoride in fruits and vegetables may then be compounded by the fact that artificial fertilizers and pesticides used in agriculture often also contain sodium fluoride to keep the level of insect activity down. This fluoride then gets washed into the soil and absorbed by the roots of our food plants as well.

Moreover, even though you may not live in a fluoridated drinking water area, you may drink common commercial beverages such as sodas, juices, beer, and wine. These beverages may have been made with fluoridated water. Keeping in mind that chromosome damage to cells can occur at fluoride amounts as low as one part per million, or 1.0 ppm, here are a few examples of the levels of fluoride in some common food and beverage products[3]:

Beverage	Fluoride in Parts Per Million
Diet Coke	2.6 ppm
Beer, Wine	15 ppm
Gerber's First Year's Juices	3 ppm
Kellogg's Fruit Loops Cereal	2.1 ppm

And of course, there are the common dental toothpastes people are using from which they may be absorbing deadly sodium fluoride on a daily basis.

The public health danger of fluoridated water is astronomical, and it will only get worse as it builds up in our environment. Americans should consider following the lead of most European countries when it comes to water fluoridation. Here is what some countries in Europe have already done:[4]

—*Sweden* banned and discontinued fluoridation in 1971.

—*Norway* and *Germany* rejected fluoridation in 1975 as '*foreign to nature, unnecessary, inefficient, irresponsible and harmful to the environment.*'

—*Holland* banned fluoridation in 1976 and changed their country's constitution so that fluoridation could never be re-introduced.

—*Denmark* rejected fluoridation in 1977. The Minister for Environment there stated that "*no adequate studies had been carried out on the long term effect on human organ systems.*"

—*France* rejected fluoridation in 1980. The Chief of Public Health in France declared it was too dangerous.

—*Finland* rejected fluoridation in 1992.

—All Councils in *Northern Ireland* have rejected fluoridation.

—*Italy, Austria, Belgium* and *Luxembourg* have all rejected water fluoridation.

Currently, less than 2 percent of the people in Europe drink fluoridated water, and studies have shown that people with the best teeth in Europe are from those countries that do *not* fluoridate their water.[5] Getting toxic fluoride out of our water, common foods and beverages, and daily toothpastes is one of the best things we can do for ourselves and our environment.

Asbestos

Another highly carcinogenic substance in our environment, that the average person has very little control over, is asbestos. Asbestos is a curious substance. It is actually a family of minerals that can *be spun* into fibers and woven into cloth. Thus, asbestos is basically a rock that has been spun into fabric. Once discovered, it became a highly sought after substance, because *asbestos will not burn!*

Around the beginning of the 1900s, the asbestos industry had become big business. Asbestos was looked at as a magical substance that gave people a sense of safety from fire. Before long, asbestos was being manufactured into thousands of different commercial products as a fire retardant. Some of these common products were potholders, floor tiles, stove linings, table paddings, coffee pots, toasters, irons, electric blankets, and hair dryers. But about 75 percent of all the asbestos produced was used in the construction of buildings. After all, what could be better than a fire-retardant building insulator?

The only problem was, and still is, that asbestos is extremely hazardous to everyone's health! The reason is that microscopic asbestos fibers are easily released into the air from the many asbestos-containing products or building insulation materials. These fibers are so microscopic, they cannot be seen by the human eye. And each of the unseen fibers can break down even further into a multitude of smaller particles, called "fibrils." These fibrils are so small, they can only be detected by an electron microscope![6]

Once released into the air, asbestos fibers and fibrils take a very long time to settle and are virtually indestructible. Anyone can breathe them into their bodies without knowing it. Once in the body, these microscopic, indestructible fibers and fibrils get caught in the sensitive membranes and linings of the lungs and other parts of the body. They irritate the tissues, cause microscopic lesions and eventually cause scar tissue to form. Finally, cancer may form in and around this scar tissue.[7]

The danger of asbestos fibers to lungs has been well known for many decades. As early as the 1920s, studies revealed that many asbestos factory workers were dying at very young ages from lung ailments. Originally, many of these ailments were classified as "asbestosis." For decades, however, the dangers of asbestos were not made public. Then, in the 1960s, studies began to reveal alarmingly high rates of lung cancer and other lung diseases among building insulation workers. These lung diseases were also surfacing in asbestos-mining workers and shipyard workers.

The reason that early studies did not show a significant lung cancer connection to asbestos was that researchers did not realize at the time that it could take *twenty years or more* for lung cancer to develop after exposure to asbestos. In the words of Dr. Irving Selikoff, a physician who studied the asbestos to lung cancer relationship among shipyard workers,

> For lung cancer the percentage of all deaths that occurred at 10 years or less was trivial; it was not until 25 years after onset of employment that deaths [from lung cancer] became common [among shipyard workers].[8]

In 1977, after completing another study—this time involving men belonging to the New York pipefitters union—Dr. Selikoff presented his conclusions to a medical meeting. After discussing the details, he summed up the cancer risk by saying, "One out of every three asbestos workers dies of lung cancer. This is simply a disaster!"[9] Selikoff also noted a small rise in deaths from esophageal, stomach, colon, and rectal cancers among the men of the pipefitters union. He attributed these intestinal tract cancer deaths to asbestos as well, pointing out that when people breathe in asbestos fibers and fibrils from the air, they also *ingest* a certain amount of them, thus contaminating the intestinal tract.[10]

In the 1970s, U.S. government agencies had finally begun to regulate permissible exposure limits to asbestos fibers in factories, construction, and shipyards, and to enact safety regulations in building demolition policies for all buildings containing asbestos. However, the danger has not gone away. Although modern appliances in the United States, such as toasters and irons, no longer contain asbestos, many buildings still do.

The use of asbestos to insulate new buildings has been banned since the mid-1970s, but millions of office workers in this country still work in asbestos-laden *older* buildings. It is difficult to know just how many buildings this is, but it has been estimated, for instance, that about *half* of the country's skyscrapers still contain asbestos insulation. And about two-thirds of all the buildings in New York City have been found to contain asbestos.[11] Air-conditioning systems in many of these buildings still circulate air right over sprayed-on asbestos insulation, which causes fibers and fibrils to be picked up and circulated directly into myriads of offices and employees' breathing spaces.[12]

Even more disturbing is the issue of asbestos in schools. In 1972 a Wyoming elementary school was ordered to be closed after the school librarian brought attention to a layer of asbestos dust that covered most of the furniture in the school! The dust turned out to be from a deteriorating ceiling that had been sprayed with asbestos 11 years before. This spraying technique was a fairly common practice from the 1950s to the 1970s. In 1977, six New Jersey elementary schools were also closed due to asbestos exposure to the children. In 1978, Harlem parents forced two New York City schools to be shut down for the same reason. Moreover, the Harlem investigation revealed that hundreds *more* schools in New York City were still contaminated with asbestos.[13]

In 1986, the "Asbestos Hazard Emergency Response Act" was passed, which provided for standards and timetables to clean up asbestos in 30,000 schools in this country. But this type of task cannot be done overnight. Meanwhile, many of these schools may be exposing about 50 million children today to the hazards of asbestos.[14] How many of these children or employees in skyscrapers will be developing cancer 20 to 25 years after exposure?

At this point in time, virtually every man, woman, and child has already been exposed to asbestos-contaminated air, even if they *have not* spent time in asbestos-laden office buildings or schools. The fibers and fibrils are already just about everywhere in our environment. The best we can do at this point is to give our support to clean-up projects and public awareness, thereby minimizing future health risks as much as possible. It is also important to know that other countries may be less aware of the dangers of asbestos. In fact some countries, such as Chile, Argentina, and parts of Brazil, do *not* have bans on asbestos and still allow the sale of many asbestos-containing household products.

Fiberglass

Similar to the issue of asbestos, but a much less studied subject at present, is the issue of fiberglass. Fiberglass shares many of the characteristics of asbestos, but instead of being rock that can be spun into fibers, it is *glass* that can be spun into fibers and then woven into material. Just like asbestos, microscopic pieces of fiberglass (which are really just needle-shaped pieces of glass) get into the air. As early as the 1970s, Dr. Mearl F. Stanton of the National Cancer Institute concluded from his experiments that glass fibers less than 3 microns across and more than 20 microns long were "potent carcinogens" in rats.[15]

The problem is that the health risks of fiberglass have not been as well studied as asbestos, and with the banning of asbestos, the production of fiberglass in the United States has been quickly increasing as an alternative. Now, fiberglass is being used for thermal and acoustic insulation in buildings and homes, in automotive parts, and in *air filters*. Tens of thousands of commercial products currently contain fiberglass, and it is estimated that *most of the homes in America now use fiberglass insulation!*

Fiberglass products can directly pollute the air around them with tiny glass fibers, just the way the asbestos can pollute the air with asbestos fibers and fibrils. Fiberglass and asbestos can also pollute the air around landfills after they have been discarded. Like asbestos, microscopic fiberglass fibers can now be measured in the air just about anywhere on the planet—whether it be in cities, rural areas, or remote mountains. As fiberglass products are being produced in ever-increasing quantities, this pollution is quickly getting worse. Yet, there is every reason to believe that the cancer-causing mechanism of fiberglass is very similar to that of asbestos.

Already, some researchers believe that a ban on fiberglass is long overdue. But despite this, and even though numerous studies have shown elevations in lung cancer rates among fiberglass factory workers, public health officials have claimed that there is *no evidence* that fiberglass is a health risk to humans. As to the truth of this claim, only time will tell.

Nuclear Radiation

The fifth big cancer-causing environmental factor of modern living is environmental radiation left over from nuclear testing and other bomb-related activities. There are many people who have filed lawsuits against the U.S. government for their exposure to nuclear radiation, and they call themselves "downwinders." These people lived in areas of the country that were downwind of nuclear testing done primarily in the 1950s and 1960s. Many of these downwinders have already died of cancer, or are currently fighting cancer as a result. Epidemiological evidence from studies on high-exposure areas of the country also indicates a strong correlation between nuclear exposure and higher incidences of cancer. Yet it still remains a problem that it is virtually impossible to *prove* any particular person's cancer was caused by nuclear fallout. Because of this difficulty, the government has been able to remain vague on the subject of how much cancer nuclear radiation from bomb testing really caused.

According to one downwinders website (www.downwinders.org), the National Cancer Institute *did* finally admit in 1997 that the fallout from atomic bomb tests carried out in the 1950s blanketed this country with much higher levels of radioactive material than was previously admitted by the government.[16] But the government report only went so far as to include the statement that ". . . there *could* be between 10,000 and 75,000 cases of thyroid cancer among those exposed."[17]

Research done by many concerned downwinders indicates that the problem is much, much bigger than the NCI is willing to admit. For one thing, many more bomb tests were conducted on land *after* the 1950s, and also offshore in the Pacific. Tiny particles of radioactive material were blown high into the atmosphere from these tests, and then carried on the wind for thousands of miles to where they could be deposited in other places. Another issue upsetting downwinders is that the government study referred to by the NCI only looked at the effects of iodine-131, which is only one of *dozens* of radioactive isotopes emitted during nuclear testing!

It is true that iodine-131 tends to cause thyroid cancer. This is because the chemical structure of this particular radioactive isotope causes it to be readily absorbed into and stored by the thyroid gland. But scores of other radioactive isotopes in the same fallout are also absorbed into the body and are equally, or even more deadly. For instance, strontium and plutonium are usually absorbed into and stored in the bone by anyone exposed to them. Once in the bone, these isotopes can damage the bone marrow and blood cell activities. Unlike radioactive iodine 131, which tends to cause thyroid cancer, radioactive strontium and plutonium can result in cancers of the bone marrow and blood, namely the multiple myelomas and leukemias.

Because of their different chemical structures, different radionuclides from nuclear fallout tend to concentrate in different organs of the body. Once there, they continue to irradiate that organ until the radiation either fully decays, or they are eliminated from the body. Unfortunately, the decay period for many of these substances is extremely long. Iodine 131 has one of the shortest time periods for decay, with a half-life of only eight days. But strontium-90 has a half-life of 30 years, and plutonium has a half-life of 24,000 years! Because strontium-90 mimics calcium storage in the bones, it generally ends up in the bones and teeth. On the other hand, radioactive plutonium may end up in the bones, liver, lungs, or other body organs and may remain there over the lifetime of the person.[18]

One downwinders organization is now making the point that, ". . . if the iodine-131 resulted in 10,000 to 75,000 cases of thyroid cancer alone, how many cases did the other isotopes produce, and of those hundreds of thousands of cases (of cancer), that they would induce, how many innocent, unwitting, and unsuspecting Americans died?"[19] Cesium-137, zirconium, and other radioactive isotopes are *also* extremely dangerous substances emitted by nuclear detonations, and they have yet to be studied!

Radioactive fallout became a known contaminant issue as early as 1945. On July 16, 1945, the first atomic bomb test was successfully carried out at Alamogordo, New Mexico. Back then, scientists knew very little about the dangers of radiation. They had the technology to create the bomb, but did not have all the technology needed to study the dangers of radioactive isotopes. Only gamma ray and X-ray radiation were understood. The more dangerous radioactive contamination issues from nuclear testing, such as beta radiation and neutrons, were a mystery. There was no technology or device that could measure some of these new radioactive particles. In fact, scientists and government officials were so naive about the dangers of fallout back then that, right after the test at Alamogordo in 1945, two physicists were sent out in a car to follow a cloud of radioactive material blowing east across the country. These physicists discovered for the first time that radioactive fallout did not fall evenly when blown by wind. Instead, it tended to fall more heavily in certain "hot spots" due to various weather and geographical conditions.

Even more far-reaching effects from the first detonation in Alamogordo were discovered three years later, in 1948. This occurred when customers of the Eastman Kodak Company complained about "fogged" film. The investigation that followed this complaint revealed that ". . . the film had been packed in paper made from straw that had been washed in water from the Wabash River, which had been contaminated by the explosion at Alamogordo, more than 1,000 miles away."[20]

On August 6, 1945, the nuclear bomb detonation occurred over Hiroshima, Japan. Three days later, on August 9, another bomb was detonated over Nagasaki. No studies on the widespread fallout of these wartime detonations were *ever* done, partly because scientists at that time did not have the technology to detect or measure many of the radioactive particles. We still do not know how much of the fallout from those two war-time bombs actually circulated via wind over the United States and other parts of the world and was deposited on land and in waterways.

Later, more was learned about the wind-blown distribution of nuclear fallout from tests done in Nevada in the 1950s and 1960s. For instance, in April 1953, *just two days* after an atomic bomb test had been conducted in the Nevada desert, a professor and his students in Troy, New York, discovered that the gamma radiation measurements on their campus suddenly shot up to 500 times the normal amount. And they found that the beta ray radiation was even higher than that in some hot spots, such as in rainspouts and puddles. This professor later discovered that the mushroom cloud created at the Nevada test site had reached 40,000 feet in the atmosphere and had then drifted 2,300 miles across the country to the northeast in just two days. The cloud of radioactive material had passed over (and mostly likely contaminated) parts of Utah, Colorado, Kansas, Missouri, Illinois, Indiana, Ohio, and Pennsylvania before it got caught up in a rain system that dropped radioactive precipitation onto upstate New York, southern Vermont and parts of Massachusetts.[21]

Over the years, about 1,000 nuclear devices were tested in Nevada, three were tested in Alaska, three in New Mexico, two in Mississippi, and two in Colorado. As early as 1953, scientists knew that a lot of the radioactive elements from these explosions were settling down to earth and contaminating not only the air and soils, but also the waterways from which we drink. From these waterways, they were then getting into our food crops and livestock. Thus, we were "eating" radioactive compounds. In fact, a 1960 study done at the University of Michigan revealed that, due to drinking milk from contaminated cows, children were getting radiation doses to their thyroid glands that were 10 to 100 times greater than doses to adult thyroid glands. This was due, in part, to the children's higher consumption of milk and also due to the higher concentration of radioactivity in the children's smaller thyroid glands.

There are two basic ways that exposure to radiation from nuclear fallout occurs: (1) externally, and (2) internally. External exposure occurs when radiation enters through the skin from the surrounding air. Internal exposure occurs when radioactive by-products are directly inhaled or ingested from food or water. It is now known that radioactive isotopes from nuclear fallout *concentrate* more and more as they move up the food chain. Algae concentrates it out of the water, plants concentrate it out of the soil, and birds, fish, and other animals concentrate it even more when they drink the water and eat the plants. The radioactive isotopes that are concentrated in dairy animals then concentrate even *more* in their milk. Even human mothers concentrate these isotopes in the milk their own bodies produce to feed their babies.

In other words, because each step up the food chain helps to accumulate and concentrate dangerous radioactive isotopes, the actual internal exposure to humans from what they eat can be *many times greater* than the external atmospheric exposure around them. And there is *no* amount of nuclear radiation that is safe. Any amount can cause cell damage!

The areas most highly contaminated by U.S. domestic nuclear testing were to the east and northeast of the Nevada desert test sites. This is because detonations were generally scheduled when wind directions were moving toward the east or northeast. The schedulers of these tests apparently knew enough about the dangers of nuclear fallout to want to avoid exposing the more densely populated areas of the south and west (such as around Las Vegas and southern California). Residents in the less populated areas subjected to the direct path of wind-blown fallout in the east and northeast (such as eastern and northern Nevada and southwestern Utah), suffered *epidemics* of cancer, infertility, miscarriages, and birth defects.

Iron County, Utah, was one of the populated areas particularly hard hit by radioactive fallout. According to the website, www.historytogo. utah.gov/ nuctest.html:

Scott M. Matheson, governor of Utah from 1977 to 1984 and a former Parowan and Cedar City resident, recalled life in Iron County during the early 1950s: "People in southern Utah were mainly concerned with making a living, and I don't recall anyone being too upset about the brilliant flashes and thunder-like blasts that were part of the 1953 atomic testing. The Upshot-Knothole series, conducted from March to June 1953, included the 'Dirty Harry' exposure that carried an enormous amount of debris downwind, over southern Utah. People were concerned about the sheep deaths that occurred in May 1953, but when the AEC said there was nothing to worry about, we all just shrugged our shoulders. No one really accepted the malnutrition rationale, but we were used to accepting whatever the government said, especially during that very nationalistic period."

As part of a test site public-relations program in March 1953, some 600 observers were invited to view a test shot and its effect on manikins, typical homes, and automobiles in an effort to get Americans more interested in civil defense. Klien Rollo represented the *Iron County Record* at the media event. Observers watched the detonation seven miles from ground zero and later were taken into the test area, after debris and dust had settled. Rollo at first thought it was "his good fortune" to be invited to the test site, but not many weeks later the newspaper began questioning the safety of nuclear fallout. It printed a long article by University of Utah student Ralph J. Hafen of St. George, in which he wrote that he felt "morally obligated to warn people of the irreparable damage that may have occurred or may in the future occur" from exposure to radiation. He also called upon the AEC to explain why cars entering St. George were washed after the shot. Predicting later problems, he cautioned that "damage done to an individual by radiation often does not make itself known for five to ten years or a generation or more . . ."

Finally, in 1982, Congress passed legislation calling for a government study on human exposure to iodine-131 caused by Nevada nuclear testing done in the 1950s and 1960s. The results of the study did not come out until 15 years later! Finally, in 1997, the National Cancer Institute released the results of their county-by-county report. Their conclusion was that *every person and animal living in the 48 contiguous states* was exposed during those two decades to iodine-131. The NCI report also concluded that the highest areas of exposure from the Nevada tests were in Iowa, Nebraska, South Dakota, Kansas, Montana, Wyoming, Colorado, Utah, Missouri, Idaho, Nevada, and Arkansas.[22]

And that study was done on just one radioactive isotope that was emitted by domestic nuclear testing. No big studies have ever been undertaken to assess the radioactive exposure caused by: (1) "Cold War" nuclear testing in the former Soviet Union that might have blown over the United States, (2) exposure from our own nuclear testing in the Pacific that might have blown back over our country, or (3) radioactive fallout from the detonation of the bombs over Hiroshima and Nagasaki which might have blown back to our country. Some researchers believe that parts of California and the Pacific Northwest may have suffered significant fallout from these three additional sources, which may have put these locations at the top of the list of most exposed U.S. areas, if these sources of nuclear radiation had been studied.

But we also need to be aware of the fact that *nuclear contamination does not only result from detonating bombs*. This is because bombs don't just create themselves. They have to be made and the nuclear explosive material used to make them has to be produced. For example, the plutonium for the bomb dropped over Nagasaki was produced at the Hanford Plutonium Nuclear Reservation in central Washington State. It is now known that the Hanford facility regularly released radioactive iodine-131 into the atmosphere from the years 1944 to 1972 as part of their process of developing nuclear bomb material. And it is a little known fact that, in 1945, the Hanford facility "accidentally" released an amount of radioactive iodine into the American skies that was equivalent to the amount released in the 1986 Chernobyl disaster![23]

The Hanford site downwinders group is a very large group of people. The areas exposed include eastern Washington, northeastern Oregon, most of Idaho, and parts of Montana and Canada. It is estimated that more than 2 million people were exposed to radioactive iodine-131, plutonium, cesium, strontium, and ruthenium.[24] One Department of Energy study, which looked at 30,000 workers at Hanford, showed cases of multiple myeloma and pancreatic cancers to be clearly correlated with exposure to radiation.[25]

Moreover, the Hanford operation used water from the Columbia River to cool its reactors. This water became contaminated with radiation and then was discharged back into the Columbia River. One researcher wrote:

> According to a formerly classified 1954 technical report by Herb Parker, former Director of the Health division at Hanford, the operators at Hanford knowingly discharged at least 8,000 curies of radioactive material per day into the Columbia River. The discharges from Hanford exposed people who ate fish and waterfowl, swam or boated on the river, irrigated their fields with water from the river, or simply drank the water from the Columbia River (such as residents of Pasco). The exposures to

radioactive materials through the water pathway increase a person's total exposure to radiation when coupled with exposure through the air emissions.[26]

We also need to be aware that radioactive contamination starts even *before* the plutonium-producing facilities are involved. Environmental contamination actually starts at the uranium mining sites. Uranium ore must be mined to fuel not only nuclear weapons, but also to fuel nuclear reactors in power plants. What happens is that when uranium ore is first extracted from the ground, it is dug up then crushed at the mining site. The problem is that the process of crushing the uranium ore, or rock, leaves behind a certain amount of pulverized material, which is approximately the consistency of flour. This is part of the uranium "tailings." These tailings are left on the ground after the mining is done, where they are free to be blown by the wind or washed into surface and ground water supplies by rain. This material is very light and can be blown a thousand miles in just a few days. It is estimated that 85 percent of the radioactivity of the uranium ore remains in these powdery tailings. And the half-life of this material is about 80,000 years!

Uranium mine sites are located in many states in the United States, including Arizona, Colorado, Idaho, New Mexico, Oregon, Pennsylvania, Texas, Utah, Wyoming, and North Dakota. Currently, investigations are going on as to how much radioactive contamination, including ground-water contamination, has occurred in these areas.

In 1990, Congress passed the "Radiation Exposure Compensation Act." This act was passed to provide millions of dollars of compensation to citizens who lived downwind of above ground atomic tests, as well as to test site workers and uranium miners. Quoting from this legislation, Congress finally declared that:

> The United States should recognize and assume responsibility for the harm done to these individuals. And Congress recognizes that the lives and health of uranium miners and of innocent individuals who lived downwind from the Nevada tests were involuntarily subjected to increased risk of injury and disease to serve the national security interests of the United States . . . The Congress apologizes on behalf of the Nation to the individuals . . . and their families for the hardship they have endured.[27]

Thus, the risk factors for cancer and other illnesses due to radioactive fallout are not gone just because we are no longer testing nuclear weapons or detonating war-time bombs. Much of this radioactive material is *still* in our environment, still contaminating all of us, and a lot of it will not go away for thousands of years. There is also a great deal of "clean up" of uranium mine sites that still needs to be done. All of the issues of radioactive fallout are important for the public to know about. Probably hundreds of thousands of people, maybe even millions of people, have already become cancer victims as a result of nuclear radioactive isotopes. Unfortunately, even though it is *known* that radiation exposure can cause virtually any type of cancer (blood, breast, lung, digestive system, and others), the National Cancer Institute continues to play down the health risks of this exposure.

References

Chapter 1 — The Cancer Reality Today

1. Moss, Ralph W., Ph.D. *The Cancer Industry*. New York: Equinox Press, 1999, p. 21.
2. *Ibid.*, p. 22.
3. *Ibid.*, p. 39.
4. *Ibid.*
5. *Ibid.*
6. Brodie, Douglas, M.D. (with Michael L. Culbert, D.Sc.). *Cancer and Common Sense: Combining Science and Nature to Control Cancer*. White Bear Lake, Minnesota: Winning Publications, 1997, p. 47.
7. Day, Lorraine, M.D. Video: "Cancer Doesn't Scare Me Anymore." (www.drday.com, or 800/574-2437).
8. Moss, *op cit.*, p. 38.
9. www.alkalizeforhealth.net

Chapter 2 — Why So Much Cancer and What Causes It?

1. Stoff, Jesse A., M.D. and Dallas Clouatre, Ph.D. *The Prostate Miracle*. New York: Kensington Books, 2000, p. 18.
2. Diamond, John W., M.D. and W. Lee Cowden, M.D. (with Burton Goldberg). *An Alternative Medicine Definitive Guide to Cancer*. California: Future Medicine Publishing, Inc., 1997, p. 570.
3. *Ibid.*, p. 571.
4. Pickrell, J. "Cancer Causer?", *Science News*. Vol. 162, no. 12, Sept. 21, 2002, pp. 179–180.
5. Diamond et al., *op cit.*, p. 579.
6. www.lightparty.com/Health/Pestacides.html.
7. Diamond et al., *op cit.*, p. 568.

8. Diamond et al., *op cit.*, p. 582.
9. *Ibid.*
10. *Ibid*, p. 585
11. *Vitamin Research News*, Aug. 2002, vol. 16, No. 8, p. 5.
12. Martini, F., et al., "Human Brain Tumors and Simian Virus 40," *Journal of the National Cancer Institute*, vol. 87, Sept. 6, 1995.
13. www.drkelley.info/articles/archive.php?artid=283.
14. Moss, Ralph, Ph.D., *WeeklyCancerDecisions.com Newsletter*, #82, 5/4/03.
15. Griffin, G. Edward. *World Without Cancer*. California: American Media, 1997, p. 83.
16. *Ibid.*, p. 84.
17. *Ibid.*, p. 78.
18. *Ibid.*, p. 112.
19. Lynes, Barry. *The Cancer Cure That Worked! Fifty Years of Suppression*. Ontario, Canada: Marcus Books, 1987, p. 17.

Chapter 3 — The Hoxsey Therapy

1. Ausubel, Kenny. *When Healing Becomes a Crime: The Amazing Story of The Hoxsey Cancer Clinics and the Return of Alternative Therapies*. Rochester, Vermont: Healing Arts Press, 2000, p. 57.
2. *Ibid.*, p. 93.
3. *Ibid.*, p. 96.
4. *Ibid.*, p. 106.
5. *Ibid.*, p. 41.
6. Walters, Richard. *Options: The Alternative Cancer Therapy Book*. Avery Penguin Putnam, 1993, pp. 98–99.
7. *Ibid.*, p. 96.
8. *Ibid.*, p. 100.
9. Ausubel, *op cit.*, p. 169.

Chapter 4 — Essiac

1. www.vegan.swinternet.co.uk/articles/health/Essiac_info.html
2. *Ibid.*
3. *Ibid.*
4. Olsen, Cynthia. *Essiac: A Native Herbal Cancer Remedy*. Pagosa Springs, Colorado: Kali Press, 1996, pp. 19–20.

Chapter 5—The Gerson Method

1. Walters, Richard. *Options: The Alternative Cancer Therapy Book*. Avery Penguin Putnam, 1993, p. 190.
2. www.gerson.org/clientservices/whatisthegersontherapy.htm
3. Haught, S.J. *Censured for Curing Cancer: The American Experience of Dr. Max Gerson*. The Gerson Institute, 1991, p. 6.
4. Carter, James P., M.D. *Racketeering in Medicine: The Suppression of Alternatives*. Virginia: Hampton Roads, 1993, p. 31.
5. www.sawilsons.com/gerson.htm
6. Carter, *op cit.*, p. 31.
7. *Ibid.*
8. www.sawilsons.com/gerson.htm

Chapter 6—Laetrile

1. Griffin, G. Edward. *World Without Cancer*. California: American Media, 1997, p.105.
2. Binzel, Philip E., M.D. *Alive and Well: One Doctor's Experience With Nutrition in the Treatment of Cancer Patients*. California: American Media, 1994, p. 114.
3. *Ibid.*, pp. 117–118.
4. *Ibid.*, p. 123.
5. *Ibid.*, p. 111
6. *Ibid.*
7. *Ibid.*, p. 113
8. Griffin, *op cit.*, p. 105.
9. *Ibid.*, p. 102.
10. *Ibid.*, p. 130.
11. Moss, Ralph W. *The Cancer Industry*. New York: Equinox Press, 1999, p. vii.
12. Griffin, *op cit.*, p. 110.
13. *Ibid.*, p. 108.
14. *Ibid.*, p. 106.
15. *Ibid.*, p. xvii.
16. Walker, Morton, "Profile of the Holistic Cancer Therapist W. Douglas Brodie, MD, HMD," *The Townsend Letter for Doctors and Patients*, February/March, 2002, p. 132.
17. Griffin, *op cit.*, p. 26.
18. Moss, *op cit.* p. 132.

Chapter 7 — Dr. Kelley's Enzyme Therapy

1. Mitchell, Terri, "War on Cancer: One Physician is Winning — Dr. Nicholas Gonzalez," *Life Extension Magazine*, October 1996.
2. *Ibid.*
3. *Ibid.*
4. *Ibid.*
5. *Ibid.*
6. *Total Health Magazine*, vol. 22, no. 5, October 2000.

Chapter 8 — Burzynski's Antineoplastons

1. Moss, Ralph W., Ph.D. *The Cancer Industry*. New York: Equinox Press, 1999, p. 290.
2. Elias, Thomas D. *The Burzynski Breakthrough*. Nevada City, California: Lexikos, 2001, p. 100.
3. *Ibid.*, p. 123.
4. *Ibid.*, p. 129.
5. Moss, *op cit.*, p.313.
6. Whitaker, Julian, M.D., *Dr. Julian Whitaker's Health and Healing Newsletter*, Mid-February 1996 Supplement, p. 3.
7. Elias, *op cit.*, p. 87.
8. *Ibid.*, p. 91.
9. Whitaker, *op cit.*, p. 3.
10. *Ibid.*, p. 4.
11. *Ibid.*
12. *Ibid.*, p. 6.
13. www.burzynskipatientgroup.org.
14. Whitaker, Julian, M.D., *Medical Alerts*, vol. 11, no. 4, 2002, p. 12.
15. www.burzynskipatientgroup.org/burdickreport.htm
16. Elias, *op cit.*, p. 76.
17. *Ibid.*
18. *Ibid.*, p. 220.
19. *Ibid.*
20. www.burzynskipatientgroup.org
21. Burzynski, Stanislaw, personal communication, April 2003.
22. Elias, *op cit.*, p. 181.
23. *Ibid.*, p. 60.
24. *Ibid.*, p. 74.

25. *Ibid.*, p. 75.
26. Whitaker, Julian, M.D., *Dr. Julian Whitaker's Health* , *Healing Newsletter*, April 1997 Supplement.

Chapter 9—Protocel: History and Theory

1. Sheridan, James Vincent. Personal Writings.
2. *Ibid.*
3. Sheridan, James Vincent and Sheridan, James Edward. "How Does Entelev/Cancell Work: A Layman's Explanation." *Journal of the Bio-Electro-Magnetics Institute*, vol. 3, no. 3. April 1992, p. 37.
4. *Ibid* , p. 40.

Chapter 11—Protocel: Suppression of the Formula

1. Galluppi, Marcello. "Entelev/Cancell: In Search of the Holy Grail." *Journal of the Bio-Electro-Magnetics Institute (BEMI)*, vol. 3, no. 3. April 1992, p. 24.
2. *Ibid.*
3. Sheridan, James Edward. "Entelev: The Latest Controversy. What Is the Significance of the NCI Graphs?." *Journal of the Bio-Electro-Magnetics Institute*, vol. 3, no. 4. March 1993, p. 9.
4. Galluppi, Marcello. "Entelev/Cancell: In Search of the Holy Grail." *Journal of the Bio-Electro-Magnetics Institute (BEMI)*, vol. 3, no. 3. April 1992, p.27.
5. Sheridan, James Edward, Personal Communication. May 2002.

Chapter 12—Protocel: How To Use Protocel Correctly

1. McKibben, Elonna, Personal Communication. July 2002.
2. Sheridan, James Vincent and Sheridan, James Edward. "How Does Entelev/Cancell Work: A Layman's Explanation." *Journal of the Bio-Electro-Magnetics Institute*, vol. 3, no. 3. April 1992, p. 41.

Chapter 13—Hospital Santa Monica

1. Altman, Nathaniel, *Oxygen Healing Therapies*. Healing Arts Press: Rochester, Vermont, 1998, pp. 19–20.

2 Donsbach, Kurt W., *Wholistic Cancer Therapy*. (Booklet) Published by Kurt Donsbach, 2000, p. 14.

3. Donsbach, Kurt W. *Oxygen As A Therapy: Hydrogen Peroxide, Hyperbaric Chamber*. Kurt W. Donsbach, 2000, p. 77.

4. Altman, *op cit.*, p. 86.

Chapter 14 — Dr. Budwig's Flaxseed Oil and Cottage Cheese Diet

1. Fischer, William L. *How To Fight Cancer and Win*. Baltimore, MD: Agora Health Books, 2000, p. 140.

2. Budwig, Dr. Johanna. *Flax Oil As a True Aid Against Arthritis, Heart Infarction, Cancer and Other Diseases*. Vancouver, Canada: Apple Publishing Co., 1994, p. 17.

3. Fischer, *op cit.*, p. 143.

4. www.mnwelldir.org/docs/cancer1/budwig.htm

5. www.houseofsteed.com/sons/budwig.htm

6. www.enviro_healthtech.com/flax.htm

7. Erasmus, Udo. *Fats That Heal, Fats That Kill*. Canada: Alive Books, 1993, p. 301.

Chapter 15 — The Rife Machine

1. Video — "The Royal Rife Story: Historical/Documentary." (Produced by AAA Production, Utah. 888/486-4420.)

2. *Ibid.*

3. *Ibid.*

4. *Ibid.*

5. Lynes, Barry. *The Cancer Cure That Worked: Fifty Years of Suppression*. Ontario, Canada: Marcus Books, 1987, pp. 17–18.

6. *Ibid.*, p. 17.

7. *Ibid.*, p. 18.

8. *Ibid.*, p. 50.

9. Video, *op cit.*

10. Lynes, *op cit.*, p. 45.

11. Video, *op cit.*

12. Lynes, *op cit.*, p. 60.

13. *Ibid.*, p. 88.

14. *Ibid.*, p. 30.

15. *Ibid.*, p. 51.

16. *Ibid.*, p. 25.

Chapter 16—714X

1. www.sonic.net/sentine/gvcon4.html
2. www.bccancer.bc.ca/pg_g_05.asp?PageID=1708&ParentID=2
3. www.sonic.net/sentinel/gvcon4.html
4. www.sph.uth.tmc.edu/utcam/therapies/714x.htm
5. www.bccancer.bc.ca/pg_g_05.asp?PageID=1708&ParentID=2
6. www.sonic.net/sentinel/gvcon4.html
7. www.essiac-resperin.com/en/report01.html
8. *Ibid.*
9. wwww.cerbe.com/en/web_review.html
10. *Ibid.*
11. www.cancerinform.freewebsites.com/naessens.html
12. *Ibid.*
13. *Ibid.*
14. www.prevention.com/cda/feature/0,1204,3847,00.html

Chapter 17—Cesium High pH Therapy

1. Brewer, A. Keith, Ph.D., "The High pH Therapy for Cancer, Tests on Mice and Humans," *Pharmacology Biochemistry and Behavior*, vol. 21, suppl. 1, 1984, pp. 1–5.
2. www.cancer-coverup.com/fighters/cesium_a.html
3. *Cancer: The Mechanism Involved and a High pH Therapy, 1978 Papers of* A. Keith Brewer, Ph.D., *and coauthors.* A. Keith Brewer Foundation, 325 N. Central Avenue, Richland Center, WI 53581.
4. Deoul, Kathleen, *Cancer Cover-Up.* Cassandra Books: Baltimore, MD, 2001, p. 37.
5. www.advancedhealthplan.com/2cesiumchlorideforcancer2.html ("Cesium Therapy in Cancer Patients," by H. E. Sartori.)
6. Deoul, *op cit.*, p. 37.
7. *Ibid.*, p. 38.
8. *Ibid.*

Chapter 18—To Alkalize or Not to Alkalize

1. Aihara, Herman. *Acid and Alkaline.* California: George Ohsawa Macrobiotic Foundation, 1986, p. 1.
2. www.cocoonnutrition.org/consult.html

3. Barefoot, Robert R. and Carl J. Reich, M.D. *The Calcium Factor: The Scientific Secret of Health and Youth.* Arizona: Deonna Enterprises Publishing, 2001, p. 137.
4. Aihara, *op cit.*, p. 17.
5. Barefoot, *op cit.*, pp. 135–136.
6. www.cocoonnutrition.org
7. www.gethealthyagain.com
8. Barefoot, *op cit.*, p. 13.
9. *Ibid.*, p. 97.
10. *Ibid.*, p. 133.
11. *Ibid.*
12. *Ibid.*, p.111.
13. *Ibid.*, p. 67.
14. *Ibid.*, p. 122.

Chapter 19—What Women *Must* Know About Hormones

1. Lee, John R., M.D., David Zava, Ph.D. and Virginia Hopkins. *What Your Doctor May Not Tell You About Breast Cancer: How Hormone Balance Can Help Save Your Life.* New York: Warner Books, 2002, p. 7.
2. Lee, John R., M.D., Jesse Hanley, M.D. and Virginia Hopkins. *What Your Doctor May Not Tell You About Premenopause.* New York: Warner Books, 1999, p. 212.
3. *Ibid.*, p. 215.
4. http://www.johnleemd.com/.
5. Lee, John R., M.D., David Zava, Ph.D. and Virginia Hopkins, *op cit.*, p. 27.
6. *Ibid.*, p. 50.
7. *Ibid.*, p. 73.
8. *Ibid.*, p. 299.
9. *Ibid.*
10. *Ibid.*, p. 99.
11. *Ibid.*, p. 35.
12. *Ibid.*, p. 78.
13. http://www.lightparty.com/Health/Pestacides.htm.
14. Lee, John R., M.D., David Zava, Ph.D. and Virginia Hopkins, *op cit.*, p. 29.
15. http://www.lightparty.com/Health/Pestacides.htm.
16. Lee, John R., M.D., David Zava, Ph.D. and Virginia Hopkins, *op cit.*, p. 53.

17. *Ibid.*, p. 53.
18. *Ibid.*
19. Moss, Ralph W., Ph.D. *Questioning Chemotherapy: A Critique of the Use of Toxic Drugs in the Treatment of Cancer.* New York: Equinox Press, 1995, p. 91.
20. Moss, Ralph W., Ph.D. *The Cancer Industry.* New York: Equinox Press, 1999, p. 51.
21. Lee, John R., M.D., David Zava, Ph.D. and Virginia Hopkins, *op cit.*, p. 5.
22. Moss, Ralph W., Ph.D. (*Questioning Chemotherapy*), *op cit.*, p. 95.
23. *Ibid.*, p. 91.
24. Brownlee, Shannon, "Bad Science + Breast Cancer," *Discover Magazine*, vol. 23, no. 8, Aug., 2002, p. 78.
25. Lee, John R., M.D., David Zava, Ph.D. and Virginia Hopkins, *op cit.*, p. 182.
26. *Ibid.*
27. *Ibid.*
28. *Ibid.*, p. 182–183.
29. *Ibid.*, p. 8.
30. *Ibid.*, p. 185.
31. *Ibid.*, p. 184.
32. *Ibid.*, p. 190.
33. Lee, John R., M.D., Jesse Hanley, M.D. and Virginia Hopkins, *op cit.*, p. 212.
34. Lee, John R., M.D. Video: "Managing Menopause."
35. Lee, John R., M.D., David Zava, Ph.D. and Virginia Hopkins, *op cit.*, p. 227.
36. Lee, John R., M.D., Jesse Hanley, M.D. and Virginia Hopkins, *op cit.*, pp. 59–60.
37. Lee, John R., M.D., David Zava, Ph.D. and Virginia Hopkins, *op cit.*, p. 198.
38. *Ibid.*, p. 132.
39. *Ibid.*, p. 134.
40. *Ibid.*
41. *Ibid.*, p. 139.

Chapter 20 — Toxic Teeth

1. www.curezone.com/diseases/cancer/cancer_dental_risk.html
2. *Ibid.*

3. Levy, M.D., Thomas, "Teeth—The Root of Most Disease?," *Extraordinary Science*, Apr./May/June, 1994.
4. *Ibid.*
5. www.curezone.com/diseases/cancer/cancer_dental_risk.html
6. *Ibid.*
7. *Ibid.*
8. Issels, M.D., Josef. *Cancer—A Second Opinion*. New York: Avery Publishing Group, 1999, p. 121.
9. Diamond, W. John., M.D. and W. Lee Cowden, M.D. (with Burton Goldberg). *An Alternative Medicine Definitive Guide to Cancer*. California: Future Medicine Publishing, Inc., 1997, p. 153.
10. Shallenberger, Frank, M.D. Personal Communication.

Chapter 21—Evaluating Conventional Methods

1. Moss, Ralph W., Ph.D. *The Cancer Industry*. New York: Equinox Press, 1999, p. 43.
2. Moss, Ralph W., Ph.D. *Questioning Chemotherapy: A Critique of the Use of Toxic Drugs in the Treatment of Cancer*. New York: Equinox Press, 1995, p. 163.
3. *Ibid.*, p. 56.
4. Diamond, W. John., M.D., W. Lee Cowden, M.D. and Burton Goldberg. *An Alternative Medicine Definitive Guide to Cancer*. Tiburon, California: Future Medicine Publishing, Inc., 1997, p. 840.
5. *Ibid.*, p. 848.
6. *Ibid.*, p. 846.
7. Moss, *op cit.* (The Cancer Industry), p. 64.
8. Moss, *op cit.* (Questioning Chemotherapy), p. 16.
9. *Ibid.*, p. 18.
10. Ausubel, Kenny. *When Healing Becomes a Crime: The Amazing Story of the Hoxsey Cancer Clinics and the Return of Alternative Therapies*. Rochester, Vermont: Healing Arts Press, 2000, p. 234.
11. *Ibid.*, p. 239.
12. Griffin, G. Edward. *World Without Cancer: The Story of Vitamin B_{17}*. California: American Media, 1997, pp. 154–155.
13. Moss, *op cit.* (Questioning Chemotherapy), p. 70.
14. www.whale.to/cancer/quotes1.html
15. *Ibid.*

16. Moss, Ralph, W., Ph.D., *Weekly CancerDecisions.com Newsletter #86*, June 7, 2003.
17. Moss, Ralph, W., Ph.D., *Weekly CancerDecisions.com Newsletter #87*, June 13, 2003.
18. Moss, Ralph, W., Ph.D., *Weekly CancerDecisions.com Newsletter #88*, June 21, 2003.

Chapter 23 — Dealing With Fear and the Mind/Body Connection

1. Diamond, W. John., M.D., W. Lee Cowden, M.D. and Burton Goldberg. *An Alternative Medicine Definitive Guide to Cancer*. Tiburon, California: Future Medicine Publishing, Inc., 1997, p. 617.
2. www.drbrodie.com
3. Mitchell, Terri, "War On Cancer: One Physician Is Winning — Dr. Nicholas Gonzalez," *Life Extension Magazine*, October, 1996.
4. Diamond, *op cit.*, p. 136.

Appendix — Five Big Environmental Cancer Triggers

1. *The John R. Lee, M.D. Medical Letter*, February 1999, p. 4.
2. www.alaskawellness.com/archives/flouride-pt3.htm
3. *Ibid.*
4. http://greenparty.ennis.ie/press/column/fluoride-poison-1_june00.html
5. *Ibid.*
6. Moss, Ralph W., Ph.D. *The Cancer Industry*. New York: Equinox Press, 1999, p. 382.
7. *Ibid.*, p. 372.
8. *Ibid.*, p. 377.
9. *Ibid.*, p. 378.
10. *Ibid.*
11. *Ibid.*, p. 386.
12. *Ibid.*, p. 385.
13. *Ibid.*, p. 384.
14. *Ibid.*, p. 386.
15. http://consumerlawpage.com/article/fiber.shtml
16. www.downwinders.org/nci/html
17. *Ibid.*

18. www.akitarescue.com/hiroshim.htm
19. www.downwinders.org/nci.html
20. www.akitarescue.com/hiroshim.htm
21. *Ibid.*
22. *Ibid.*
23. Diamond, W. John., M.D., W. Lee Cowden, M.D. and Burton Goldberg. *An Alternative Medicine Definitive Guide to Cancer.* Tiburon, California: Future Medicine Publishing, Inc., 1997, pp. 567–568.
24. www.akitarescue.com/hiroshim.htm
25. *Ibid.*
26. www.downwinders.com/pathways.htm
27. http://historytogo.utah.gov/nuctest.html

Index

Give the Gift of

Outsmart Your Cancer

To Family, Friends and Colleagues

Order Form

To order copies of *Outsmart Your Cancer* by phone, call **(800) 266-5564**

To order copies online, go to: www.OutsmartYourCancer.com

To order by fax, copy this form and fax it to: (775) 588-0385

To order by mail, copy this form and mail it to:
Thoughtworks Publishing, P.O. Box 4949, Stateline, NV 89449

☐ My check or money order is enclosed. (Payable to "Thoughtworks Publishing")

Please charge my ☐ Visa ☐ Mastercard ☐ Discover ☐ American Express

Name _____

Organization _____

Address _____

City/State/Zip _____

Phone _____ E-mail _____

Card # _____

Exp. Date _____ Signature _____

Retail Discounts:	1–2 books	no discount ($19.95 ea)
	3–5 books	15% off ($16.95 ea)
	6–10 books	25% off ($14.95 ea)

For *Larger or Wholesale Orders:* Call Thoughtworks Publishing at (888) 679-2669

Please send me _____ copies of *Outsmart Your Cancer: Alternative Non-Toxic Treatments That Work* at $ _____ each for a total of $ _____

Sales Tax: (Nevada residents only) multiply by 7.25% $ _____

Shipping: Add $5.95 shipping for the first book $ ___5.95___

Plus $1.50 for each additional book $ _____

(All books shipped by U.S. Priority Mail)

TOTAL: $ _____

[all prices in U.S. dollars]